WOMEN'S HEALTH
NURSE
PRACTITIONER

Certification Review

WOMEN'S HEALTH NURSE PRACTITIONER

Certification Review

JoAnn Zerwekh, EdD, RN, FNP, CS

University of Phoenix
Carondelet Health Network Community Services
Tucson, Arizona
Nursing Education Consultants
Dallas, Texas

Jo Carol Claborn, MS, RN, CNS

El Centro College
Nursing Education Consultants
Dallas, Texas

W.B. SAUNDERS COMPANY

A Division of Harcourt Brace & Company

Philadelphia   London   Toronto   Montreal   Sydney   Tokyo

W.B. SAUNDERS COMPANY
A Division of Harcourt Brace & Company

The Curtis Center
Independence Square West
Philadelphia, Pennsylvania 19106

Library of Congress Cataloging-in-Publication Data

Zerwekh, JoAnn Graham.
    Women's health nurse practitioner certification review / JoAnn
Zerwekh, Jo Carol Claborn.
        p.   cm.
    ISBN 0–7216–7740–1
    1. Nurse practitioners—Examinations, questions, etc.   2. Women—
Diseases—Examinations, questions, etc.   3. Women—Health and
hygiene—Examinations, questions, etc.   4. Gynecologic nursing—
Examinations, questions, etc.   5. Maternity nursing—Examinations,
questions, etc.   I. Claborn, Jo Carol.   II. Title.
    [DNLM: 1. Nursing Care examination questions.   2. Nursing Process
examination questions.   3. Genital Diseases, Female—nursing
examination questions.   4. Obstetrical Nursing examination
questions.   5. Women's Health examination questions.   6. Nurse
Practitioners examination questions.   WY 18.2Z58W   1999]
RT82.8.Z47   1999
610.73′076—dc21
DNLM/DLC   98-34770

WOMEN'S HEALTH NURSE PRACTITIONER CERTIFICATION REVIEW
                                        ISBN 0–7216–7740–1

Printed in the United States of America

Last digit is the print number: 9   8   7   6   5   4   3   2   1

To Tom, my soul mate,
who brings a smile to my face and
a warm glow in my heart.
                    JoAnn

To Robert, my friend and partner,
whose love and patience keeps me going.
                    Jo

Series Contributors

Susan E. Chaney, EdD, MS, BSN
Professor, Family Nurse Practitioner
  Coordinator
Texas Woman's University
Family Nurse Practitioner
Homeless Outreach Medical Services
Parkland Health and Hospital System
Dallas, Texas

Cynthia Churgin, RN, FNP, CNM
Casa Blanca Medical Group
Mesa, Arizona

Sharon I. Decker, RN, CS, MSN,
  CCRN
Professor of Clinical Nursing
Director, Clinical Simulation Center
Texas Tech University Health Sciences
  Center
Lubbock, Texas

Nicolette Estrada, RN, MS, FNP-C
Chief Research Coordinator
Carl T. Hayden VA Medical Center
Phoenix, Arizona

Mary Jo Gagan, RNCS, FNP, PhD
Assistant Professor
University of Arizona College of Nursing
Nurse Practitioner
Campus Health
University of Arizona College of Nursing
Tucson, Arizona

Ela-Joy Lehrman, MS, MAEd, PhD
Program Manager for Nursing, Counseling,
  and General Studies
University of Phoenix
Tucson, Arizona

Beverly McCoy, BSN, MS, FNP
Clinical Director/Family Nurse Practitioner
Breaking the Circle Children's Health Care
Arizona State University
College of Nursing
Tempe, Arizona

Jacquelyn McGlamery, BSN, FNP
Family Nurse Practitioner
Sierra Tucson
Tucson, Arizona

Loretta Manning, RNC, MSN, GNP
Educational Consultant, Sylvia Rayfield &
  Associates
Executive Director, I CAN, Inc. Publishing
Atlanta, Georgia

Kathleen T. Ogle, RN, MS, CFNP
Instructor
Bowie State University
Department of Nursing
Bowie, Maryland;
Family Nurse Practitioner
Maryland Primary Care Physicians
Arnold, Maryland

Alice B. Pappas, BSN, MSN, PhD
Associate Dean for Academic Affairs
Baylor University School of Nursing
Dallas Texas

Jodi Pelusi, RN, MS, FNP
University of Phoenix
Phoenix, Arizona

Patricia J. Pinckard, MS, ANP
Adult Nurse Practitioner
Occupational Health
Desert Samaritan Medical Center
Mesa, Arizona

Sylvia M. Root, EdD, RNC, FNP
Associate Professor
Arizona State University
Tempe, Arizona

Patricia Scully, RN, MS, JD
Nurse Attorney Consultant
Tucson, Arizona

Patricia A. Shannon, RN, MS, CS, PNP
Faculty, University of Phoenix;
Director of Nurses and Nurse Practitioners
North Valley Pediatrics PC
Phoenix, Arizona;
Adjunct Faculty
Arizona State University
Tempe, Arizona;
President/Consultant
Pediatric Nursing . . . PLUS
Phoenix, Arizona

Linda Stevenson, RN, PhD
Baylor University School of Nursing
Dallas, Texas

Gail Tucker, RN, MS, FNP
BMT Nurse Practitioner
Good Samaritan Regional Medical Center;
City of Hope/Samaritan Bone Marrow
    Transplant
Phoenix, Arizona

Gayle P. Varnell, RN, CPNP, PhD
Assistant Professor
Nurse Practitioner Program Coordinator
The University of Texas at Tyler
Tyler, Texas

John Walter, RN, BS, CPNP
Guest Lecturer
Family Nurse Practitioner Program
University of Arizona College of Nursing;
Pediatric Nurse Practitioner
University Physicians
Tucson, Arizona

Pamela Becker Weilitz, AD, BSN,
    MSN(R)
Assistant Clinical Professor, Graduate
    Program
St. Louis University School of Nursing;
Adult Nurse Practitioner
Washington University School of Medicine
University Care
St. Louis, Missouri

Margaret "Pegi" Yancy, RN, MS,
    OGNP
Faculty Associate
Arizona State University
Tempe, Arizona;
Women's Health Nurse Practitioner
Department of Reproductive Medicine
St. Joseph's Hospital and Medical Center
Phoenix, Arizona

Preface

With the dawn of the role of the nurse practitioner, there is an increasing need for additional reference information and study materials for the certification examinations. Nurse practitioners are playing a vital role in the changing health care delivery system in the United States. The numbers of candidates for the certification examinations is rapidly increasing as more nursing programs implement the nurse practitioner curriculum in their graduate programs. *Women's Health Nurse Practitioner Certification Review* has been developed to assist the advanced practice nurse to prepare for the WHNP certification examination. Extensive efforts have been made to include current information that is representative of the content based on the blueprints for the certification exams. This book of questions is not intended to be an exhaustive review of the content, but an adjunct to the review process. Over 900 review questions are included in all.

Test-taking strategies are included in Chapter 1. As a candidate prepares for the examination, it is vitally important to be familiar with and to practice good testing strategies. Testing strategies can prevent the candidate from making mistakes and selecting the wrong answer. As the review process begins, a review of the testing strategies chapter and the practice of good testing strategies is critical. With many years experience in the field of testing, we have consistently identified the importance practice testing plays in the review process. Practice questions give the candidate an opportunity to review questions written from different perspectives. To enhance the review process, answers with complete rationales are provided at the end of each chapter. Not only does the candidate increase their knowledge of the subject area, but with more practice, testing skills become fine tuned. Good testing skills make the candidate more comfortable and help to decrease the stress associated with certification exams.

This book also includes chapters reviewing important concepts related to Growth and Development and Health Promotion and Maintenance. These chapters provide questions that test information related to growth and development, general health supervision, and health maintenance. The clinical chapters are developed using a systems approach, i.e., cardiovascular, respiratory, endocrine, etc. In each of these chapters, the test questions are divided into three areas: Physical Examination and Diagnostic Tests, Disorders, and Pharmacology. This format assists the candidate to easily locate specific questions. The last three chapters in the text are on Theory and Research; Issues and Trends; and Legal and Ethical aspects of nurse practitioner practice. The test questions in these chapters focus on professional competencies inherent in the role and function of the WHNP.

Our thanks to the many nurse practitioners across the country who provided questions and insight into the role of the nurse practitioner. We wish to thank Robin Carter, our editor at W.B. Saunders, for her support and suggestions in our preparation of the manuscript. Thank you also goes to all the nurse practitioners who took time from their busy schedules to review the questions for content and clarity.

Acknowledgments

We are continually grateful for the contributions and efforts of our test item contributors who provided their expertise and knowledge for this nurse practitioner certification review series.

We thank the manuscript reviewers for their suggestions and insights as we tackled this large project:

Harvey Baker, RNCS, ARNP
Oswego Family Medical Clinic
Oswego, Kansas

Susan Appel, RN, MN, CCRN, CS
Carolinas College of Health Sciences
Charlotte, North Carolina

Genell Lee, BSN, MSN, JD
Hauth & Lee, LLC
Birmingham, Alabama

Stephanie A. Batalo, RN, BSN, MSN, FNP
Trinity Health System
Steubenville, Ohio

Dorothy J. Stuppy, RN, PhD
University of Texas at Arlington
Arlington, Texas

Lynette M. Wachholz, MN, RN, ARNP, IBCLC
The Everett Clinic
Everett, Washington

We thank the staff at W.B. Saunders Company: Robin Carter, Senior Editor, and Marie Pelcin and Ross Landy, editorial assistants for their calmness and patience. Joan Sinclair, who managed the book's production. It was such a pleasure to work with you again on another publication. Berta Steiner for copyediting and typesetting the manuscript. What a job to keep track of thousands of questions!

Last, but certainly not least, we want to thank: Our children, Tyler and Ashley Zerwekh, Jaelyn Claborn, Michael Brown, and Kim Aultman, for teasing their mothers about writing 5 books!! Our parents, Charles Graham and Hazel Cooper, for their continued support and encouragement. Tom Gaglione and Robert Claborn for their encouragement, support, and love. We love you all.

Contents

Test-Taking Strategies

Testing Strategies

Knowing how to take an examination is a skill that is developed through practice and experience. Being able to take an examination effectively is almost as important as the basic knowledge required to answer the question. Everyone has taken an examination only to find in the review of the exam that questions were missed due to inadequate testing skills. Nurse practitioner programs provide the graduate student with a comprehensive base of knowledge; how you utilize this knowledge will determine your success on a certification examination. The certification examination is an objective test that covers knowledge, understanding, and application of professional nursing theory and practice. When you register for the examination, you will receive a "Candidate Handbook" or information materials from the Certification Board administering the examination.

Read the information in this chapter carefully and make sure you understand the strategies discussed. This chapter is designed to help you identify problem areas in testing skills and learn how to use strategy and judgment in selecting correct answers. It is important for you to practice testing skills if you are going to be able to utilize these skills on the certification examination.

Question Characteristics

A. Multiple-choice questions
   1. Scene or scenario—establishes the setting of the question. Not all questions will have a scenario, if a scenario is included, consider the appropriateness of the answer to the information provided.
   2. Stem—states the question that is being asked.
   3. Options—there are four options from which to choose an answer.
      a. Distractors—designed to distract you from the correct answer.
      b. Correct answer—correctly answers the question asked in the stem.
      c. There are only four options in any item; there are no combinations of options to consider.
      d. There is only one correct response; no partial credit is given for another answer.
B. Questions are derived from clinical situations common in the practice setting.

Strategies for Multiple-Choice Questions

1. Cover the options with your hand or a piece of scratch paper.* This strategy makes you focus on the content of the question and prevents your eyes from "darting" to look at the distractors. If you peruse the distractors before you completely understand the question, key words in the distractors will influence your interpretation of the question.

2. Do not read extra meaning into the question. The question is asking for specific information; if it appears to be simple "common sense," then assume it is simple. Do not look for a hidden meaning in what appears to be an easy question.

EXAMPLE:

The nurse practitioner understands that the most common form of facial paralysis in the adult client is:

1. Facial nerve fasciitis.
2. Trigeminal neuralgia.
3. Bell's palsy.
4. Herpes zoster.

The correct answer is Option #3. Be careful not to "read into" the question and add pain to the facial paralysis symptom. The most common form of facial paralysis is Bell's palsy, which is a disorder affecting the facial nerve and characterized by muscle flaccidity of the affected side of the face. Trigeminal neuralgia is a disorder of cranial nerve V characterized by an abrupt onset of pain in the lower and upper jaw, cheek, and lips. Herpes zoster affects the dermatomes and does not cause a paralysis, but pain is possible with postherpetic neuralgia.

EXAMPLE:

When administering skin tests to an immunocompromised client, the nurse practitioner must consider:

1. The importance of not applying more than one skin test at a time.
2. The skin test may react more aggressively than expected.

3. The use of a known allergen for the client and utilize it as a control.
4. The immunocompromised client should not be skin tested.

The correct answer is Option #3. Do not read into the question and make it more difficult by trying to make the client sicker (i.e., full-blown acquired immunodeficiency syndrome [AIDS]). It is important to remember to apply controls when skin testing the immunocompromised client. Ask clients what diseases they believe they have immunity to, such as measles. Apply the "known" allergen and the skin test to be tested. If the client is unable to mount an immune response at all, the known allergen will not react. By not applying the controls, the nurse practitioner may assume a skin test is negative, when in fact the client's immune system is unable to respond.

3. Read the stem correctly. Make sure you understand exactly what information the question is asking.

EXAMPLE:

A client with a history of Parkinson' disease has a positive tuberculosis (TB) skin test and isoniazid (INH) is ordered as a prophylactic medication. Prior to beginning INH, it is important for the nurse practitioner to determine:

1. Is the client's Parkinson's condition being treated with levodopa (Larodopa)?
2. How long the client has been diagnosed with Parkinson's disease?
3. How much respiratory compromise is the client currently experiencing?
4. Is the urinary output and renal function adequate?

The question asks you to determine if giving the INH to a client with Parkinson's disease is a problem. The correct answer is Option #1. This question requires the nurse practitioner to critically think about possible medications the client may be on and whether they would interfere with the ordering of INH. In this case, INH requires concurrent administration of vitamin B_6 to prevent problems of optic neuritis. Vitamin B_6 will decrease the effectiveness of levodopa. If the client is to receive the INH, his antiparkinson medication needs to be re-evaluated.

---

*This testing strategy of covering the distractors is from Phoebe K. Helm, Ed.D.

4. Before considering the options, formulate in your mind possible answers to the question. If none of the options fit in the pool of answers you anticipated, go back and re-evaluate the question. Assess each of the options with regard to your pool of possible answers.

E X A M P L E :

The usual clinical presentation of an adult client with cystitis is:

1. No chills, fever, headache, malaise, or discomfort noted.
2. Acute onset of chills, fever, flank pain, headache, malaise, and costovertebral angle tenderness.
3. Complaints of dysuria, urgency, frequency, nocturia, and suprapubic heaviness.
4. Signs and symptoms of fever, irritability, decreased appetite, vomiting, diarrhea, constipation, dehydration, and jaundice.

Formulate in your mind possible answers to the question. Think to yourself, "Which of these symptoms are normally seen with cystitis? What is different about pyelonephritis? Is the usual presentation without symptoms? Is there involvement of the gastrointestinal tract (as eluded to in Option #4). If you are unsure, go back and reassess the question. In this instance, Option #3 is correct. An adult with cystitis usually presents with dysuria, urgency, frequency, nocturia, and suprapubic heaviness. Acute onset of chills, fever, flank pain, headache, malaise, and costovertebral angle tenderness are common adult symptoms of pyelonephritis.

---

5. Identify what type of response the question is asking. A positive stem requires identification of three false items and one positive as the correct answer.

E X A M P L E :

Clients who believe they have been exposed to human immunodeficiency virus (HIV) should have an HIV antibody test how soon after the exposure?

1. The next day and 2 months later.
2. 6 months after exposure and again at twelve months.
3. 6–12 weeks after exposure and again at 6 months.
4. 4 weeks and 12 weeks.

The correct answer is Option #3. This question requires you to identify three incorrect responses and one correct response. The HIV antibody develops between 6 and 12 weeks after exposure. Because of the variability of antibody development, it is recommended that the test be repeated in 6 months to confirm the findings.

6. Identify questions that require identification of something the practitioner should not or would not do (i.e., unsafe action, contraindication, inappropriate action).

E X A M P L E :

The nurse practitioner is prescribing astemizole (Hismanal) for a geriatric client's allergy problems. When considering the client's current medications, which medication would be a contraindication to the administration of astemizole (Hismanal)?

1. Erythromycin ethylsuccinate (E.E.S).
2. Verapamil (Calan).
3. Propanolol (Inderal).
4. Captopril (Captoten).

The correct answer is Option #1. Macrolides and Hismanal should not be administered concurrently. The nurse practitioner is required to identify a medication that should not be ordered.

7. Questions may also be analytical. These questions may ask the nurse practitioner to identify findings, statements, and the like that are consistent/inconsistent with the client's presenting problem and/or differentiate between them.

E X A M P L E :

Dementia can be distinguished from delirium by:

1. Dementia lasts days to weeks compared to delirium, which lasts months to years.
2. Dementia is often associated with medications or systemic illness.
3. Dementia exhibits a disturbance in attention that is not present in delirium.
4. Dementia does not include altered perception, such as illusions.

Before you examine the options in this question, it is important to think about the difference between dementia and delirium. The correct answer is Option #4. Adults with dementia do not usually have altered perceptions that include illusions.

They may experience hallucinations and delusions. Dementia does last months to years. Delirium is often associated with medications or systemic illness and a disturbance in the ability to pay attention.

8. Identify key words that affect your understanding of the question. Make sure you understand exactly what information the question is asking. Be aware of questions in which the stem includes words such as *except, contraindicated, avoid, least, not applicable,* and *does not occur.* These words change the direction of the question. It may help to rephrase the question in your own words in order to better understand what information is being requested.

E X A M P L E :

Clients with arteriosclerotic heart disease (ASHD) go through several stages before becoming severely compromised. Which **does not occur** in the early stages of ASHD?

1. Decreased urine output.
2. Dyspnea on exercise.
3. Anginal pain relieved by rest.
4. Increased serum triglyceride levels.

Rephrase the question: In early stages of ASHD, which of the following does not occur? It is important that you identify the key point "early stages of ASHD" and the key words "does not occur." If you miss these essential points, you do not understand the question, and chances are you will not choose the correct answer. The correct answer is Option #1: a decrease in urine output occurs when cardiac disease is advanced enough to cause a severe decrease in cardiac output and renal perfusion.

---

9. As you read the options, eliminate those you know are not correct. This will help narrow the field of choice. When you select an answer or eliminate a distractor, you should have a specific reason for doing so.

E X A M P L E :

A 45-year-old female complains of knee pain when kneeling and a "clicking" noise when walking up steps. On exam, there is a slight knee effusion and tenderness when palpating the patella against the condyles. The diagnosis for this client is:

1. Anterior cruciate tear. (*No, the client generally cannot bear weight on the extremity without it buckling or giving way.*)
2. Dislocated patella. (*No, there would be considerable effusion and locking of the knee in flexion.*)
3. Chondromalacia patella. (*Yes, there is clicking and anterior knee pain around or under the kneecap aggravated by knee extensor stress.*)
4. Tendinitis. (*No, there would be no clicking sound with movement.*)

After systematically evaluating the options, Option #3 is the correct answer.

---

10. Identify similarities in the distractors. Frequently, three distractors will contain similar information, and one will be different. The different one may be the correct answer.

E X A M P L E :

An elderly client is to be encouraged to increase her intake of protein. The addition of which of these foods to 100 ml of milk will provide the greatest amount of protein?

1. 50 ml light cream and 2 tbsp corn syrup.
2. 30 gm powdered skim milk and 1 egg.
3. One small scoop (90 gms) ice cream and 1 tbsp chocolate syrup.
4. Two egg yolks and 1 tbsp sugar.

Options #1, #3, and #4 all contain a simple sugar. The correct answer, Option #2, has more protein. Notice that three of the options are similar; the one that is different may be the correct answer. This strategy is not a substitute for basic knowledge but may help you figure out the question.

---

11. Select the most comprehensive answer. All of the options may be correct, but **one** will include the other three options or need to be considered first.

E X A M P L E :

Diagnostic studies used in the differential diagnosis of systemic lupus erythematosus (SLE) include:

1. Complete blood count (CBC), SMA-12, and erythrocyte sedimentation rate (ESR).
2. Chest radiograph and coagulation profile.

3. Antinuclear antibodies (ANA), ESR, and C-reactive protein.
4. CBC, urinalysis, and chest radiograph.

The correct answer is Option #3. Although all of the tests included in the answer may be included in a complete physical examination, laboratory tests specific or inclusive for the diagnosis of SLE include the ANA, ESR, and C-reactive protein. During flares the ESR and C-reactive protein are elevated. The ANA titer in a client with SLE is positive at a 1:80 ratio.

12. Select the best answer that is most specific to what the question asks. All of the options may be correct, but **one** is more specific or essential.

E X A M P L E :

When taking the history of a client with known allergies, what is the most important information to determine?

1. Reaction associated with each allergen.
2. Drug allergies.
3. Food allergies.
4. Environmental exposure.

It is absolutely essential that the reaction to each allergen is known. The other options are important but are not most important during the taking of the history. Recognize key words that identify the question that is asking for a priority of care—first, initial, best, most. The correct answer is Option #1. The other alternatives may be correct but should be prioritized. Often clients will indicate they have discomfort with a particular food or medication, such as nausea, stomach pain, or diarrhea, and consider it an allergy. The signs and symptoms of the reaction, speed of onset, how long it lasts, and what successful treatment has been used in the past are important information. Both drug and food allergies should be explored.

13. Watch questions in which the options contain several items to consider. After you are sure you understand what information the question is requesting, evaluate each part of the option. Is it appropriate to what the question is asking? If an option contains one incorrect item, the entire option is incorrect. All of the items listed in the selection must be correct if it is to be the answer to the question.

E X A M P L E :

When evaluating an electrocardiogram (ECG), what characteristics most clearly indicate atrial tachycardia?

1. Heart rate of 96, P waves present on each QRS complex, T wave every other beat.
2. P waves present on every other beat, heart rate of 100, and irregular.
3. Heart rate of 110, P waves present prior to each QRS complex, and regular.
4. P waves for every third QRS complex, adequate P-R interval, rate of 90.

The correct answer is Option #3. In a methodical evaluation of the items in the distractors, you can eliminate items in Options #1, #2, and #4. Sinus or atrial tachycardia is characterized by a rate at or above 100, P waves are present for each QRS complex, the P-R interval is below 0.20, the T wave occurs after each QRS complex, and the beat is regular.

14. Be alert to relevant information contained in previous questions. Sometimes, as you are answering questions, you will find information similar to the information being tested in previous test questions. Previous questions may assist you in identifying relevant information in the current question.

E X A M P L E :

The American College of Physicians (ACP) recommends that healthy adults receive a tetanus-diphtheria (Td) booster vaccination:

1. Every 5 years.
2. At age 75.
3. At age 65.
4. Every 10 years.

The ACP recommends that adults receive a Td booster every 10 years or a single booster at age 50 for clients who have completed full pediatric series, including teenage and young adult boosters. The correct answer to this question is Option #4. In another question involving immunizations, you read the following question.

E X A M P L E :

In taking the history of an alert, older adult, the nurse practitioner determines the client is an avid gardener and spends a great deal of time outside. He had a pneumococcal vaccination last year and states he cannot remember when he had a tetanus vaccination. A health maintenance recommendation for this client would be to obtain:

1. Pneumococcal vaccine.
2. Tetanus vaccine.
3. Hepatitis B vaccine.
4. No recommendation.

The correct answer is Option #2. A clue to the answer to this question may be found in the previous question. Older adults who enjoy gardening and outdoor activities should have a Td booster once every 10 years, as the ACP recommends this practice.

15. Multiple-choice mathematical computations may be included in the exam. Mathematical computations may include calculations of IM, PO, and IV dosages; calculations of pediatric dosage; determining creatinine clearance; and conversion of units of measurement.

EXAMPLE:

The nurse practitioner is ordering digoxin (Lanoxin) 0.25 mg for a client who has difficulty swallowing pills. How would the order be written?

1. Digoxin 0.25 mg Sig: 5 ml elixir PO qd.
2. Digoxin 0.25 mg Sig: 1 tab PO qd.
3. Digoxin 0.25 mg Sig: 2.5 ml PO elixir qd.
4. Digoxin 0.025 mg/5 ml Sig: 5 ml PO qd.

First, you must obtain the typical dispensing of oral digoxin, which is 0.05 mg/ml for the elixir. To receive a dose of 0.25 mg, the correct answer would be Option #1.

16. Evaluate priority questions carefully. Frequently all of the answers are appropriate to the situation. You need to decide which of the actions you should do first.

FIGURE 1–1 PERITONITIS "HOT BELLY"
From Zerwekh J, Claborn J, Miller CJ: Memory Notebook of Nursing, Vol I. Dallas, TX: Nursing Education Consultants Publishing, Inc, 1994, p 85, with permission.

EXAMPLE:

While working in her garden, an older adult was bitten on the hand by a raccoon. Her last Td booster was 4 years ago. At the rural clinic, the nurse practitioner cleansed the wound. The next action is:

1. Administer tetanus antitoxin.
2. Contact local animal control authorities.
3. Administer rabies immune globulin (RIG) and human diploid cell vaccine (HDCV).
4. Teach the client how to do hourly soaks to the hand using normal saline and peroxide.

The correct answer is Option #3. Any type of animal bite that might be associated with an animal that may potentially harbor rabies (skunks, bats, raccoons, foxes, coyotes, rats) should be treated with both active and passive rabies immunization. The priority action is to prevent rabies. Tetanus antitoxin would be indicated, if the adult was not current on the Td immunization. Animal authorities would be called after the initial treatment to locate the animal and sacrifice it, so that the brain can be examined for rabies.

Techniques to Increase Critical Thinking Skills

Memory aids and mindmapping are tools that assist in drawing associations from other ideas with the use of visual images. Mnemonics are words, phrases, or other techniques that help you remember information. Imagery is a tool that helps you identify a problem and visualize a mental picture. Learning content utilizing these techniques will assist you in recalling information more effectively.

Mindmapping™ is a method of organizing important information that is in sharp contrast to the traditional outline format. A thought or concept is written in the center of the page, and images and color are added to information as ideas begin to flow from the center focus (see Fig. 1–1).

Acronyms help you to recall information via word association or arrangements of letters to recall specific information. Examples of these are the 6-Ps of dyspnea (see Fig. 1–2), the 5-Ps of circulatory assessment (see Fig. 1–3), and the ABCs of malignant melanoma (see Fig. 1–4).

Acrostics are catchy phrases in which the first letter of each word stands for something to recall. For example, in remembering the use of canes

FIGURE 1–2 6 Ps OF DYSPNEA
From Zerwekh J, Claborn J, Miller CJ: Memory Notebook of Nursing, Vol II. Dallas, TX: Nursing Education Consultants Publishing, Inc, 1997, p 22, with permission.

FIGURE 1–3 CIRCULATION ASSESSMENT: THE 5 Ps
From Zerwekh J, Claborn J, Miller CJ: Memory Notebook of Nursing, Vol II. Dallas, TX: Nursing Education Consultants Publishing, Inc, 1997, p 27, with permission.

and walkers (see Fig. 1–5) think of "Wandering Wilma's Always Late" (**W**alker **W**ith **A**ffected **L**eg). Everyone remembers the cranial nerve mnemonic (see Fig. 1–6).

Memory aids or images are pictures or caricatures that help you to recall information more effectively (see Fig. 1–7).

Rhymes are phrases or words spoken in a rhythmic or musical manner that increase recall. A helpful musical rhyme for hypoglycemia versus hyperglycemia is "hot and dry, sugar high; cold and clammy, need some candy" (see Fig. 1–8). Another rhyme, "fingers, nose, penis, toes," identifies the areas where lidocaine with epinephrine is contraindicated as a local anesthetic. Or, "two is too much," may help you remember toxic levels of the following three drugs, which have a narrow margin of safety—lithium, digoxin, theophylline (see Fig. 1–9).

Note: These are just examples. There are entire books on these helpful aids (see the list of references).

Testing Skills for Paper-and-Pencil Tests

1. Go through the exam and mark all the answers that you know are correct. This ensures you have adequate time to answer the questions you know. Go back and evaluate those questions for which you did not readily recognize the answer.

2. Do not indiscriminately change answers. If you go back and change an answer, you should have a specific reason for doing so. Sometimes you remember information and

HINTS TO MALIGNANT MELANOMA

FIGURE 1–4 HINTS TO MALIGNANT MELANOMA (ABCD)
From Zerwekh J, Claborn J, Miller CJ: Memory Notebook of Nursing, Vol I. Dallas, TX: Nursing Education Consultants Publishing, Inc, 1997, p 137, with permission.

realize you answered the question incorrectly. Frequently, test-takers "talk themselves out of" the correct answer and change it to the incorrect one.

3. After you have completed the exam, go back and check your booklet and make sure all of the questions are answered. Answer all of the questions, even if you must guess.

Testing Skills that Apply to Both Paper-and-Pencil Tests and Computer Testing

1. Listen carefully to the instructions given at the beginning of the examination. Make sure you understand all of the information given and exactly how to mark your answers, and/or how to use the keyboard.

2. Watch your timing. Do not spend too much time on one question. It is very important that you practice your timing on the sample exams. When you being to take a paper-and-pencil test, plan on finishing within the first three fourths of the allocated time. It is not necessary to review all of the questions after you have completed the test. Do it right the first time and there is no need to review the entire test again. Go back and answer the questions that you left blank. Watch your timing on computer tests—make use of a computer clock, if it is available.

3. Be aware of your "first hunch." It is frequently the correct answer. Sometimes information is processed by the brain without you being aware of it. If something about an answer "feels right" or you have a "gut-level feeling," pay attention to it.

4. Eliminate distractors that assume the client

FIGURE 1–5 CANES AND WALKERS
From Zerwekh J, Claborn J, Miller CJ: Memory Notebook of Nursing, Vol II. Dallas, TX: Nursing Education Consultants Publishing, Inc, 1997, p 8, with permission.

"would not understand," or "is ignorant" of the situation, or those that "protect them from worry." For example, "The client should not be told she has cancer because it would upset her too much."

5. Be aware of distractors that contain the words *always* and *never*.

6. There is no pattern of correct answers. Both computer and paper-and-pencil examinations are compiled by a computer and the position of the correct answers is selected at random.

Decrease Anxiety

Your activities on the day of the examination strongly influence your level of anxiety. By care-fully planning ahead, you will be able to eliminate some anxiety-provoking situations.

1. Visit the examination site prior to the day of the exam. Evaluate travel time, parking, and time to get to the designated area. Get an early start to allow extra time.

2. If you have to travel some distance to the examination site, try to spend the night in the immediate vicinity.

3. Do something pleasant the evening prior to the examination. This is not the time to "crash study."

4. Anxiety is contagious. If those around you are extremely anxious, avoid contact with them prior to the examination.

5. Make your meal before the test a light, healthy one.

CRANIAL NERVE MNEMONIC

| S = Sensory | M = Motor | B = Both |

O	Olfactory	O	On	S	Some
O	Optic	O	Old	S	Say
O	Oculomotor	O	Olympus'	M	Marry
T	Trochlear	T	Tiny	M	Money
T	Trigeminal	T	Tops	B	But
A	Abducens	A	A	M	My
F	Facial	F	Finn	B	Brother
A	Acoustic	A	And	S	Says
G	Glossopharyngeal	G	German	B	Bad
V	Vagus nerve	V	Viewed	B	Business
S	Spinal	S	Some	M	Marry
H	Hypoglossal	H	Hops	M	Money

© 1994 Nursing Education Consultants

FIGURE 1–6 CRANIAL NERVE MNEMONIC
From Zerwekh J, Claborn J, Miller CJ: Memory Notebook of Nursing, Vol II. Dallas, TX: Nursing Education Consultants Publishing, Inc. 1994, p 91, with permission.

HYPERTHYROIDISM

INTOLERANCE TO HEAT
FINE-STRAIGHT HAIR
BULGING EYES
FACIAL FLUSHING
ENLARGED THYROID
TACHYCARDIA
↑ SYSTOLIC BP
BREAST ENLARGEMENT
WEIGHT LOSS
MUSCLE WASTING
FINGER CLUBBING
TREMORS
↑ DIARRHEA
MENSTRUAL CHANGES (AMENORRHEA)
LOCALIZED EDEMA
© 1994 Nursing Education Consultants
C.J. MILLER

FIGURE 1–7 HYPERTHYROIDISM
From Zerwekh J, Claborn J, Miller CJ: Memory Notebook of Nursing, Vol I. Dallas, TX: Nursing Education Consultants Publishing, Inc, 1994, p 46, with permission.

BLOOD SUGAR MNEMONIC

Hot & Dry = Sugar High

Cold & Clammy = Need Some Candy

© 1994
Nursing
Education
Consultants

FIGURE 1–8 BLOOD SUGAR MNEMONIC
From Zerwekh J, Claborn J, Miller CJ: Memory Notebook of Nursing, Vol I. Dallas, TX: Nursing Education Consultants Publishing, Inc, 1994, p 50, with permission.

6. Avoid eating highly spiced or different foods. This is not the time for a gastrointestinal upset.

7. Wear comfortable clothes. This is not a good time to wear tight clothing or new shoes.

8. Wear clothing of moderate weight. It is difficult to control the temperature to keep everyone comfortable. Take a sweater or wear layered clothes that can be removed if you get too warm.

9. Wear soft-soled shoes; this decreases the noise in the testing area.

10. Make sure you have the papers that are required to gain admission to the exam site. Do not forget your reading glasses, if you wear them.

11. Do not take study material to the exam site. You cannot take it into the exam area and it is too late to study.

12. Do not panic when you encounter content with which you are unfamiliar in a question. Use good test-taking strategies, select an answer, and continue. Remember, you are not going to know all of the right answers.

13. Reaffirm to yourself that you know the material. It is not time for any self-defeating behavior or negative self-talk. **YOU WILL PASS!!** Build your confidence by visualizing yourself in 6 months working in the area you desire. Create that mental picture of where you want to be and who you want to be—certified nurse practitioner. Use your past successes to bring positive energy and "vibes" to your certification. **WE KNOW YOU CAN DO IT!**

Study Habits

Enhancing Study Skills

* Decide on a study schedule—write it down and stick with it.

* Divide the review material into segments—pediatrics, well-woman, geriatric, and so forth.

FIGURE 1–9   TOXIC LEVELS OF LITHIUM, DIGOXIN, AND THEOPHYLLINE
From Zerwekh J, Claborn J, Miller CJ: Memory Notebook of Nursing, Vol II. Dallas, TX: Nursing Education Consultants Publishing, Inc, 1997, p 43, with permission.

- Prioritize the segments; review first the areas in which you feel you are deficient and/or weak.
- Identify areas that will require additional review.
- Establish a realistic schedule—study in short segments or "bursts." Avoid marathon sessions.
- Plan on achieving your study goal several days prior to the examination.
- Do not study when you are tired or when there are frequent distractions or interruptions.
- Review general concepts of practice from a variety of resources.

Group Study

- Keep the group limited to four or five people.
- Group members should be mature and serious about studying.

- The group should agree on the planned study schedule.
- If the group makes you anxious or you do not feel it meets your study needs, do not continue to participate.

Testing Practice

- Include the testing practice in your schedule.
- Select about 50 questions for a practice testing session of 1 hour. This will allow you to evaluate the pace of the exam (i.e., approximately a question per minute).
- Try to answer the questions as if you were taking the real examination. Do not look up the right answer immediately after answering the question.
- Utilize the testing strategies described in this section.
- Evaluate the practice exams for problem areas: testing skills and knowledge base.

- Evaluate the questions you answer incorrectly. Review the rationale for the right answer and understand why you missed it.
- Utilize the questions at a later point to review the information again.

References

Beitz J: Unleashing the power of memory: The mighty mnemonic. *Nurse Educator*, 22(2), 25–28, 1997.

Bloomingfield R: Mnemonics, Rhetorics, and Poetics for Medics. Salem NC: Harbinger Medical Press, 1982.

Rayfield S, Manning L: Nursing Made Insanely Easy. Shreveport, LA: ICAN, Inc, Publishing, 1997.

Zerwekh J, Claborn J: Test-taking strategies. In NCLEX-RN™: A comprehensive Study Guide, 3rd ed. Dallas, TX: Nursing Education Consultants Publishing, Inc, 1997.

Zerwekh J, Claborn J, Miller CJ: Memory Notebook of Nursing, Vol I. Dallas, TX: Nursing Education Consultants Publishing, Inc, 1994.

Zerwekh J, Claborn J, Miller CJ: Memory Notebook of Nursing, Vol II. Dallas, TX: Nursing Education Consultants Publishing, Inc, 1997.

Growth & Development

Physical Assessment

1. Growth hormone secretion tests along with a history and physical exam have indicated a positive diagnosis for delayed puberty. The next step for the nurse practitioner is to:

    1. Treat with hormone replacement.

    2. Refer to pediatric endocrinologist.

    3. Treat with hormone stimulation therapy.

    4. Refer for possible pituitary tumor.

2. An 11-year-old girl who has just begun to show signs of breast development asks the nurse practitioner when she will start having periods like her friends? The practitioner's response is based on the knowledge that:

    1. The average age of menarche is 12.8 years.

    2. Most girls will have a growth spurt following the onset of menarche.

    3. Menarche usually occurs about 3–6 months after the onset of breast development.

4. Menarche usually occurs about 18–24 months after the onset of breast development.

3. A teenage girl with curly pubic hair on the mons pubis and breast enlargement without secondary contour would be classified on the Tanner Scale as:

    1. Tanner stage I.

    2. Tanner stage II.

    3. Tanner stage III.

    4. Tanner stage IV.

4. During the physical examination of a 13-year-old female, it is developmentally important that the nurse practitioner:

    1. Maintain a comfortable silence.

    2. Verbally affirm normalcy.

    3. Discuss only the major areas of abnormality.

    4. Verbally address problems of sexually transmitted diseases.

5. At a school clinic an adolescent girl comes in complaining of dizziness midmorning and a second episode in class that morning. The practitioner should question the adolescent regarding diet/nutrition, drug use, and:

    1. Asthma.

    2. Pregnancy.

    3. Heart disease.

    4. Stress.

6. A 14-year-old girl is seen in the clinic by the nurse practitioner because she has not achieved menarche. Examination reveals axillary and pubic hair and breast buds with increased size of areola. Based on these findings the most appropriate intervention would be:

    1. Bone age studies.

    2. Labs for luteinizing hormone (LH) and follicle-stimulating hormone (FSH) levels.

    3. Chromosome analysis to rule out Turner's syndrome.

    4. Reassurance that she is developing normally.

7. The nurse practitioner understands the following about birth defects and growth and development problems in mothers with prenatal alcohol exposure:

    1. If alcohol is ingested late in the pregnancy, there is a higher incidence of postmaturity syndrome.

    2. The practice of drinking alcohol while eating a meal significantly reduces the risk of fully expressed fetal alcohol syndrome.

    3. If alcohol is ingested in large amounts early in the pregnancy, there is an increased incidence of fully expressed clinical features.

    4. Growth retardation is associated with early trimester alcohol consumption and postmaturity syndrome.

8. Precocious puberty is defined as:

    1. Onset of puberty before age 8 in females and 9 in males.

    2. Onset of puberty before age 5 in females and 7 in males.

    3. Onset of puberty before age 10 in females and 12 in males.

    4. Onset of puberty for either sex before older siblings enter puberty.

9. The major influence on the timing of puberty is:

    1. Exposure to light.

    2. Genetics.

    3. General health.

    4. Nutrition.

Aging

10. As an individual ages, which physiologic change would affect responses to pharmacologic agents?

    1. Increased gastric emptying.

    2. Increased glomerular filtration rate.

    3. Decreased percentage of body fat.

    4. Decreased albumin concentration.

11. The number one cause of accidental death in clients older than 65 years of age is:

    1. Motor vehicle accidents.

    2. Poisoning.

    3. Falls.

    4. Drowning.

12. The nurse practitioner is assessing the nutritional status of an elderly client. The nurse practitioner identifies the common physiologic changes in the gastrointestinal system to be:

    1. Increased peristalsis.

    2. Decreased absorption of iron.

    3. Maintenance of normal fat metabolism.

    4. Increased drug metabolism.

13. The aging process causes what normal physiologic changes in the heart?

1. Heart size stays the same, the valves thicken and become rigid secondary to fibrosis and sclerosis.

2. Cardiomegaly occurs along with prolapse of the mitral valve and regurgitation.

3. Dilatation of the right ventricle with sclerosis of pulmonic and tricuspid valves.

4. Hypertrophy of the right ventricle with decreasing capacity and compromised efficiency of the coronary arteries.

14. During a teaching session, the nurse practitioner instructs the client regarding normal skin lesions in the older population. These would include:

1. Seborrheic dermatitis.

2. Senile keratosis.

3. Senile lentigo.

4. Squamous cell.

15. Which assessment is a normal physiologic change of the respiratory system that occurs with aging?

1. Decreased residual lung volume (RV).

2. Hyperresonance.

3. Increased forced vital capacity (FVC).

4. Increased tactile fremitus.

16. The nurse practitioner indicates an understanding of the normal aging process with which documentation of the gastrointestinal system in the physical examination?

1. Increase in the size of the liver (16 cm).

2. Absent bowel sounds.

3. Femoral bruit.

4. Increased adipose tissue.

17. Which physiologic factor of aging contributes to incontinence in the elderly?

1. Decreased vascularity of the bladder mucosa.

2. Increased urethral closing pressure.

3. Increased ability to concentrate urine.

4. Decreased bladder capacity.

2   Answers & Rationales

Physical Assessment

1. **(2)** Once the tentative diagnosis is made the nurse practitioner should refer to a pediatric endocrinologist for further work-up. It is beyond the scope of the nurse practitioner's practice to treat at this point.

2. **(4)** Menarche usually occurs about 18–24 months after the onset of breast development. The average age of menarche is 12.8 years, but that is not what the practitioner should base her response on. Most girls have a growth spurt at Tanner stage IV.

3. **(3)**

Stage	Pubic Hair
I	None
II	Countable; straight; increased pigmentation and length
III	Darker; begins to curl; increased quantity on mons pubis
IV	Increased quantity; coarser texture; labia and mons well covered
V	Adult distribution; with feminine triangle and spread to medial thighs

	Breast Development
I	None
II	Breast bud present; increased areolar size
III	Further enlargement of breast; no secondary contour
IV	Areolar area forms secondary mound on breast contour
V	Mature; areolar area is part of breast contour; nipple project

4. **(2)** Early adolescence is a time when the child undergoing great physical changes continually wonders if they are normal. To verbally affirm areas of normalcy during the exam can decrease anxiety.

5. **(2)** Although all areas would be assessed, pregnancy is a common reason for midmorning syncope in adolescents, and is associated with altered nutrition.

6. **(4)** Menarche usually occurs about 18–24 months after the onset of breast development. Bone age and labs are not necessary, since development is within the normal limits. The findings are not indicative of a chromosomal abnormality; therefore, chromosome analysis is unnecessary.

7. **(3)** Large amounts of alcohol early in the pregnancy have the most devastating effects on the maturing fetus. There is no safe, established dose for alcohol in pregnancy. Food consumption along with alcohol intake does not reduce the risk of defects. Ingesting alcohol in the later months of pregnancy is associated with an increased incidence of premature and small-for-gestational age neonates.

8. **(1)** Precocious puberty is defined as that which begins at age 8 for females and age 9 for males.

9. **(2)** Genetics is the primary determinant of the timing of puberty. Other factors including geographic location, exposure to light, nutritional status, and health status all play a role, but genetics is the major influence.

Aging

10. **(4)** Medications are often protein bound (not fat); albumin decreases with age. A low albumin level decreases the number of protein-binding sites, causing an increase in the amount of free drug in the plasma. Drug overdose may occur in the elderly. Gastric emptying and glomerular filtration rate *decrease* with the aging process.

11. **(3)** Falls are the major cause of morbidity and mortality in the elderly. It is often the precipitating event for a cascade of problems leading to death. Complications from falls include fractures, pneumonia, pressure ulcers, pain, and immobility.

12. **(2)** Decreased hydrochloric acid, which occurs with aging, leads to decreased absorption of iron and vitamin B_{12}. Fat absorption would decrease, as would peristalsis and drug metabolism.

13. **(1)** The heart does not increase in size with normal aging. An enlarged heart is a result of cardiac dysfunction. Dilatation of the left ventricle occurs with myocardial infarctions and altered cardiac functioning secondary to cardiac disease, not normal aging. The aging process does cause fibrosis and sclerosis of the cardiac valves; all valves are equally affected.

14. **(3)** The senile lentigine is a gray-brown, irregular, macular lesion on sun-exposed areas of the face, arms, and hands that are normal skin lesions. The other lesions are commonly occurring abnormal skin lesions in the older adult.

15. **(2)** A normal age-related change is an increase in the anteroposterior diameter, which results in hyperresonance. Age-related changes result in an increase in the RV and decrease in the FVC. An increased tactile fremitus is a deviation that is of diagnostic significance.

16. **(4)** Common age-related changes of the gastrointestinal system include an increase in adipose tissue, a decrease in liver size, reduced motility and peristalsis, a decrease in acid secretions and motor activity of stomach, and a decrease in the glomerular filtration rate. Absence of bowel sounds after full 5 minutes and bruits are deviations of clinical significance.

17. **(4)** A decreased bladder capacity along with the decreased ability to concentrate urine and the decreased urethral closing pressure following menopause lead to incontinence. Other factors are depression, decreased mobility, decreased vision, lack of attention to bladder cues of fullness, and so forth.

Health Promotion & Maintenance

1. The current American Cancer Society dietary recommendations for cancer prevention include:

   1. Maintaining a desirable body weight and eating a variety of foods, including fruits and vegetables, and foods that are high in fiber.

   2. Increasing the amount of protein in the diet.

   3. Including a moderate amount of alcohol in the diet.

   4. There are no dietary recommendations for the prevention of cancer.

2. In the presence of dyslipidemia and diabetes, the National Cholesterol Education Program guidelines set the goal for lipid levels as:

   1. LDL <130 mg/dl and triglyceride levels <200 mg/dl.

   2. LDL <160 mg/dl and triglyceride levels <240 mg/dl.

   3. LDL <100 mg/dl and triglyceride levels <180 mg/dl.

   4. LDL <150 mg/dl and triglyceride levels <220 mg/dl.

3. The American Diabetes Association recommends screening adults starting at age 45 with a fasting plasma glucose (FPG) test every:

   1. 1 year.

   2. 3 years.

   3. 5 years.

   4. 10 years.

4. A client is continuing her recovery at home after an extensive surgery. The nurse practitioner would instruct the client to increase her intake of what foods to promote healing?

   1. Tomatoes, rice, whole bran cereal.

   2. Milk, poultry, yellow vegetables.

   3. Red meat, oranges, green beans.

   4. Liver, corn, eggs.

5. Which of the health promotion screenings should be implemented annually for the elderly client over 65?

   1. Chest x-ray.

   2. Pneumococcal vaccination.

   3. Sigmoidoscopy.

   4. Stool guaiac.

6. While teaching a class to a senior women's group, which would be most important for the nurse practitioner to consider during the presentation?

   1. Provide a lot of overhead lighting in order to enhance visualization.

   2. Provide handouts on blue paper with black print.

   3. Review a video narrated by a woman.

   4. Recognize that the clients' past life experiences are beneficial in learning new information.

7. The newest recommendations from the American Cancer Society for yearly mammography to begin is at age:

   1. 50.

   2. 45.

   3. 60.

   4. 40.

8. In teaching a client who is to have a test for colon-rectal screening, the nurse practitioner should instruct the client to:

   1. Eat at least 2 servings of rare meat daily prior to collecting samples.

   2. Avoid antibiotics, aspirin, iron, and anti-inflammatory medications.

   3. Take extra vitamin C to avoid a subsequent bladder infection that would make collecting samples difficult.

   4. Eat extra servings of foods such as broccoli, cabbage, potatoes, cantaloupe, and turnips to increase the fiber and ensure good samples.

9. The recommended number of servings of the bread/cereal/pasta/rice group is how many servings per day?

   1. 6–11 servings.

   2. 2–4 servings.

   3. 3–5 servings.

   4. 2–3 servings.

10. The age at which a *screening* mammogram is recommended as part of a woman's periodic health evaluation, if the woman is not at increased risk for breast cancer, is:

    1. 30 years old.

    2. 35 years old.

    3. Before the age of 40.

    4. Before the age of 50.

11. The history collected on a new client who enters a practice is to include:

    1. Interval history, past medical and surgical history, family medical and surgical histories, psychosocial history, usual dietary habits, physical activity, tobacco and other substance use, sexual practices, and a review of systems.

    2. Interval history, past medical history, family medical history, dietary habits, substance use, and sexual practices.

    3. Past medical and surgical histories, family medical history, psychosocial history, physical activity, tobacco and other substance use, and sexual practices.

    4. The history listed on the form provided to clients for completion prior to the physical examination is sufficient and no interview needs to be done.

12. The most common occupationally related disease is:

    1. Repetitive motion injury.

    2. Hearing loss.

    3. Lung disease.

    4. Cancer.

13. The nurse practitioner is discussing lifestyle changes and decreasing risk factors for cardiovascular diseases with a group of geriatric clients. What is most important to include in this discussion?

    1. Decrease smoking, increase vitamin supplements, increase protein intake.

2. Control hypertension, stop smoking, maintain normal weight, exercise regularly.

3. Maintain normal levels of serum blood sugar, decrease cholesterol intake.

4. Get a yearly physical examination, increase fiber in diet, exercise regularly.

14. What lifestyle modifications are most effective in controlling hypertension in the older client?

    1. Maintain normal weight, decreased sodium diet, exercise regularly.

    2. Increase dietary protein, decrease weight, learn stress reduction techniques.

    3. Consume a high-complex carbohydrate, low-sodium diet, decrease stress.

    4. Reduce weight, increase vitamin supplements, and exercise regularly.

15. The nurse practitioner is developing written materials on health care information for parents. Guidelines for developing education materials at an acceptable reading level include all **except**:

    1. Present the most important material first.

    2. Use all capital letters.

    3. Keep sentences short and to the point.

    4. Add visual graphic images to clarify information.

16. In explaining the purpose of primary prevention programs to a group of nursing students, the nurse practitioner relates that primary prevention programs:

    1. Work to lower the incidence of birth defects.

    2. Emphasize early diagnosis and treatment of pediatric anomalies.

    3. Minimize the handicapping effect of mental retardation.

    4. Focus on the prevention of complications and rehabilitation.

17. A new mother asks about the differences between human milk and cow's milk. The nurse practitioner explains:

    1. Human milk has more lipase and linoleic acid.

    2. Human milk has more calcium (Ca), phosphorus (P, sodium (Na), and potassium (K).

    3. Cow's milk has low protein and casein content.

    4. Cow's milk has high linoleic acid and low saturated fatty acids.

18. According to the American Academy of Pediatrics (AAP), infants may be fed whole cow's milk once they reach:

    1. 6 months of age.

    2. 8 months of age.

    3. 12 months of age.

    4. 18 months of age.

19. In the preparation of reading and education materials for clients, the nurse practitioner is aware that the reading level of most adults is at the:

    1. Twelfth-grade level.

    2. Tenth-grade level.

    3. Sixth-grade level.

    4. Fourth-grade level.

Immunizations

20. The nurse practitioner understands that the following is considered an attenuated live-virus vaccination:

    1. Rubella and measles.

    2. Mumps and hepatitis B.

    3. Poliomyelitis and hepatitis B.

    4. Rubella and rabies.

21. In taking the history of a healthy 50-year-old adult, the nurse practitioner determines the client is an avid gardener and spends a great deal of time enjoying the out-of-doors. A health maintenance recommendation for this client is to obtain a:

    1. Pneumococcal vaccine.

    2. Tetanus vaccine.

    3. Hepatitis B vaccine.

    4. Varicella vaccine.

22. Which statement describing the polyvalent pneumococcal vaccine is **incorrect**?

    1. It is recommended for those with chronic respiratory illness.

    2. It can be given on the same visit as the influenza vaccine.

    3. It should be given yearly.

    4. It is never recommended for children.

23. The influenza vaccination is recommended annually for high-risk groups. The nurse practitioner knows that the greatest need for this vaccination would be for:

    1. Adults with chronic disease.

    2. Residents of long-term care facilities.

    3. Dialysis clients.

    4. Health care employees.

24. The nurse practitioner understands that the only contraindication to hepatitis B vaccination is:

    1. Pregnancy and lactation.

    2. History of poliomyelitis.

    3. Prior anaphylaxis or severe hypersensitivity.

    4. Mild viral illness.

25. Immunizations and chemoprophylaxis offered routinely to clients who are 65 years of age and older are:

    1. Diphtheria-tetanus-pertussis absorbed (DTP), influenza, and Pneumovax.

    2. Tetanus-diphtheria (Td), influenza, and pneumococcal vaccine.

    3. Td and influenza; to those with chronic diseases offer the pneumococcal vaccine.

    4. Influenza and pneumococcal pneumonia and Td to those who have not had one in the last 10 years.

26. The American College of Physicians (ACP) recommends that healthy adults receive a Td booster vaccination:

    1. Every 5 years.

    2. Every 8 years.

    3. At age 60.

    4. Every 10 years.

27. Which statement most correctly describes tetanus toxoid?

    1. Tetanus toxoid (T) induces more persistent antitoxin antibody titers.

    2. DPT and diphtheria and tetanus toxoids absorbed (DT) are safe to give to adults.

    3. The recommended dose for the adult is 0.75 ml IM.

    4. Tetanus toxoid fluid provides the same antitoxin antibody titers as tetanus toxoid.

28. Immunizations recommended for healthy young adults include:

    1. Measles, rubella, varicella, and hepatitis B.

    2. Penumovax, influenza, and rubella.

    3. Tetanus, influenza, varicella, Pneumovax and hepatitis B.

    4. Influenza, hepatitis B, rubella, measles, and tetanus.

3

Answers & Rationales

1. **(1)** The American Cancer Society does recommend the maintenance of a desirable body weight; research has shown an association between increased deaths from various cancers and varying degrees of being overweight. Another recommendation is to eat a wide variety of foods, consistent with the Food Guide Pyramid put out by the U.S. Department of Agriculture and the U.S. Department of Health and Human Services. A variety of fruits and vegetables should be included in the daily diet (5–9 servings/day), as research has shown that there is an association between lower cancer rates and high fruit and vegetable consumption. High-fiber foods are also recommended; a lower risk of colon cancer is seen in those individuals who consume a high-fiber diet. There are no recommendations to increase the amount of protein in the diet at this time; due to the high consumption of red meat in the American diet, many people are already getting large quantities in their current diets. The American Cancer Society recommends limiting the daily consumption of alcohol to two drinks for males, one drink for females, and no drinks for pregnant females. They also state that ideally, no alcohol should be consumed; regular alcohol consumption has been shown to increase the risk of various cancers.

2. **(1)** The recommendation for low-density lipoprotein (LDL) is <130 mg/dl and for triglyceride levels <200 mg/dl. All other choices have inaccuracies of goals.

3. **(2)** The American Diabetes Association recommends screening adults starting at the age of 45 every 3 years.

4. **(3)** The client needs an increased intake in protein and vitamin C to promote healing. Red meat, citrus fruits, and green vegetables will give the highest amounts of these elements from the selections offered.

5. **(4)** This evaluation will assist in identifying any problems with bleeding. Option #1 is not necessary. Option #2 is not a screening and would not be administered annually. A sigmoidoscopy is recommended every 3–5 years for clients over 50.

6. **(4)** This applies the concept of adult educational principles. Overhead lighting may produce an increase in the glare, which can decrease visualization. There is an alteration of color perception (e.g., blue appears green-blue) as an individual ages. As individuals age the ability to hear women's and children's voices decreases, since these are high-pitched voices. This video would not enhance the program if these clients frequently have presbycusis as a result of the normal aging process.

7. **(4)** In the summer of 1997, the National Institutes of Health and the American Cancer Society changed the recommendation to begin yearly mammography at age 40.

8. **(2)** Screening for colon-rectal cancer includes annual fecal occult blood screening for individuals over age 50. Avoiding medications that can cause gastrointestinal irritation and bleeding can help avoid false-positive results. Rare meat and vegetables that are high in peroxidase (like the ones listed) will cause false-positive results, whereas vitamin C can cause false-negative results.

9. **(1)** The recommended servings for each of the food groups are as follows:

Food Group	Servings
Bread/cereal/rice/pasta	6–11 servings
Fruits	2–4 servings
Vegetables	3–5 servings
Meat/poultry/fish, dry beans, eggs, & nuts	2–3 servings
Fats/oils/sweets	Sparing uses

10. **(3)** A screening mammogram is recommended before the age of 40.

11. **(1)** All of these areas are important to probe in the initial interview of a new client. The history will help determine the necessary components of the physical examination and laboratory or radiologic studies that are ordered and the counseling that is done during the appointment.

12. **(3)** All of these disorders can be associated with workplace exposure but currently, lung disease is still the most common occupationally related disease. Musculoskeletal injuries are on the rise.

13. **(2)** Hypertension, smoking, and hyperlipidemia are the major risk factors for the development of cardiovascular disease. Controlling hyperglycemia, high dietary fiber intake, and vitamin supplements assist in maintaining a healthy lifestyle; however, they are not as important in preventing cardiovascular disease.

14. **(1)** These three modifications are the most effective in maintaining normal blood pressure.

15. **(2)** Printed materials must be written to a level of readability so that they can be understood. Do not use all capital letters, as it is difficult to read. Also, it is helpful to write in the active versus the passive voice, to use one- and two-syllable words, to avoid complex grammatical structures, and to express only one idea in each sentence.

16. **(1)** Primary prevention programs exist to prevent disease, malfunctioning, or maladaption from ever occurring. Examples of these types of programs include promoting consumption of a healthy diet, the practice of safe sex, the avoidance of alcohol and tobacco use, and so forth. Secondary prevention is early diagnosis and treatment (i.e., screening for tuberculosis or sickle cell disease, and breast and testicular self-examination). Tertiary prevention is the prevention of complications and rehabilitation after the disease or condition has already occurred (i.e., cardiac rehabilitation, having blood for a complete blood count [CBC] drawn before chemotherapy).

17. **(1)** Cow's milk is not as good of a nutritional source as human milk, because it has more mineral content (Ca, P, Na, K), which causes a larger renal solute load. In addition, cow's milk is high in protein, casein, and saturated fat and lower in carbohydrates.

18. **(3)** At 1 year of age, infants may be fed whole cow's milk. The purpose for waiting is that it has been shown that cow's milk is low in iron, linoleic acid, and vitamin E, as well as being high in protein, sodium, and potassium.

19. **(3)** The reading level of most American adults is at the sixth-grade level.

Immunizations

20. **(1)** Attenuated live-virus vaccines are available for the following communicable diseases: measles, mumps, rubella, poliomyelitis, yellow fever, and smallpox. Rabies vaccine is a killed virus and hepatitis B is a purified viral antigen obtained from the blood of an infected client and then inactivated when manufactured into a vaccination.

21. **(2)** Adults who enjoy gardening and outdoor activities should have a tetanus vaccine at least every ten years due to the high risk activities. A pneumococcal vaccine is recommended for adults age 65 or older, or for those who have a chronic illness or who are immunosuppressed. Most older adults have had chicken pox as a child and do not require the vaccine.

22. **(3)** It is not given more often than every 10 years and may be effective for longer periods.

23. **(2)** Influenza outbreaks may affect 60% of those in long-term care and fatality rates are high. All the other groups listed are appropriate for the influenza vaccine but are not as high a priority.

24. **(3)** Prior anaphylaxis and severe hypersensitivity would be considered a contraindication; a mild viral illness would not. The client who is pregnant or lactating may be immunized.

25. **(4)** Pneumococcal and annual influenza immunizations are recommended for those who are 65 years of age and older. Adult Td is offered to those who have not had a booster in the last 10 years.

26. **(4)** The ACP recommends that adults receive a Td booster every 10 years or a single booster at age 50 for clients who have completed a full pediatric series, including teenage and young adult boosters.

27. **(1)** Tetanus toxoid induces more persistent antitoxin antibody titers than tetanus toxoid fluid. DPT and DT are for use in children under the age of 7 years; however, they should *not* be used in adults. The recommended dose of DT for an adult is 0.5 ml IM.

28. **(4)** Five to 20% of young adults are susceptible to measles and/or rubella. Influenza and hepatitis B immunizations are recommended for students who have exposure to a large number of people. Tetanus immunization is recommended every 10 years, especially in high-risk situations (young adults that participate in outdoor sports). Pneumovax is indicated in a young adult who has a chronic disease, such as diabetes, chronic pulmonary disease, or chronic cardiovascular disease, and is also indicated for young adults who are immunocompromised.

Cardiovascular

Physical Examination & Diagnostic Tests

1. The nurse practitioner is performing a physical examination on a healthy female adult. On auscultation the stethoscope would be placed in what areas to best hear the characteristic sounds of S_1 and S_2?

   1. S_1 is best heard at the apex and S_2 at the base of the heart.

   2. Both are heard equally well on the right side at the midclavicular line.

   3. On the left side, S_1 is at the area of pulmonic valve and S_2 at the aortic valve.

   4. Both sounds are heard best at Erb's point at the third intercostal space at the sternal margin.

2. On the general assessment of an adult client, the nurse practitioner determines the presence of the apical impulse at the point of maximal impulse (PMI) on the client's chest wall. Where on the chest wall is the PMI normally found?

   1. Second intercostal space at the midclavicular line on the left side.

   2. Right lower sternal border, fifth intercostal space.

   3. Left side at the fifth intercostal space on the midclavicular line.

   4. Left fifth intercostal space, lateral to the midclavicular line.

3. The nurse practitioner is auscultating the carotids for a whooshing sound. The correct procedure is:

   1. Use the diaphragm of the stethoscope.

   2. Use the bell of the stethoscope.

   3. Place the stethoscope 1 inch off the area above the sternocleidomastoid muscle.

   4. Position the client at a 30-degree angle, press firmly with the bell of the stethoscope.

4. When inspecting the precordium, the nurse practitioner is checking for:

   1. Scars and anatomic landmarks.

   2. Pulsations and retractions.

   3. Heaves and cardiac dullness.

   4. Pericardial friction rub and lifts.

5. While examining a client in the left lateral decubitus position, the nurse practitioner auscultates a third heart sound (S_3). The nurse practitioner knows:

   1. This sound is normally heard in children and young adults and is considered a physiologic S_3.

   2. This rarely is associated with myocardial failure in the older adult.

   3. This client should be immediately referred to a cardiologist for evaluation.

   4. This is considered a normal splitting of the S_2 during inspiration and is accentuated by positioning.

6. The nurse practitioner knows the correct auscultatory site for the aortic area is:

   1. Midclavicular line, fifth interspace, left side.

   2. Left fourth interspace close to the sternum.

   3. Right second interspace close to the sternum.

   4. Midclavicular line, second interspace, left side.

7. The nurse practitioner should include the following in his/her teaching when ordering a lipid profile on a client:

   1. A normal breakfast should be consumed the morning of the exam.

   2. The client should be fasting for 12 hours prior to the exam, with the client's typical diet being ingested for the 7 days prior to the exam.

   3. There are no alcohol or diet restrictions for this test.

   4. The client may take any current medications with a few sips of water before the test.

8. When auscultating the heart sounds of a 72-year-old client with a history of hypertension, the nurse practitioner notes an S_4. This finding could indicate:

   1. A normal variant in people 65 years or older.

   2. The beginning of ventricular failure.

   3. A decreased resistance to ventricular filling.

   4. A severely failing heart.

9. A 55-year-old client has a blood pressure of 168/100. This is classified as:

   1. Moderate hypertension.

   2. Mild hypertension.

   3. High normal blood pressure

   4. Severe hypertension.

10. The nurse practitioner is examining a client with a history of rheumatic fever and who is being followed for the development of carditis. During the cardiac auscultation, where on the chest wall is the stethoscope placed to determine the most common murmurs associated with this condition?

    1. At the left sternal border, fourth left intercostal space.

    2. Fifth intercostal space, left side at the midclavicular line.

    3. Second or third intercostal space at the left of the sternal border.

    4. Second intercostal space on the right of the sternal border.

11. A client presents with unusual coolness in the left hand as compared to the right hand. What is the next step in the examination?

    1. Palpate the radial pulse on both hands for a full minute.

    2. Feel the forehead with the backs of the fingers.

    3. Feel the forearms with the backs of the fingers.

    4. Hold the hand in a dependent position and re-examine in 3 minutes.

12. S_1 and S_2 are identified when the nurse practitioner auscultates for cardiac sounds. The physiology responsible for the production of these heart sounds is:

    1. Contraction of the ventricles and closure of the atrioventricular (AV) valves produces S_1, closure of the semilunar valves forms S_2.

2. Closure of the aortic valve produces S_2, opening of the mitral valve and filling of the left ventricle forms S_1.

3. The opening of the AV valves produces S_1, closure of the semilunar valves produces S_2.

4. Opening of the tricuspid produces S_1, closure of the pulmonic forms S_2.

13. The nurse practitioner is assessing a cardiac client who is experiencing an atrial dysrhythmia. The pulse rate is irregular at 110 bpm and there is concern regarding a pulse deficit. How is a pulse deficit determined in this client?

1. A 12-lead electrocardiogram (ECG) is necessary to determine the presence and length of the P-R intervals.

2. The apical pulse is counted and then the radial pulse is counted; the pulse deficit is determined by the difference in the two rates.

3. The apical pulse is counted, and an increase or decrease is correlated with the phases of the respiratory cycle.

4. The apical pulse and radial pulse are determined simultaneously; the pulse deficit established if the apical rate is higher than the radial rate.

14. The nurse practitioner notes a grade V systolic murmur while examining a client's precordium. Which describes this type of murmur?

1. Barely audible, faint with the bell of the stethoscope.

2. Heard only with the diaphragm of the stethoscope.

3. Heard with the stethoscope partly off the chest.

4. Heard without the aid of the stethoscope.

15. When assessing temperature of an extremity as part of a peripheral vascular assessment on a client, which part of the hand is the most sensitive?

1. Palm.

2. Fingertips.

3. Back of the wrist.

4. Backs of the fingers.

16. A 45-year-old female's lipid profile results are sent to the nurse practitioner. They are as follows: total cholesterol = 287 mmol/L; high-density lipoprotein (HDL) = 30 mg/dl; low-density lipoprotein (LDL) = 165 mg/dl; triglycerides = 238 mg/dl. The nurse practitioner interprets these results as:

1. Abnormal; the elevated triglyceride level is of the most concern and should be treated immediately.

2. Borderline, this is considered to be a borderline-risk lipid profile.

3. Abnormal; the total cholesterol and LDL levels are elevated, and the HDL is too low.

4. Normal; these results are of no concern; follow-up with client in 1 year.

17. On assessment of a geriatric client, the nurse practitioner notes bilateral pulsations and distention of the jugular veins when the client's head is elevated 45 degrees. What further assessment information needs to be obtained at this time?

1. Estimate the level of venous pressure by measuring from the sternal angle to the highest level of venous pulsations.

2. Place the client in the supine position and determine the effect of position change on distention and pulsations of the jugular vein.

3. Carotid pulses should be measured due to the increased left ventricular pressure.

4. Have the client hold her breath to facilitate evaluation for the presence of carotid bruits.

18. The nurse practitioner is examining a woman with a known history of mitral valve disease. What type of murmur heard on auscultation supports a history of mitral stenosis?

    1. Diastolic murmur, heard loudest at the apex with the client on her left side.

    2. Midsystolic ejection murmur, heard loudest over the left lower sternal border.

    3. Holosystolic murmur, heard loudest over the apex and left axillary area.

    4. Diastolic murmur, heard loudest with her in sitting position leaning forward.

19. Which symptoms would indicate to the nurse practitioner that the client is experiencing intermittent claudication?

    1. Petechiae and itching of the lower part of the leg.

    2. Extensive discoloration and edema of the upper leg.

    3. Profuse rash and discoloration from trunk down to feet.

    4. Complaints of pain on walking, relieved by sitting down.

20. A 52-year-old woman with a history of heart disease presents to the clinic with a significant bradycardia. The nurse practitioner orders a stat EKG which shows a complete A-V disassociation. What is the next best action for the nurse practitioner to take?

    1. Arrange for the client to see a cardiologist immediately.

    2. Evaluate the apical radial pulse to determine a pulse deficit.

    3. Refer the client to a cardiologist for a stress test.

    4. Order a 24 hour Holter monitor and evaluate changes.

Disorders

21. The diagnosis of hypertension (HTN) should be established on the basis of:

    1. At least three readings with an average systolic blood pressure (BP) of 140 mm Hg and diastolic pressure of 90 mm Hg.

    2. At least five readings 1 month apart.

    3. One reading of 140 mm Hg systolic and 90 mm Hg diastolic or above.

    4. One reading taken in three different positions.

22. A client has a 2-year history of hypertensive heart disease. The nurse practitioner expects the major pathophysiologic change to be:

    1. Right ventricular hypertrophy.

    2. Left atrial dilation.

    3. Left ventricular hypertrophy.

    4. Right atrial dilation.

23. From the following description, what data most clearly describes atrial tachycardia?

    1. Heart rate of 96, P waves present on each QRS complex, T wave every other beat.

    2. P waves present on every other beat, heart rate of 100, and irregular.

    3. Heart rate of 110, P waves present prior to each QRS complex, and regular.

    4. P waves for every third QRS complex, adequate P-R interval, rate of 90.

24. The nurse practitioner is performing an assessment on a client who is having difficulty controlling his left-sided congestive heart failure (CHF). The nurse practitioner understands that the primary symptoms associated with this type of failure are:

    1. Systemic venous congestion.

    2. Dyspnea and pulmonary congestion.

    3. Increased peripheral edema and anorexia.

    4. Atrial fibrillation with a rate around 110.

25. A geriatric client has a diagnosis of left-sided CHF. The nurse practitioner would identify what common condition frequently associated with CHF?

    1. History of peripheral vascular disease.

2. History of untreated hypertension.

3. Current treatment for ventricular dysrhythmias.

4. History of chronic obstructive pulmonary disease (COPD).

26. In evaluating the effectiveness of cardiopulmonary resuscitation (CPR) on the adult client, the nurse practitioner would note:

1. Dilated pupils.

2. Palpable carotid pulse.

3. Capillary refill within 2 seconds.

4. Pink and warm skin.

27. The nurse practitioner is evaluating an ECG. The client presented at the clinic with complaints of weakness and fainting. Her ECG reveals a cardiac rate of 68, absent P waves, regular QRS complex, T-waves are present after each QRS complex. The best interpretation of this information is:

1. A normal ECG; need to further evaluate client's complaints of weakness.

2. Third-degree block with junctional rhythm; keep client at rest and transfer to emergency room for cardiology consult.

3. First-degree block; need to further evaluate possibility of digitalis toxicity and/or levels of cardiac antiarrhythmic medications.

4. Administer sublingual nitroglycerin and refer client for a cardiology consult.

28. Cardiovascular risk factors predisposing females to cardiovascular disease include:

1. Absence of estrogen adversely affects lipoprotein metabolism.

2. Fat deposited on hips mobilizes, raising serum cholesterol.

3. Coronary arteries are longer and wider in diameter.

4. Resting ejection fraction is lower.

29. When assessing the carotid pulse of a 72-year-old indigent client at a community-based clinic, the nurse practitioner notes a bounding pulse with rapid rise and sudden collapse. The nurse practitioner would include which additional assessment to support this finding?

1. Auscultation for a diastolic murmur.

2. Auscultation for paradoxical pulse.

3. Blood pressure in both arms lying, sitting, and standing.

4. Blood pressure for an auscultatory gap.

30. The nurse practitioner understands that the pain experienced with angina pectoris or a myocardial infarction is caused by irritation of the myocardial nerve fibers by the increase in:

1. Blood glucose.

2. Lactic acid.

3. Serum potassium.

4. Serum magnesium.

31. New York Heart Association Functional Class III for clients with cardiac disease is characterized by:

1. Symptoms are present at rest; any activity leads to increased discomfort.

2. Slight limitation in ordinary physical activity, resulting in fatigue, palpitations, dyspnea, or angina.

3. No physical limitation in activity.

4. Marked limitation in activity; clients are comfortable at rest, but ordinary activity leads to symptoms.

32. During the history and physical examination of a client with suspected early CHF, which is the most prominent finding?

1. Moist crackles in the lung bases bilaterally.

2. Anorexia with weight loss of 3 lb in 1 week.

3. Increased urinary output, peripheral edema.

4. Facial edema and distended neck veins.

33. Chest pain that is sudden and severe, described as tearing and accompanied by a decrease in peripheral pulses, may indicate a diagnosis of:

    1. Angina.

    2. Acute myocardial infarction (MI).

    3. Aortic dissection.

    4. Pericarditis.

34. Dietary therapy for hyperlipidemia occurs in two steps, a Step I and a Step II diet. A Step I diet includes, as daily intake:

    1. Total fat ≤30% of total calories, <300 mg cholesterol, 8–10% saturated fat.

    2. Total fat ≤30% of total calories, <200 mg cholesterol, <7% saturated fat.

    3. Total fat ≤40% of total calories, <400 mg cholesterol, <15% saturated fat.

    4. Total fat ≤30% of total calories, <2000 total calories, <3 gm sodium.

35. In an overweight, older adult female client with an elevated cholesterol level and abnormal lipoprotein profile, the first step in treatment includes:

    1. Prescribing a bile acid sequestrant agent.

    2. Initiation of a diet and exercise program.

    3. Estrogen replacement therapy.

    4. Referral to a cardiologist.

36. The nurse practitioner understands that the most common symptom of CHF in adults is:

    1. Anorexia.

    2. Dependent edema.

    3. Dyspnea.

    4. Weakness.

37. The nurse practitioner teaches the cardiac client to avoid foods high in saturated fats, which include:

    1. Nuts, legumes, and seeds.

    2. Fish, shellfish, and mussels.

    3. Palm oil, coconut oil, and butter.

    4. Peanut oil, soybean oil, and olive oil.

38. An elderly female client is complaining of chest pain. A parameter to assist the nurse practitioner to differentiate the chest pain of angina from that of an infarction is:

    1. Myocardial pain with an infarction is more severe.

    2. Anginal pain is more substernal and does not radiate to other areas.

    3. Anginal pain is frequently relieved by nitroglycerin.

    4. Pain from an infarction is always associated with other symptoms.

39. The nurse practitioner is evaluating a client in the office who is complaining of chest pain. The ECG shows some signs of ischemia, and the client is to be transferred to the emergency department. What drug might the nurse practitioner give the client while awaiting transport to the emergency department?

    1. Furosemide (Lasix) 40 mg IV.

    2. Morphine sulfate 25 mg IV.

    3. Streptokinase IV.

    4. Acetylsalicylic acid (aspirin) 81 mg PO.

40. An elderly client is being evaluated for a complaint of dizziness. The symptom that will make the nurse practitioner consider that this is a life-threatening event as opposed to a disease that is not life threatening is:

    1. The onset of the dizziness occurs in certain positions.

    2. It is accompanied by tinnitus.

    3. The symptoms worsen when standing and improve when lying down.

    4. It is preceded by rapid breathing.

41. A 28-year-old female presents to the nurse practitioner with a history of chest pain that has been increasing over the past several days. The client states that the pain worsens upon lying down. She denies any shortness of breath, cough, or radiation of the pain. She does give a history of a recent coxsackievirus infection. On exam, it is

noted that the client has a cardiac friction rub. One probable diagnosis considered by the nurse practitioner is:

1. Acute myocardial infarction.

2. Pleural effusion.

3. Pericarditis.

4. Esophageal reflux.

42. The nurse practitioner would most likely suspect which differential diagnosis for an elderly client presenting with atrial fibrillation and functional decline?

1. Hyperthyroidism.

2. Hypothyroidism.

3. Sick-sinus syndrome.

4. Congestive heart failure.

43. During the cardiac auscultation of an older adult, a grade II/VI murmur, heard best at the second right intercostal space, is noted. The murmur is auscultated louder with squatting. There is a small carotid pulse with a delayed upstroke. The client's history is benign, and his activity tolerance is within normal limits for his age. The nurse practitioner would interpret this murmur to be indicative of:

1. Aortic regurgitation.

2. Aortic stenosis.

3. Mitral valve prolapse.

4. Mitral regurgitation.

44. A middle-aged female with no known coronary artery risk factors presents with a cholesterol level of 255 mg/dl. The nurse practitioner would:

1. Start her on an HMG-CoA reductase inhibitor (statins), the most potent lipid-lowering agents.

2. Start her on a Step I diet, since all clients should be given a trial on a diet.

3. Repeat cholesterol and obtain HDL and calculated LDL levels.

4. Do nothing, since she has no coronary risks.

45. A client has a history of mitral valve stenosis and comes to the clinic for an annual checkup. What findings on the physical exam would correlate with the beginning of complications often seen with these clients?

1. History of chest pain relieved by rest, increase in peripheral edema.

2. Chest pain with deep inspiration and low-grade fever for 3 weeks.

3. History of dyspnea on exertion, increasing fatigue, presence of diastolic murmur.

4. Orthostatic hypotension, tachycardia but regular pulse, 15-point pulse deficit.

Pharmacology

46. A 49-year-old female was started on a thiazide diuretic for hypertension 1 month ago. She arrives in the clinic complaining of muscle cramps and dizziness. Physical exam findings are:

- BP 132/88 mm Hg (previous 186/112)
- Pulse 112
- Respirations 24
- Tenting positive
- Skin turgor decreased
- Neck veins flat
- STAT serum electrolytes
  Sodium 114 mEq/L
  Chloride 92 mEq/L
  Potassium 3.0 mEq/L
- STAT blood glucose 201 mg/dl

Initial treatment for this client should include fluid replacement:

1. Orally with free water and a potassium supplement.

2. Intravenously with normal saline and regular insulin subcutaneously.

3. Intravenously with 1000 ml of normal saline with 40 mEq potassium chloride (KCl) at 50 ml/hr.

4. Intravenously with 1000 ml of Ringer's lactate at 250 ml/hr.

47. A client is recovering from an acute episode of thrombophlebitis and is being treated with warfarin (Coumadin) 5 mg PO daily. In reviewing medication information, the nurse practitioner would include what information in her teaching?

    1. Decrease the servings of green leafy vegetables and do not take a multivitamin supplement.

    2. Limit dairy products, since they tend to decrease medication effectiveness.

    3. Don't walk for exercise; aerobic exercises are more effective.

    4. Maintain a daily record of intake and output to evaluate renal function.

48. The nurse practitioner is evaluating a client who is complaining of "not feeling good." She has a history of coronary artery disease (CAD) and CHF. Vital signs are pulse 72, respirations 20, blood pressure 130/88, temperature is normal. There are no complaints of chest pain or difficulty breathing, some nausea but no vomiting over the past 2 days, and lower extremities are negative for edema. The client states she has been able to take her medications. Her current medications are digoxin (Lanoxin) 0.25 bid, hydrochlorothiazide (Hydrodiuril) 100 mg bid, potassium (Micro-K) 10 mEq daily, and nitroglycerin transdermal patches. What is the priority of care for this client?

    1. Obtain a STAT ECG and white blood cell (WBC) count.

    2. Obtain arterial blood gases and supply oxygen at 4 L/min.

    3. Obtain serum digoxin and potassium levels.

    4. Obtain serial cardiac enzymes now and q6h × 2.

49. The nurse practitioner has prescribed losartan (Cozaar) 50 mg PO qd. This medication promotes vasodilation by:

    1. Inhibiting conversion of angiotensin I to angiotensin II.

    2. Promoting the release of aldosterone.

    3. Promoting the synthesis of prostaglandin.

    4. Inhibiting calcium influx into smooth muscle cells.

50. A client with a history of hypertension is started on Aldactone 50 mg PO qd. The nurse practitioner instructs the client to call the clinic if which symptoms are experienced?

    1. Muscle weakness, fatigue, and paresthesias.

    2. Decreased reflex response, nausea, and vomiting.

    3. Muscle twitching, numbness of the limbs, and depression.

    4. Weight gain, excessive thirst, and fever.

51. A client with a serum cholesterol of 256 mg/dl, HDL of 38 mg/dl, and LDL of 172 mg/dl is instructed on dietary modifications and niacin (nicotinic acid) 1 gm PO tid. Specific instructions include:

    1. Limiting fluid intake.

    2. Taking measures to minimize orthostatic hypotension.

    3. Administering the drug an hour after eating.

    4. Making slight modifications in diet are required with drug therapy.

52. When monitoring for the therapeutic effects of verapamil (Calan SR), the nurse practitioner would assess for a(an):

    1. Increase in heart rate.

    2. Decrease in systemic vascular resistance.

    3. Increase in blood pressure.

    4. Decrease in ventricular premature beats.

53. An adult female client with essential hypertension was treated by the nurse practitioner with enalapril (Vasotec) 5 mg daily. After 6 months of therapy, the blood pressure was measured at 150/100 mm Hg. The nurse practitioner recommended sodium restriction and increased the enalapril to 10 mg daily. The client's blood pressure was unchanged after 3 additional

months. At this point, the nurse practitioner should:

1. Double the dose of enalapril (Vasotec).
2. Add 25 mg of hydrochlorothiazide (Hydrodiuril) daily.
3. Double the dose of enalapril and add 25 mg of hydrochlorothiazide daily.
4. Switch to captopril (Capoten) 50 mg tid.

54. When prescribing antihypertensive drug therapy for elderly clients, the nurse practitioner recognizes that elderly clients have decreased receptor sensitivity and a changing baroreceptor response. Which class of antihypertensive agents should be avoided with elderly clients?

1. Calcium entry antagonists.
2. Diuretics.
3. β-Blockers.
4. Angiotensin converting enzyme (ACE) inhibitors.

55. Medications used in managing ischemic heart disease include:

1. β-Blockers, sedatives, aspirin.
2. Nitrates, β-blockers, calcium channel blockers, aspirin.
3. Vasoconstrictors, aspirin, anxiolytics.
4. Nitrates, ACE inhibitors, aspirin, lipid-lowering drugs.

56. The nurse practitioner initiates antihypertensive therapy for a middle-aged nonsmoking female. One week later, the client returns for a follow-up visit and complains of a recurrent dry cough since initiating the medications. This is most likely a side effect of a(an):

1. β-Blocker.
2. Thiazide diuretic.
3. ACE inhibitor.
4. Calcium channel blocker.

57. The role of digoxin in the management of CHF is still being defined, but is definitely indicated in CHF:

1. With atrial fibrillation.
2. With mitral stenosis.
3. With normal ejection fraction and sinus rhythm.
4. Due to acute pericardial disease.

58. The nurse practitioner should monitor the elderly client for which of the most common adverse reactions of digoxin?

1. Blurred vision.
2. Confusion.
3. Diarrhea.
4. Eating disorder.

59. A geriatric client has been on procainamide (Pronestyl) for 4 years to control her cardiac dysrhythmias. The nurse practitioner would evaluate for what side effect in the chronic use of this medication.

1. Elevated liver functions.
2. Appearance of antinuclear antibodies.
3. Shortened AV interval.
4. Tachycardia.

60. Secondary prophylaxis for acute rheumatic fever (ARF) in a 25-year-old school teacher includes:

1. Penicillin V 125–250 mg PO bid indefinitely.
2. Erythromycin 800 mg PO bid.
3. One-time dose of 2.0 million units benzathine penicillin G combined with penicillin G procaine (Bicillin C-R) IM.
4. No medication prophylaxis is needed after the client reaches the early twenties.

4 Answers & Rationales

Physical Examination & Diagnostic Tests

1. **(1)** S$_1$ is heard loudest at the apex, S$_2$ at the base. Each sound should be carefully assessed as to the intensity of the sound in each area.

2. **(3)** The PMI represents the thrust and contraction of the left ventricle. The left ventricle lies behind the right ventricle and extends to the left, forming the left border of the heart.

3. **(2)** The correct procedure is to listen for carotid bruits with the bell of the stethoscope, which brings out low-frequency sound and filters out high-frequency sound. It should be placed very lightly on the neck with just enough pressure to seal the edge.

4. **(2)** The purpose of inspection and palpation of the precordium is to determine the presence and extent of normal and abnormal pulsations. A slight retraction of the chest wall just medial to the midclavicular line in the fifth interspace is a normal finding, while marked actions or retraction of the rib is abnormal and may indicate pericardial disease. Pericardial friction rubs are heard by auscultation.

5. **(1)** The splitting during inspiration refers to S$_1$ and S$_2$. The S$_3$ is normal in children, young adults, and pregnant women. In the older adult with heart disease, this often signifies myocardial failure.

6. **(3)** The right side of the chest close to the sternal border at the second intercostal space is the correct area to auscultate the aortic valve. The mitral valve is auscultated at the fifth left intercostal space at the midclavicular line. The tricuspid value is auscultated at the fourth left intercostal space at the sternal border. The pulmonic valve is auscultated at the second left intercostal space at the sternal border.

7. **(2)** A 12-hour fast is recommended, due to the influence of intake on cholesterol levels (they may increase). A normal diet for the 7 days prior to the exam is recommended so that an accurate picture of the client's normal life is obtained. Alcohol should not be consumed 48 hours before the test—it may increase cholesterol, HDL, LDL, and triglyceride levels. If possible, all medication should be withheld until the test is over, especially corticosteroids, diuretics, β-blockers, oral contraceptives, and estrogens.

8. **(1)** An S$_4$ is a normal variant in people 65 years or older and may result from increased resistance to ventricular filling during atrial contraction.

9. **(1)** According to the classification of hypertension, this is within the moderate range.

10. **(2)** The fifth intercostal space at the midclavicular line on the left side is the best place to auscultate the closure sounds of the mitral valve. Option #1 describes the area of the tricuspid valve, Option #3 describes the area of the pulmonic valve,

and Option #4 describes the aortic valve area.

11. **(3)** It is important to determine if the coolness extends proximally from the hand. Then, palpation of pulses would be appropriate.

12. **(1)** Closure of the AV valves, which allows the filling of both ventricles simultaneously, produces the first heart sound (S_1), closure of the aortic and pulmonic valves produces the second heart sound (S_2).

13. **(4)** The apical and peripheral pulse (radial) must be evaluated simultaneously in order to determine if all of the apical beats are being reflected in the radial pulse. If there is an apical rate of 100 and a radial rate of 90, the client is said to have a pulse deficit of 10 points. This is usually done with two people counting over the same time period.

14. **(3)** A grade V heart murmur is very loud and can be heard with the stethoscope partly off the chest wall. A grade VI murmur is the loudest and is audible with the stethoscope just removed from contact with the chest wall and accompanied by a thrill. A grade I murmur is barely audible or very faint with the bell of the stethoscope.

15. **(4)** The most sensitive area on the examiner's hand is the backs of the fingers.

16. **(3)** Desired levels for a lipid profile are total cholesterol <200 mg/dl, HDL >35 mg/dl, LDL <130 mg/dl, and triglycerides <250 mg/dl. A high total cholesterol, coupled with a low HDL, is a positive risk factor for coronary heart disease (CHD), and is of the most concern for this client. In addition, this client has an elevated LDL level. These parameters, taken as a whole, would mandate intervention in this client.

17. **(1)** Jugular vein distention is common in geriatric clients. When it is present with the client's head elevated at a 45-degree angle, further examination needs to be conducted regarding the venous pressure, which is reflective of pressure in the right heart chambers. The supine position will increase venous pressure and does not provide valid information in this situation. Auscultation for carotid bruits is an important part of

assessment but does not have significant value in evaluating jugular vein distention.

18. **(1)** Mitral valve stenosis is a diastolic murmur of low intensity heard at the apex of the heart. Option #2 describes characteristics of a murmur with aortic stenosis. Option #3, a holosystolic murmur, is characteristic of mitral regurgitation, which allows for backflow of blood from ventricles into the atrium. Option #4 best describes aortic regurgitation.

19. **(4)** Classically, intermittent claudication is described as pain on activity that is relieved by stopping the activity.

20. **(1)** A complete A-V dissociation is a complete or 3rd degree block and must be addressed immediately. It is a very unstable rhythm, medications will not increase the rate since it is not atrial in origin. Evaluating for a pulse deficit or ordering a Holter monitor are not appropriate and will not provide useful information for the dysrhythmia. The client does not need to be referred, she needs to be seen immediately.

Disorders

21. **(1)** A diagnosis of HTN from a single measurement of BP elevation should not be done. A minimum of three readings with an average systolic BP of 140 mm Hg and a diastolic BP of 90 mm Hg establishes the diagnosis. An average of two or more readings taken at each of two or more visits should follow an initial screening. The client should be seated with arm at heart level. No caffeine or nicotine ingestion should be allowed 30 minutes prior to the reading. The room should be quiet a minimum of 5 minutes, and an appropriate cuff should be used. One high reading should be confirmed within 2 months.

22. **(3)** In the early stages of hypertensive heart disease, where there is an increased peripheral resistance to blood flow, the most significant change occurring to the heart is the left ventricular hypertrophy with an increase in the size of the myocardial cells without a corresponding increase in cell number (i.e., hyperplasia). After a period of time, all of the other options listed occur in the heart.

23. **(3)** Sinus or atrial tachycardia is characterized by a rate at or above 100, P waves are present for each QRS complex, the P-R interval is below 0.20, the T wave occurs after each QRS complex, and the beat is regular.

24. **(2)** Respiratory symptoms are predominant with clients in left-sided heart failure. Venous congestion and peripheral edema are associated with right-sided failure.

25. **(2)** Untreated hypertension causes significant increased work on the left ventricle, eventually causing CHF.

26. **(2)** Palpable carotid pulse with each compression is the best sign of effective CPR. The other answers are appropriate but not the best indicator of effective resuscitation efforts.

27. **(2)** This is a description of complete block with hemodynamic consequences. The client should be seen immediately by a cardiologist for the possibility of pacemaker insertion. First-degree block has characteristic P waves and long P-R interval. The client should not just be referred for follow-up, he should be seen by a cardiologist as soon as possible.

28. **(1)** Cardiovascular risk factors predisposing females to cardiovascular disease include smaller body size, declining estrogen level, heart and thoracic cavity that is smaller and lighter in size, coronary arteries that are smaller in diameter, shorter P-R interval, higher resting ejection fraction, increased body fat percentage, and fat distributed in the abdomen may be mobilized more easily in response to stress and raise serum cholesterol and blood glucose levels.

29. **(1)** Waterhammer pulse (bounding with a rapid rise and sudden collapse) is produced by an increase in pulse pressure and may be caused by an increased stroke volume, a decrease in peripheral resistance, or both. Because the nurse practitioner is suspecting either aortic regurgitation or a patent ductus arteriosus (primarily in children), auscultation for a diastolic murmur is indicated.

30. **(2)** Occlusion of the coronary arteries deprives the myocardial cells of glucose needed for aerobic metabolism. Anaerobic metabolism occurs, which causes the accumulation of lactic acid. Lactic acid irritates the myocardial nerve fibers, sending pain messages to the cardiac nerves and upper thoracic posterior roots located in the left shoulder and arm.

31. **(4)** Option #1 is Functional Class IV. Option #2 is Functional Class II. Option #3 is Functional Class I. Option #4, the correct response, is Functional Class III.

32. **(1)** The moist crackles (rales) heard in the bases of the lung are the most prominent physical examination findings of early CHF. They are caused by transudation of fluid into the alveoli and into the airways. Later findings include distended neck veins, peripheral edema, hepatomegaly, and ascites (rather than weight loss).

33. **(3)** Aortic dissection almost invariably begins with sudden onset of severe chest pain that is tearing or ripping in quality and is accompanied by loss or decrease in peripheral pulses and neurologic deficits. The pain of angina and acute MI is usually described as a pressure. Pericarditis produces pain that is more gradual in onset.

34. **(1)** A Step I diet involves daily intake of ≤30% total calorie intake made up of fat, <300 mg/day cholesterol intake, and 8−10% daily saturated fat intake. A decrease to <200 mg/day of cholesterol and 7% saturated fat is a Step II diet, prescribed if Step I is ineffective. The third selection is closer to the current average American's diet. Although watching calorie and sodium intake is important for weight and BP control, it is not part of a Step I diet plan for hyperlipidemia.

35. **(2)** Diet and exercise are the mainstays of any treatment program and would be used initially in all cases. A bile acid sequestrant agent or estrogen replacement therapy may eventually be necessary if no improvement is seen with diet/exercise therapy. Referral to a cardiologist is not necessary, unless the client develops symptoms or shows resistance to treatment.

36. **(3)** Dyspnea is the most common symptom of CHF. Initially, it is present only with moderate exertion, but as severity of CHF increases, the dyspnea may occur with mild exertion or at rest. Fatigue is another common complaint. Right-sided heart failure is associated with weakness, anorexia, nausea, and dependent edema. Chronic left ventricular failure usually leads to right ventricular failure.

37. **(3)** Palm and coconut oils, along with butter, are very high in saturated fats and should be avoided. The other selections are moderately high in fat content, but consist of mostly unsaturated fats.

38. **(3)** Anginal pain is difficult to differentiate from that of an infarction. One of the most characteristic symptoms is the relief of the anginal pain with the administration of sublingual nitroglycerin.

39. **(4)** Aspirin helps prevent the formation of platelet-aggregating substances and may help the occlusion of narrowed coronary arteries. While Lasix, morphine, and streptokinase all have their place in treating acute MI, it is unlikely that they are available in the average primary-care office.

40. **(3)** Dizziness that improves when lying down and worsens when standing is symptomatic of cardiac involvement and may indicate serious cardiac dysrhythmias. If dizziness occurs in certain positions, it is indicative of benign positional vertigo, which is common in the elderly. Dizziness accompanied by tinnitus is common in acute labyrinthitis and, if preceded by rapid breathing, may be caused by hyperventilation.

41. **(3)** The stated history of a recent coxsackievirus infection, pain that worsens when supine, and a friction rub is classic for viral pericarditis. The client's age makes an acute MI unlikely and the pain is not typical for pleural effusion or reflux.

42. **(1)** Signs and symptoms of hyperthyroidism in the older adult include progressive functional decline, atrial fibrillation, MI, tachycardia, weakness, fatigue, weight loss, anorexia, diarrhea, nervousness, tremor, pruritus, memory loss, and heat intolerance.

Symptoms of hypothyroidism include arthralgia, weakness, decreased mental function, depression, constipation, weight loss, dry coarse skin with yellowish cast, dry sparse hair, and mask-like puffy face with periorbital edema. Bradycardia would be assessed with both sick-sinus syndrome and CHF. Sick-sinus syndrome is often associated with the "bradycardia-tachycardia" syndrome.

43. **(2)** This assessment is consistent with aortic stenosis. Aortic regurgitation is a diastolic murmur and secondary to rheumatic heart disease. There is no history given of rheumatic heart disease. Mitral valve disease is one of the most common valvular disorders. A small percentage of mitral valve prolapse clients do suffer from autonomic dysfunction and complain of palpitations, atypical chest pain, orthostatic dizziness, near-syncope, cold extremities, throbbing headaches, and neurasthenia and manifest tachyarrhythmias. Mitral regurgitation may remain asymptomatic for many years, because the left ventricle dilates and adjusts well to the increase in volume load. Onset of dyspnea and fatigue may not occur for decades.

44. **(3)** The nurse practitioner needs to repeat the cholesterol and obtain HDL and LDL levels before initiating any treatment. The HDL and LDL will help stratify risks and guide aggressiveness of intervention.

45. **(3)** Mitral stenosis most often results in CHF, there is generally no chest pain or fever. Atrial fibrillation is not uncommon however it is very irregular, the irregular pulse may result in a pulse deficit.

Pharmacology

46. **(3)** Thiazide diuretics inhibit sodium reabsorption, promoting the excretion of sodium, chloride, and water. As the extracellular fluid volume decreases, plasma renin activity and aldosterone levels increase, resulting in potassium loss. Treatment is to restore the volume with normal saline and correct the potassium depletion. If the sodium is increased too rapidly, irreversible neurologic damage can occur.

47. **(1)** Vitamin K is an antidote for Coumadin. Increased intake of green leafy vegetables could cause an increase in vitamin K levels and decrease the effectiveness of the medication. Also, multivitamin supplements may contain additional vitamin K.

48. **(3)** The client presents with the classic profile of digitalis toxicity, which is frequently related to hypokalemia, especially since the potassium replacement is rather low for an adult and there is history of poor eating and nausea. Other options may be done; however, it is important to determine the presence of hypokalemia and digitalis toxicity, so it may be addressed immediately.

49. **(1)** ACE inhibitors, such as losartan (Cozaar), decrease the conversion of angiotensin I to angiotensin II, a potent vasoconstrictor, and inhibit the release of aldosterone.

50. **(1)** Aldactone is a potassium-sparing diuretic. Clients should be instructed on signs of hyperkalemia.

51. **(2)** Niacin can cause vasodilatation, leading to orthostatic hypotension. Antihyperlipidemic drugs may cause constipation. The effectiveness of antihyperlipidemics is enhanced when taken before or with meals.

52. **(2)** Calcium channel blockers depress the rate of discharge from the sinoatrial node and conduction velocity through the AV node causing a decrease in heart rate; relax the coronary and systemic arteries producing vasodilation (decrease in afterload and blood pressure); and decrease myocardial contractility (negative inotropic effect).

53. **(2)** The dose of the client's medication had been doubled by the nurse practitioner according to the recommended protocols. The aim of therapy is to use the drugs alone or in combination to return arterial pressure to normal levels with minimal side effects. Since the therapy had been continued, doubled, the next step is to add a low-dose thiazide diuretic. Therefore, the hydrochlorothiazide addition is the correct choice. Because of reduced side effects, the ACE inhibitors are used alone first, with a slight preference for certain ACE inhibitors (enalapril over captopril, and losartan [Cozaar] over both of them).

54. **(3)** Blood pressure should be lowered cautiously, using smaller doses of calcium entry antagonists, ACE inhibitors, or diuretics in the elderly. β-Blockers are not appropriate in normal doses for the elderly because of decreased β-receptor sensitivity in these clients. Larger doses also result in depression, impotence, fatigue, and declining mental function. Elderly clients are especially likely to experience CHF and peripheral vascular insufficiency from β-adrenergic blocker toxicity.

55. **(2)** Nitrates are venous and arterial dilators that decrease myocardial oxygen demand. β-Blockers have an antianginal effect and reduce myocardial oxygen demand. Calcium channel blockers relieve myocardial ischemia by reducing myocardial oxygen demand and dilating coronary arteries. Aspirin is effective for primary and secondary prevention of MI. Unless contraindicated, small doses of aspirin (162–325 mg daily) should be prescribed for clients with angina. Clients remaining symptomatic when treated with nitrates, β-blockers, or calcium channel blocking drugs should be treated with a β-blocker plus a combination of another agent. Appropriate combinations are a nitrate or a β-blocker plus a calcium channel blocker other than verapamil. Combination therapy does not include sedatives, vasoconstrictors, ACE inhibitors, or lipid-lowering drugs.

56. **(3)** Adverse side effects of ACE inhibitors include cough (1–30%), headache, and dizziness. Adverse effects of calcium channel blockers include peripheral edema, dizziness, headache, nausea, and tachycardia. Adverse effects of thiazide diuretics include nausea, vomiting, diarrhea, dizziness, and headache. Side effects of β-blockers include fatigue, impotence, depression, and shortness of breath.

57. **(1)** Digoxin, once a first-line drug on all clients with CHF, is now used in clients with atrial fibrillation, other tachycardias, and clients with left ventricular dysfunction. By controlling the ventricular rate in the client with atrial fibrillation or

tachycardias, cardiac output increases. In cases of diastolic dysfunction with a sinus rhythm, digitalis is of no benefit. Digoxin is of relatively little value in most forms of cardiomyopathy, myocarditis, mitral stenosis, and chronic constrictive pericarditis.

58. **(2)** Noncardiac adverse reactions include a change in the mental status. While visual disturbances; diarrhea; and anorexia, nausea, or vomiting are also adverse reactions, they are not the most common in the elderly.

59. **(2)** Eighty per cent of the clients who chronically use procainamide develop antinuclear antibodies. Twenty per cent of these clients develop a lupus-like syndrome.

60. **(1)** Secondary prevention or preventing the recurrent attacks of acute rheumatic fever is controversial. Some authorities identify the early 20s and 5 years since last ARF attack as the criteria to stop the use of prophylactic penicillin, unless the client is at increased risk of exposure to streptococcal infections, such as school teachers or health professionals. Other authorities recommend lifelong prophylactic drug therapy. Although erythromycin is an alternative medication for penicillin-sensitive individuals, the dose in Option #2 is for a client having a dental or surgical procedure. The secondary prophylaxis dose for erythromycin is 250 mg PO bid.

Respiratory

Physical Examination & Diagnostic Tests

1. The nurse practitioner knows that normal breath sounds that have a low pitch and soft intensity and that are heard better on inspiration are called:

    1. Bronchial.

    2. Vesicular.

    3. Bronchovesicular.

    4. Rhonchi.

2. When auscultating for vocal resonance in a client with possible consolidation of lung tissue, the nurse practitioner hears "a-a-a" when the client says "e-e-e." This is called:

    1. Tactile fremitus.

    2. Bronchophony.

    3. Whispered pectoriloquy.

    4. Egophony.

3. The nurse practitioner understands the following about hyperresonance in percussion of the lungs:

    1. It is a normal finding in the adult client.

    2. It occurs commonly in pediatric clients.

    3. It is characterized by soft intensity, high pitch, short duration, and extreme dullness quality.

    4. It is characterized by loud intensity, high pitch, medium duration, and dull quality.

4. What is the correct procedure when percussing the chest?

    1. Start at the right upper side of the anterior chest and move to the left side.

    2. Begin at the upper left side of the posterior chest and compare to the respective anterior side, moving from front to back.

    3. Percuss systematically and symmetrically the anterior chest, moving from the left to right side, then do the posterior chest.

    4. Percuss the posterior chest and then measure for diaphragmatic excursion on the anterior chest.

5. The nurse practitioner understands that pleural friction rubs are:

   1. Auscultated in the lower anterolateral chest.

   2. Heard best at the end of expiration.

   3. Characterized by a continuous low-pitched snoring sound heard early in inspiration.

   4. Noted when the client says "e-e-e" and the examiner hears through the stethoscope "a-a-a".

6. Normal physiologic changes in the respiratory system of the geriatric client include:

   1. Increased rigidity of the rib cage and an increase in the anteroposterior (AP) diameter of the chest.

   2. Increased ciliary action resulting in a more forceful and recurrent cough.

   3. Increase in number of smaller alveoli with a decrease in residual capacity.

   4. Decrease in AP diameter of the rib cage with a decrease in lung expansion.

7. When assessing for tactile fremitus, the nurse practitioner would place her hands over what area of the client's chest?

   1. On the anterior chest at the level of the sixth intercostal space.

   2. At the level of bifurcation of the bronchi on the posterior chest wall.

   3. At the apex on the anterior chest wall.

   4. At the level of the diaphragm on the posterior chest wall.

8. On assessment of the client's respiratory status, crepitation is felt over the third rib at the midaxillary line on the left side. The interpretation of this finding is:

   1. There is a consolidation of fluid in the left lower lobe of the lung.

   2. Severe inflammation is present on the visceral pleural surfaces of the left lung.

   3. An increase in pressure has occurred in the pleural cavity on the right lung.

   4. Air is present in the subcutaneous tissue from an air leak in the respiratory system.

9. An important anatomic landmark on the anterior thoracic wall is the angle of Louis. Where on the thorax is this landmark present?

   1. The midnipple line on either side of the manubrium.

   2. Bilaterally at the manubriosternal junction.

   3. Midline at the base of the suprasternal notch.

   4. Just below the clavicle, but above the manubrium.

10. During the assessment of a geriatric client's respiratory status, the nurse practitioner determines the presence of coarse tactile fremitus posteriorly at the second intercostal space. The best interpretation of this finding is:

    1. Increased air trapping in the alveoli on the affected side.

    2. Presence of fluid or solid mass within the lungs.

    3. Increased pressure in the bronchial tree.

    4. Presence of hyperactive airway disease.

11. When the lateral diameter of the chest is the same size as the AP diameter, the nurse practitioner correctly documents this finding as a:

    1. Biot deviated chest.

    2. Pigeon chest.

    3. Funnel chest.

    4. Barrel chest.

12. An adult female client comes to the clinic with the chief complaint of "coughing up blood." She has no history of respiratory or cardiac problems. Her vital signs are pulse 96, respirations 28, blood pressure 140/92, temperature 99°F orally. The initial diagnostic evaluation of this client includes:

    1. Electrocardiogram (ECG), pulmonary function studies, sputum cytology.

2. Purified protein derivative (PPD) skin test, chest x-ray, sputum smear for acid-fast bacillus.

3. Arterial blood-gas (ABG) studies, complete blood count (CBC), chest x-ray.

4. Direct bronchoscopy with biopsy and complement fixation antibody titer.

13. When assessing the pulmonary function studies of a client, which assessment finding is seen in chronic air flow limitation such as emphysema?

    1. Decrease in forced vital capacity (FVC) and forced expiratory volume timed (FEV_1).

    2. Increase functional residual capacity (FRC) and residual volumes (RV).

    3. Decrease residual volume (RV) and increase in total lung capacity (TLC).

    4. Increase in forced expiratory volume timed (FEV_1) and total lung capacity (TLC).

14. A client comes to the clinic complaining of difficulty breathing, lethargy, and coughing up blood in his sputum. She has no history of chronic illness or major health problems. The nurse practitioner orders diagnostic tests to determine the problem. What diagnostic test results would require immediate treatment of this client?

    1. Positive sputum smear for acid-fast bacillus.

    2. Sputum culture positive for *Pneumocystis carinii*.

    3. Presence of hemolysis on complement fixation test.

    4. Oxygen saturation 94%, leukocyte count >5000 white blood cells (WBCs)/mm³.

15. The nurse practitioner is planning a community screening program for lung cancer in geriatric clients. Which examination is best to use for this program?

    1. Bronchoscopy with biopsy for cytology.

    2. Arterial blood-gas studies.

    3. Pulmonary function test.

    4. Chest x-ray and compare with previous x-ray.

16. An adult client arrives at the clinic complaining of difficulty breathing, a cough, and chest pain. History indicates the client was discharged from the hospital 2 days ago after a cesarean section and a 15-pack-year smoking history. Diagnostic studies should include:

    1. Sputum for culture and sensitivity.

    2. Cardiac troponin proteins.

    3. Pulse oximetry.

    4. Arterial blood-gas studies.

17. When interpreting PPD skin tests in clients at a long-term care facility, the nurse practitioner identifies positive results in individuals with:

    1. Redness or erythema at the site.

    2. An induration reaction of ≥5 mm.

    3. An induration reaction of ≥10 mm.

    4. An induration reaction extending to 15 mm.

Disorders

18. A client has received a blunt trauma injury to his chest. An assessment finding that would be most indicative of further respiratory complications would be:

    1. Complaints of increased pain over the affected area.

    2. Oximetry readings consistently around 90%.

    3. Decreased breath sounds on the affected side.

    4. Fever of 102°F and increased sputum production.

19. The nurse practitioner understands that the following characteristic is more likely to occur when the adult client has pneumonia (due to *Streptococcus pneumoniae*) rather than bronchitis:

    1. Rusty sputum.

    2. Cough.

    3. Dyspnea.

    4. Wheezing.

20. What would be a priority intervention for a client experiencing a respiratory arrest?

    1. Start chest compressions at 15 compressions and two breaths.

    2. Open the airway with a head tilt and chin lift.

    3. Give oxygen via a rebreathing mask at 10 L/min.

    4. Pinch the nose and give two breaths.

21. A client comes to the emergency room complaining of difficulty breathing. What is most important to establish initially on this client?

    1. What type of activity produces the dyspnea.

    2. The presence of consolidation via a chest x-ray.

    3. Arterial blood-gas levels with respect to oxygen pressures.

    4. Presence of bilateral breath sounds over the lower lobes.

22. A client is severely dyspneic and the history strongly suggests the possibility of a foreign body in the bronchi. What observation would contribute to the documentation of this problem?

    1. Unilateral retraction of the right chest wall.

    2. The presence of crepitation on the anterior chest wall.

    3. Retraction of the lower chest wall.

    4. A friction rub heard over the area of the bronchi.

23. The nurse practitioner is assessing a client who is complaining of shortness of breath and chest discomfort. His respirations are shallow and at a rate of 26. When evaluating the diaphragmatic excursion, it is determined that the diaphragm on the right is slightly higher than on the left side. The best interpretation of these findings is:

    1. This is normal due to the liver on the right side.

    2. There may be atelectasis in the right lower lobe.

    3. Consolidation is present in the right lower lobe.

    4. This indicates the presence of early stages of chronic obstructive lung disease.

24. A 22-year-old female comes to the office complaining of chest pain and shortness of breath. She states the problems started suddenly after running two miles. She states she has no past history of pulmonary problems. She is about 68 inches tall and weighes approximately 120 lb, her pulse rate is 118, her respiratory rate is 30, there are decreased breath sounds, and there is hyperresonance over the left lung. The best diagnosis for this client is:

    1. Spontaneous pneumothorax.

    2. Exercise-induced asthma.

    3. Pulmonary edema.

    4. Acute bronchiectasis.

25. A young woman presents at the clinic with complaints of tingling in her face and hands, sudden shortness of breath, and vague chest discomfort. She appears very anxious and denies any history of respiratory problems. On examination her hands are cool to touch and her vital signs are respirations 34, pulse regular at a rate of 100, blood pressure 110/76, and normal temperature. Respiratory examination reveals bilateral breath sounds with tachypnea, no adventitious sounds, and normal percussion and visual examination of the chest. The best immediate treatment is:

    1. Rebreathing into a paper bag and encouraging controlled diaphragmatic breathing.

    2. Albuterol (Proventil) two puffs with a metered-dose inhaler (MDI).

    3. Oxygen at 4 L and arterial blood gases after 30 minutes.

    4. Establish an IV and infuse 500 ml normal saline for volume depletion.

26. A newly diagnosed COPD client is being discharged from the hospital. The nurse practitioner is discussing home care with the client. What information is important

for the nurse practitioner to include in the home care teaching?

1. Use the bronchodilator prior to exercising.

2. Maintain bed rest for the first few days at home.

3. Decrease amount of fluid intake to prevent fluid overload.

4. Maintain flow rate on oxygen around 5–7 L.

27. A client is admitted to a rural emergency department by ambulance. Primary assessment reveals:

   • Respirations: 38/min with use of accessory muscles, prolonged expiration and wheezes
   • ECG: Sinus tachycardia rate 140
   • Blood pressure: 192/98
   • Lethargic: Responds to name only by opening eyes
   • Cyanosis of lips

Therapeutic interventions initiated by emergency medical technicians include:
   • Intravenous therapy of D_5W at 30 ml/hr
   • Oxygen therapy at 48% by venturi mask

STAT arterial blood gases indicate:
   • pH = 7.24
   • Pa_{CO_2} = 82 mm Hg
   • HCO_3 = 36
   • Pa_{O_2} = 76 mm Hg

Prior to obtaining a second set of arterial blood gases, the nurse practitioner would:

1. Assist respirations with bag valve mask with 100% oxygen.

2. Administer 1 ampule of sodium bicarbonate.

3. Change oxygen delivery to nasal cannula at 2 L.

4. Disconnect the supplemental oxygen.

28. Instructions to the elderly client with COPD concerning nutritional therapy would include foods that are:

1. High caloric, high protein, low carbohydrate.

2. High caloric, low protein, high carbohydrate.

3. Low caloric, high protein, low carbohydrate.

4. Low caloric, low protein, high carbohydrate.

29. Age-associated changes that increase the risk for pneumonia in the elderly client include an increase in:

1. Compliance of the chest wall.

2. Diameter of the trachea and bronchi.

3. Lung parenchyma.

4. Cough forcefulness.

30. The nurse practitioner is aware that the flu or influenza:

1. Can be caused by receiving a flu vaccine when your resistance is low.

2. Is characterized by a slow, insidious onset of chills, fever, and muscle aches.

3. In older adults may persist for several weeks with symptoms of lack of energy and extreme tiredness.

4. Is primarily contagious in the early autumn and spring.

31. An older adult client presents with complaints of dyspnea, cough, fatigue, and dependent edema that has been worsening over the past few days. In planning the treatment for this client, the nurse practitioner considers:

1. Streptokinase therapy.

2. Hospitalization for evaluation of heart function.

3. Prescription for Lasix 40 mg PO qd.

4. Addition of a calcium channel blocker to the client's medications.

32. An adult client with a history of asthma calls to tell the nurse practitioner that she is "blowing 55%" on the peak flowmeter. What advice would the nurse practitioner give this client?

1. Call an ambulance immediately.

2. Use the bronchodilator now and come in to the office today.

3. Office evaluation this week.

4. Refer to a pulmonary physician.

33. An elderly client is evaluated by the nurse practitioner for a complaint of cough, fever, chest pain, and sputum production. In gathering a history on this client, it is important to know if the client has:

    1. Received the pneumococcal vaccine.

    2. Traveled out of the country.

    3. Pets in the household.

    4. Recently started new medications.

34. An elderly client presents with signs and symptoms that make the nurse practitioner suspect the diagnosis of pneumonia. Which assessment would the nurse practitioner most likely evaluate during the examination?

    1. Chest pain with inspiration.

    2. Confusion with a low-grade temperature.

    3. Congested, productive cough.

    4. Fever with leukocytosis.

35. In developing a plan for an older client with pneumonia, the nurse practitioner understands that 30–40% of community-acquired pneumonia is caused by which organism?

    1. *Haemophilus influenzae*.

    2. *Klebsiella pneumoniae*.

    3. *Mycobacterium tuberculosis*.

    4. *Streptococcus pneumoniae*.

36. Which plan would be most appropriate to include in the health promotion plan for an older client who is at risk for developing pneumonia?

    1. Administer the pneumococcal vaccination annually.

    2. Administer the pneumococcal vaccination and yearly influenza immunization.

    3. Perform sputum culture annually along with a chest x-ray.

    4. Perform PPD every 3–5 years.

37. The nurse practitioner evaluates an older client with a current history of alcoholism. The client presents with an elevated temperature, congested cough producing rusty sputum, and occasional chills. The suspected diagnosis is bacterial pneumonia. The Gram-stained sputum smear would most likely reveal which organism?

    1. *Haemophilus influenzae*.

    2. *Klebsiella pneumoniae*.

    3. *Staphylococcus aureus*.

    4. *Streptococcus pneumoniae*.

38. An elderly client residing in a nursing home has recently been exposed to tuberculosis. The nurse practitioner interprets the initial PPD test to be negative. Which plan would be most appropriate at this time?

    1. Evaluate the client in another year.

    2. Repeat PPD test in 1 week.

    3. Ignore results and immediately begin ethambutol.

    4. Evaluate the client in 6 months, since she is asymptomatic at this time.

39. The nurse practitioner knows that Horner's syndrome is commonly associated with:

    1. Chronic bronchitis.

    2. Pulmonary tuberculosis.

    3. Pancoast's syndrome of lung cancer.

    4. Pulmonary embolism.

40. An adult client who smokes presents with complaints of breathlessness. The nurse practitioner notes on examination dilated blood vessels on the chest, and mild edema of the head and supraclavicular area. She recognizes this condition as:

    1. Thyroid abnormality.

    2. Chronic bronchitis with mild congestive failure.

    3. Asthma with fluid retention.

    4. Superior vena cava obstruction.

41. An elderly client presents with postural hypotension, and laboratory studies reveal hyponatremia. The most likely cause of this is:

    1. Diabetic ketoacidosis.

    2. Severe trauma.

    3. Bronchogenic carcinoma.

    4. Antacid overuse.

42. The nurse practitioner knows the following about asthma in the elderly:

    1. Subcutaneous epinephrine is standard therapy.

    2. It is usually of the allergic type.

    3. Attacks are usually preceded by viral infections.

    4. The clinical presentation is usually dyspnea, costal retraction, and fever.

43. Clinical signs and symptoms of late-phase asthma include:

    1. Bronchoconstriction refractory to bronchodilator therapy.

    2. Sneezing, watery eyes, and cough.

    3. Wheezing and increased sputum production.

    4. Bronchodilation secondary to release of histamine.

44. The nurse practitioner is assessing a client for asthma. What is a common clinical manifestation of asthma?

    1. Pruritis.

    2. Diffuse crackles.

    3. Nocturnal exacerbation.

    4. Chronic hypoxemia.

45. During a routine follow-up visit for a client with asthma, the client states that she has been doing fine except that when she goes out for dinner she notices she has increased bronchospasm and wheezing. Which would be an appropriate response?

    1. "Have you been taking your medication?"

    2. "Do you usually have wine with dinner?"

    3. "I recommend you not go out for dinner."

    4. "Does going out to dinner make you stressed?"

Pharmacology

46. The nurse practitioner is following up on a client who is experiencing acute asthmatic problems. Albuterol (Proventil) by MDI has been ordered as treatment. Which client response would indicate to the nurse practitioner that the client understands how to take her medication?

    1. "I will take one puff of the medication and then wait a minute before taking the second puff."

    2. "I will take two puffs of the medication every 4 hours, even if I am not short of breath."

    3. "It is important for me to take this medication on a regular cycle to prevent future attacks."

    4. "I will take two puffs, one right after the other, whenever I begin to get short of breath."

47. A client who was recently diagnosed with tuberculosis calls the clinic because her urine is reddish orange. She is taking isoniazid (INH; Laniazid), rifampin (Rifadin), and pyrazinamide. An appropriate response for the nurse practitioner to make would be:

    1. "These are urinary tract infection symptoms; drink plenty of fluids."

    2. "This is a normal response to the rifampin."

    3. "Often this is an indication of liver toxicity. Stop the medications."

    4. "This is probably bleeding and you should see a physician immediately."

48. A 25-year-old females comes into the emergency room with complaints of extreme shortness of breath. She is confused and her past medical history is not available. Her vital signs are pulse 124, respirations 32, blood pressure 124/80, temperature normal. Physical examination reveals diffuse expiratory wheezes, hyperresonance on percussion, and a prolonged expiratory phase. The best treatment for this client includes:

    1. Aminophylline by mouth.

    2. Beclomethasone (Beclovent) inhaler.

    3. Epinephrine by injection.

    4. Albuterol (Proventil) metered-dose inhaler.

49. A client with a history of bronchial asthma is seen in the clinic for increased episodes of difficulty breathing. The client has been taking theophylline 100 mg PO tid. The client is a 40-year-old obese female with an 18-pack-year history of cigarette smoking and an excessive intake of coffee daily, and he eats a low-carbohydrate, high-protein diet. Which identified factors decrease the therapeutic effects of the theophylline?

   1. Age and gender.

   2. Coffee intake and weight.

   3. Age and weight.

   4. Smoking history and diet.

50. A 70-year-old female comes to the clinic complaining that she has been experiencing increased difficulty breathing over the past few days. She has a history of chronic obstructive lung disease and coronary artery disease. She was recently diagnosed with hypertension. Examination reveals no jugular vein distention, slight increase in the AP diameter of the chest, and no productive cough; her breath sounds are present but expiratory wheezes are noted bilaterally, and she denies complaints of chest pain. Her vital signs are pulse 72, respirations 34, and blood pressure 170/100. Her current medications are ipratropium bromide (Atrovent) inhaler two puffs every 6 hours, nitroglycerin transdermal patches, and propranolol (Inderal) 60 mg PO bid. The best treatment for this client is:

   1. Discontinue the propranolol (Inderal) and begin verapamil (Calan) 80 mg PO tid qd.

   2. Begin theophylline (Theo-Dur) 200 mg q12h PO.

   3. Discontinue the propranolol (Inderal) and begin atenolol (Tenormin) 50 mg PO qd.

   4. Start beclomethasone (Beclovent) inhaler two puffs three or four times daily.

51. The recommended range for maintaining serum theophylline levels is:

   1. 0.05–2 μg/ml.

   2. 5–15 μg/ml.

   3. 20–25 μg/ml.

   4. 30–40 μg/ml.

52. A client in a long-term facility whose roommate has been diagnosed as having active tuberculosis should be started on chemoprophylaxis:

   1. As soon as possible and initiated at the time of screening skin testing.

   2. In 72 hours after PPD skin test results are obtained.

   3. Only if PPD skin test results are positive.

   4. In 3 months if the repeated skin test is positive.

53. In adults with asthma, the most common reason why outpatient treatment fails and results in hospitalization is:

   1. Exposure to allergens.

   2. Increased use of steroids.

   3. Improper inhaler technique.

   4. Use of cromolyn inhalers.

54. Which can elevate theophylline levels?

   1. Concomitant treatment with cimetidine (Tagamet).

   2. Intravenous ampicillin.

   3. Heavy smoking.

   4. History of seizure disorder.

55. A client with a long history of chronic airflow limitation has noticed a change in sputum over the past few days (e.g., increased amount of thick, yellow-green mucous, and congestion). Appropriate therapy is:

   1. Hismanal 10 mg PO qd.

   2. Augmentin 500 mg PO tid × 10 days.

   3. Tylenol with codeine.

   4. Vancenase MDI 2 puffs.

56. Which medication is most effective in promoting a decrease in airway inflammation as well as providing long-term medication coverage in a client with asthma?

   1. Isoetharine (Bronkometer).

2. Beclomethasone dipropionate (Vanceril, Beclovent).

3. Albuterol (Proventil, Ventolin).

4. Pirbuterol (Maxair).

57. The nurse practitioner is planning prophylactic treatment for a client with asthma. What is the best medication to use for the asthmatic client who is not currently experiencing an exacerbation?

1. Antibiotics.

2. Inhaled glucocorticoids.

3. B_1-Agonist.

4. Methacholine challenge.

58. Clients with asthma need to be instructed to:

1. Begin their inhaled steroids as soon as symptoms appear.

2. Using the MDI, take two puffs of the β_2 agonist prn.

3. Use their inhaled steroids when they experience bronchospasm.

4. Start their antibiotic regimen when they experience bronchospasm.

59. A client presents in the clinic with a dry hacking, nonproductive cough that is interfering with her sleep. The nurse practitioner would encourage the client to purchase an over-the-counter preparation that contains:

1. Pseudoephedrine.

2. Phenylpropanolamine.

3. Guaifenesin.

4. Dextromethorphan.

60. A geriatric client is seen for an upper respiratory infection and the nurse practitioner decides to prescribe erythromycin. On review of the client's history, what current medication would be a contraindication to the administration of erythromycin?

1. Cisapride (Propulsid).

2. Lisinopril (Zestril).

3. Moexipril (Univasc).

4. Atenolol (Tenormin).

61. A client with chronic asthma is seen in the clinic complaining of vomiting and stomach cramps. She is confused and is unsure what medications he is currently taking. Her vital signs are blood pressure 158/92, pulse 152 and irregular, respirations 28 and shallow. What STAT diagnostic study should be obtained?

1. Serum electrolytes.

2. Digoxin level.

3. Theophylline level.

4. Arterial blood gases.

62. A client is seen in the clinic complaining of increased difficulty breathing and an intermittent productive cough that worsens in the evening. The history reveals that the client has a 20-pack-year history of smoking. Breath sounds are clear to auscultation, there is no evidence of fever, and chest radiography is within normal limits. The nurse practitioner instructs the client concerning the importance of smoking cessation and fluid therapy and prescribes:

1. Erythromycin 500 mg PO qid × 14 days.

2. Albuterol 2 mg PO tid.

3. Mucomyst inhalation 10 ml of 10% solution q4h prn.

4. Tetracycline 100 mg q12h × 14 days.

63. When initiating preventative care to decrease the incidence of pneumonia in clients in an extended-care facility, the nurse practitioner would identify clients receiving immunosuppressive therapy, repeated antibiotic use, sedation, and:

1. β_1-Adrenergic blocking agents.

2. Calcium channel blockers.

3. Diuretics.

4. Histamine$_2$ (H$_2$) antagonists.

■■■

5 Answers & Rationales

Physical Examination & Diagnostic Tests

1. **(2)** The sounds heard over normal lung tissue are called vesicular breath sounds. The inspiratory phase of the vesicular breath sound is heard better than the expiratory phase and is about 2.5 times longer for these low-pitched, soft sounds. Bronchial breath sounds are normally heard over the trachea and usually indicate pathology. Bronchial breath sounds are high-pitched, loud sounds with a shortened inspiratory and lengthened expiratory phase. Bronchovesicular breath sounds have an intermediate pitch and intensity, with equal duration of expiratory and inspiratory sounds heard mainly over the second interspace anteriorly and between the scapulae posteriorly. Rhonchi are abnormal breath sounds that are low-pitched with a snoring quality.

2. **(4)** Tactile fremitus is a palpable vibration of the thoracic wall that is produced when the client speaks. Bronchophony is the increase in loudness and clarity of vocal resonance. Whispered pectoriloquy is exaggerated bronchophony and is heard through a stethoscope when the client whispers a series of words (i.e., "ninety-nine"). In egophony, the spoken voice has a nasal or bleating quality when heard through a stethoscope, and the spoken "e-e-e" sounds like "a-a-a."

3. **(2)** Hyperresonance is an abnormal percussion tone in adults, but normally occurs in a child's lung. It is characterized by very loud intensity, very low pitch, and long duration, and has a booming quality.

4. **(3)** Both anterior and posterior chest is to be percussed systematically and symmetrically, moving from left to right. Diaphragmatic excursion is usually only measured on the posterior chest.

5. **(1)** Most often heard in the lower anterolateral thorax, pleural friction rubs are loud, dry, creaking or grating sounds produced by the rubbing together of inflamed and roughened pleural surfaces that are heard best during the latter part of inspiration and the beginning of expiration. Option #3 is characteristic of sonorous rhonchi.

6. **(1)** There is a decrease in the number of alveoli, and the alveoli become rigid and lose the ability to recoil. The loss of alveolar elasticity affects the ability of the client to exhale effectively and there is an increase in the residual volume. There is also a decrease in basilar inflation and a decrease in the ability to expel foreign matter. The AP diameter of the chest increases as see in clients with kyphosis.

7. **(2)** The bifurcation of the trachea or bronchi on the posterior chest wall is the best area for assessment of tactile fremitus. Care should be taken to avoid the area over the scapula.

8. **(4)** Crepitation or crepitus (also called subcutaneous emphysema) is air bubbles

under the skin from a rupture somewhere in the respiratory system, less common from an infection by a gas-producing organism. Crepitation always requires attention.

9. **(2)** This landmark can be used to determine the position of the second rib and intercostal space and corresponding spaces below that level. It is a visible and palpable angle of the sternum at the point where the second rib attaches to the sternum.

10. **(2)** Fluid or solid mass transmits the vibrations so that tactile fremitus may be felt on the exterior chest wall. Increased air trapping will cause a decreased or absent fremitus. A reactive airway results in wheezing due to edematous airway.

11. **(4)** The adult chest is somewhat asymmetrical and the AP diameter is often one half that of the transverse diameter.

12. **(2)** The client should be initially evaluated for tuberculosis. Pulmonary function studies, ABG studies, and bronchoscopy are not indicated at this time. Complement fixation studies are done to diagnose atypical pneumonia.

13. **(1)** Hyperinflation due to air trapping causes an increase in FRC, RV, and TLC (which may be twice normal). A corresponding decrease in FVC and FEV_1 occurs. This causes a flattening of the diaphragm, decreased inspiratory efficiency, and increased work of breathing.

14. **(1)** The positive sputum for acid-fast bacillus is indicative of active tuberculosis. *P. carinii* is a common organism in healthy respiratory tracts; it becomes a problem if the client is immunocompromised. Hemolysis on a complement fixation test is a negative finding. Oxygen saturation is low, the leukocyte count is within normal ranges, and treatment of this is not as important here as for the tuberculosis.

15. **(4)** For preliminary screening, the chest x-ray is the best, since it is less expensive and less invasive. It is even more beneficial if it can be compared to previous chest x-rays. All of the other options are beneficial in diagnosing the malignancy, but the x-ray is best for a screening program.

16. **(4)** This client is at risk for a pulmonary embolism due to hypercoagulation related to giving birth, smoking, and vascular injury (recent surgery). Assessment reveals common symptoms of pulmonary embolism: dyspnea, cough, and pleuritic pain. Diagnostic tests include ABGs, 12-lead ECG, chest x-ray, and echocardiogram. ABGs reflect a PaO_2 of <80 mm Hg and a $PaCO_2$ <36 mm Hg.

17. **(3)** Positive interpretation of PPD skin test results are as follows:

Induration	Positive in:
≥5 mm	Individuals with human immunodeficiency virus (HIV) infection
	Recent close contact with individuals with active tuberculosis (TB)
	Individuals with chest x-ray indicating healed TB
≥10 mm	Medically underserved individuals
	IV drug users
	Clients in long-term care facilities
≥15 mm	All individuals

Disorders

18. **(3)** The most common respiratory complication after a traumatic injury to the chest is pneumothorax caused by a fractured rib. Oximetry readings at 90% and increased pain are expected at this point and may not be indicative of a problem.

19. **(1)** Pneumococcal pneumonia due to *S. pneumoniae* often presents abruptly with high fever, shaking chills (rigor), cough productive of purulent or rusty sputum, headache, and pleuritic chest pain. In acute bronchitis, cough is the primary symptom and initially is dry and nonproductive. Fever, dyspnea, wheezing, and possible mucoid sputum production are also characteristic of acute bronchitis.

20. **(2)** According to the American Heart Association, the protocol for cardiopulmonary resuscitation (CPR; rescue breathing) due to respiratory arrest would be to open the airway by tilting the head and lifting the chin.

21. **(1)** It is most important to determine what precipitates the dyspnea. Is it present during rest or does it occur with activity? What level of activity precipitates the problem? This is important information necessary in order to determine the severity of the client's complaint.

22. **(1)** The most common area for a foreign body obstruction is the right bronchi; this will produce a unilateral retraction of the right chest wall. Retraction of the lower chest occurs with lower respiratory problems such as asthma. A pleural friction rub is heard when there is inflammation between the visceral and parietal pleura. Crepitation is present when air is leaking into the subcutaneous tissue.

23. **(1)** This is a normal finding due to the bulk of the liver. Atelectasis and consolidation will present with normal diaphragmatic movement but with dullness to percussion over the affected area. Obstructive lung disease will result in hyperresonance and limited diaphragmatic excursion, but it will be bilateral.

24. **(1)** Spontaneous pneumothorax occurs in healthy, thin, young adults, especially after strenuous exercise; predominant symptoms include sudden pain and dyspnea. The clinical hallmark of asthma is wheezing; with pulmonary edema there is frequently coughing, frothy sputum, and crackles heard on auscultation. Bronchiectasis is most often chronic and is characterized by moist crackles and wheezing on auscultation; cough is usually present.

25. **(1)** The situation described is hyperventilation; by slowing the breathing and breathing into a paper bag the carbon dioxide levels will be restored and the acid-base problem resolved. Albuterol, oxygen, ABGs, and IV fluids are not appropriate initial treatment.

26. **(1)** In order to prevent dyspnea on activity, the bronchodilator should be used prior to walking or increased physical activity. The client should not stay in bed but should be encouraged to gradually increase activity. Fluid intake of 2–3 L/day should be encouraged, unless there are cardiac problems. The oxygen level should not exceed 3- to 4-L flow.

27. **(3)** Elevated bicarbonate levels of blood are expected in clients with chronic hypercapnia. Hypoventilation and acidemia can result when too much oxygen is delivered. Supplemental oxygen should not be discontinued, because the PaO_2 levels decrease faster than the stimulus to breathe returns to eliminate the accumulated store of carbon dioxide (CO_2). Discontinuing supplemental oxygen, even for a short period of time, could cause serious complications.

28. **(1)** Nutritional needs are met by high-caloric, high-protein foods. High-carbohydrate foods need to be avoided in clients who retain CO_2 because carbohydrates metabolize into CO_2 as a waste product.

29. **(2)** Age-associated physiologic changes include the following: a decreased compliance of the chest wall, making deep inspiration difficult; the trachea and bronchi increase in diameter, increasing dead space, resulting in a decrease of volume of air reaching the alveoli; the lung parenchyma become less elastic, which decreases the function of the alveoli; and breathing becomes more shallow and cough forcefulness decreases due to respiratory muscles weakening.

30. **(3)** The flu, or influenza, is a highly contagious respiratory infection that occurs epidemically during the winter cold months. It is characterized by a sudden onset of chills, elevated temperature (101°–104°F), headache, fatigue, muscle pain, dry cough, laryngitis, rhinorrhea, and red eyes following a waiting period of 24–48 hours from time of exposure via respiratory droplets from an infected person or indirectly by drinking from a contaminated glass. Flu vaccines do not cause the flu, as they are made with a killed virus.

31. **(2)** Worsening dyspnea and fatigue with increasing cough may be indicative of early pulmonary edema. Clients with pulmonary edema require hospitalization with oxygen therapy, IV furosemide (Lasix), and morphine. Clients who are suspected to be in pulmonary edema *should not* be treated on an outpatient basis. Calcium channel blockers are of little benefit in heart failure.

32. **(2)** This client is considered to be in the "yellow" zone of personal best peak flow but is close to the "red" zone (50% or less of personal best). The client should use her bronchodilator immediately and, if not improved, may need emergency intervention by the nurse practitioner.

33. **(1)** The pneumococcal vaccine is recommended for elderly clients, since their immune systems are less efficient. The symptoms of fever, chest pain, and sputum production are suggestive of pneumonia.

34. **(2)** Confusion may be the first sign that the elderly client is septic. The client may not have a temperature or leukocytosis. The client may not experience any discomfort or a cough.

35. **(4)** *Streptococcus pneumoniae* is the most common cause of community- and nursing home–acquired pneumonia. *Haemophilus influenzae* is common in elderly clients with underlying chronic diseases (e.g., COPD, diabetes). *Klebsiella pneumoniae* and other gram-negative bacteria are pathogens in alcoholics, immunocompromised hosts, and hospitalized clients. *Mycobacterium tuberculosis* in an infrequent cause of pneumonia.

36. **(2)** This will decrease complications and hospitalizations for the older client. The pneumococcal vaccination is not administered annually. Options #3 and #4 are not recommended. The PPD should be done annually for high-risk clients.

37. **(2)** *Klebsiella pneumoniae* and other gram-negative bacteria are important pathogens in alcoholics, immunocompromised hosts, and hospitalized clients. *Haemophilus influenzae* is common in elderly clients with underlying chronic diseases (e.g., COPD, diabetes mellitus). *Staphylococcus aureus* generally affects elderly clients recovering from influenza, and is also frequent in hospitalized clients and diabetics. *Streptococcus pneumoniae* is the most common bacterial pathogen (30–40% of pneumonia cases), and most common cause of community- and nursing home–acquired pneumonia.

38. **(2)** Up to 25% of elderly clients with newly diagnosed TB have a negative tuberculin skin test due to waning cellular immunity with senescence. If the initial PPD test is negative, a repeat PPD test 1 week later is recommended in elderly clients. The repeat test is useful to stimulate a booster phenomenon in clients whose initial infection occurred many years in the past. The other options contain incorrect information.

39. **(3)** Horner's syndrome, which is paralysis of the cervical sympathetic nerves resulting in ptosis, loss of sweating, and constriction of the pupil and sinking of the eyeball on one side, is very commonly associated with malignant tumors in the upper lung leading to nerve compression.

40. **(40)** Superior vena cava obstruction is a complication of malignancy involving the mediastinum and rapidly progresses into an oncologic emergency.

41. **(3)** Hyponatremia results from an overproduction of antidiuretic hormone caused by an ectopic production from the bronchogenic tumor. Ketoacidosis and trauma result in fluid loss, causing hypernatremia, as does overuse of sodium-containing antacids.

42. **(3)** In older individuals the asthma is usually accompanied by infection. It is rarely allergic and costal retraction and fever are not usually seen. Subcutaneous epinephrine is not standard treatment but is sometimes indicated in emergent situations.

43. **(1)** Late-phase asthma occurs at 6–12 hours after the initial or acute bronchoconstrictive phase. The inflammatory response is the result of mast cell degranulation and release of histamine. Histamine acts on the lung by causing bronchoconstriction, vascular permeability, and vasodilatation. In late-phase asthma, bronchoconstriction is refractory to most bronchodilator therapy.

44. **(3)** Nocturnal exacerbation of asthma is a common clinical sign. It is linked to the variation in circulating catecholamines and vagal tone. Chronic hypoxemia and diffuse crackles are seen in the client with chronic bronchitis. Pruritus is often seen in contact allergic reactions.

45. **(2)** Asking the client about the consumption of wine with dinner is the most appropriate response. Many wines, especially white wines, contain sulfites that can trigger a mild allergic response.

Pharmacology

46. **(1)** In order for the medication to be most effective, there needs to be a 1-minute lapse time between the two puffs of medication. The first puff will open the upper airways. This will allow more effective penetration of the lower tract with the second puff of medication.

47. **(2)** The client would not stop taking the medications, as this is a common side effect of rifampin. Also, soft contact lenses may become discolored.

48. **(4)** β-Agonist (albuterol) MDI is the first line of treatment to decrease airflow obstruction. Aminophylline by mouth would take too long to be effective. Epinephrine is used predominantly for anaphylactic reaction. Beclovent is a steroid inhaler that is most effective when used prophylactically rather than in acute episodes.

49. **(4)** The use of tobacco increases the metabolism of theophylline, causing a need for greater dosage than required in nonsmokers. A high-protein, low-carbohydrate diet increases the metabolism of theophylline and decreases serum concentrations. Coffee (and other xanthine-containing beverages) may increase the central nervous system effects of xanthine derivatives.

50. **(1)** β-Blockers (Inderal and Tenormin) are known to cause exacerbation of chronic respiratory problems. Another antihypertensive such as a calcium channel blocker should be considered. The client's pulse is at 74, and his blood pressure remains elevated, which indicates the β-blocker is probably not effective in decreasing the blood pressure in this client. Theophylline derivatives are not indicated unless other medications are not effective. Drug interactions and increased levels of toxicity present problems in the elderly client.

51. **(2)** Therapeutic plasma levels range from 5–15 μg/ml. Drug levels of 20 μg/ml or greater are associated with toxicity.

52. **(1)** Chemoprophylaxis is initiated at the time of the screening skin testing. Skin testing should be repeated in 3 months, if initial test results are negative. If the second skin test is negative, chemoprophylaxis can be stopped.

53. **(3)** One of the most common causes of outpatient treatment failure is improper inhaler technique. While exposure to allergens may trigger an asthma attack, the proper use of inhalers will control those attacks. Use of both steroids and cromolyn inhalers has decreased the severity of asthma attacks.

54. **(1)** Theophylline is used in the treatment of chronic lung disease and can accumulate in toxic levels. Cimetidine decreases the hepatic clearance of theophylline. Nicotine and some antiseizure drugs may actually increase clearance, and ampicillin does not change the clearance.

55. **(2)** Antibiotic therapy is indicated when there is a change in color, consistency, or amount of sputum. Cough suppressants and antihistamines should be avoided.

56. **(2)** Beclomethasone dipropionate is a long-acting corticosteroid that stabilizes mast cells and greatly reduces mast cell degranulation when exposed to allergens. All of the other medications are bronchodilators used for rapid reversal of bronchospasm.

57. **(2)** Treatment of the client with asthma includes inhaled glucocorticoids for their anti-inflammatory effects. Antibiotics are indicated if there is a concurrent infection such as acute bronchitis. β$_2$-Agonist are used for their bronchodilator effects and rapid onset of action. Methacholine challenge is used in the diagnosis of asthma.

58. **(2)** The client with asthma should be instructed to keep their inhaled β$_2$-agonist with them at all times in case of

bronchospasm and use them as needed. The β_2-agonists are effective in reversing bronchospasm. Inhaled steroids are long acting and will not give immediate relief; therefore, the client should be instructed to use them regularly as prescribed and use their inhaled β_2-agonist as needed. Beginning antibiotics is not indicated for acute bronchospasm.

59. **(4)** Dextromethorphan is specific for control of coughing. Guaifenesin is an expectorant, and Options #1 and #2 are decongestants to decrease nasal and upper respiratory congestion.

60. **(1)** The combination of cisapride (Propulsid) and erythromycin-based antibiotics can precipitate fatal dysrhythmias. Another antibiotic should be considered. (*Testing tip: three of the selection of distractors are antihypertensive medications; only one is different and it is the correct answer.*)

61. **(3)** The drug therapy regimen for chronic asthma usually includes theophylline. Symptoms of toxicity include anorexia, nausea, vomiting, confusion, restlessness, tachycardia, dysrhythmias, and seizures.

62. **(2)** The hallmark clinical presentation of acute bronchitis is a productive cough. The nurse practitioner should rule out pneumonia. This was accomplished with this client through the normal chest x-ray and breath sounds. Bronchodilators (Albuterol) have been found to eliminate the cough of acute bronchitis. Antibiotic therapy (erythromycin and tetracycline) is not recommended. Research has demonstrated that antibiotic-susceptible organisms rarely cause acute bronchitis.

63. **(4)** H_2 antagonists neutralize the normal gastric acid barrier, allowing for an increased colonization of gram-negative bacilli and *Staphylococcus aureus*.

Immune & Allergy

Physical Examination & Diagnostic Tests

1. When taking the history of a client with known allergies, what is the most important information to determine?

   1. Reaction associated with each allergen.

   2. Drug allergies.

   3. Food allergies.

   4. Environmental exposure.

2. Diagnostic studies used in the differential diagnosis of systemic lupus erythematosus (SLE) include:

   1. Complete blood count (CBC), SMA-12, and erythrocyte sedimentation rate (ESR).

   2. Chest radiograph and coagulation profile.

   3. Antinuclear antibodies (ANA), ESR, and C-reactive protein.

   4. CBC, urinalysis, and chest radiograph.

3. Which tests are appropriate for the nurse practitioner to order in an initial work-up for asymptomatic clients at risk for human immunodeficiency virus (HIV)?

   1. CD4 count, HIV enzyme-linked immunosorbent assay (ELISA).

   2. Serology for cytomegalovirus, herpes simplex virus, and Epstein-Barr virus.

   3. HIV ELISA and Western blot.

   4. Hepatitis screen and Western blot.

4. The nurse practitioner would anticipate which laboratory finding in a client with joint pain, "butterfly rash," photosensitivity, weight loss, and fever?

   1. Presence of antinuclear antibodies.

   2. Negative serum complement level.

   3. Increased red blood cell (RBC) and white blood cell (WBC) count.

   4. Glycosuria.

5. When assessing a client for angioedema, the nurse practitioner would examine the:

   1. Neck and ears.

   2. Heart sounds.

   3. Abdomen.

   4. Eyes and mouth.

6. Clients who believe they have been exposed to HIV should have an HIV antibody test how soon after the exposure?

   1. The next day and 2 months later.

   2. 6 months after exposure and again at 12 months.

   3. 6–12 weeks after exposure and again at 6 months.

   4. 4 weeks and 12 weeks.

7. The most reliable test for the presence of specific immunoglobulin E (IgE) antibody is:

   1. Skin testing.

   2. Radioallergosorbent testing (RAST).

   3. Smears for eosinophils.

   4. Complete blood count.

8. To diagnose allergic rhinitis in the primary care office setting the nurse practitioner would consider performing?

   1. A nasal smear for eosinophils.

   2. A total serum IgE.

   3. Skin testing.

   4. Radioallergosorbent testing (RAST).

Disorders

9. Client education regarding common antigens of anaphylaxis includes:

   1. Extreme weather.

   2. Egg albumin.

   3. Pungent odors.

   4. Animal dandruff.

10. The nurse practitioner understands that an HIV infection results in a reduction of:

    1. Helper T cells.

    2. Suppressor T cells.

    3. Killer T cells.

    4. Suppressor B cells.

11. Which assessment finding is commonly associated with a diagnosis of systemic lupus erythematous (SLE)?

    1. Excitability, diarrhea, vomiting.

    2. High fever, measles-like rash on limbs, weight gain.

    3. Joint pain, malar rash, photosensitivity.

    4. Weight loss, diarrhea, epigastric pain.

12. After a repeat HIV antibody test, a client continues to test positive but is asymptomatic. The nurse practitioner understands which of the following about possible transmission of the virus by the client?

    1. The client is infectious when symptoms are active.

    2. The client is infectious for life.

    3. The dormant virus is not infectious while the client is asymptomatic and the T cell count is high.

    4. Laboratory tests should be done monthly to identify the infectious periods of the disease process.

13. A young woman has just received news of a positive HIV test. She does not want her sexual partner to be informed. What is the most appropriate response to her decision?

    1. Respect for her decision, since she is the client.

    2. Letting her know that you have a legal responsibility to inform her partner.

    3. Counseling her about your ethical responsibility to inform all sexual partners.

    4. Noting her decision in the record for future reference.

14. A client presenting with complaint of fatigue, malaise, arthralgias, oral ulcers, malar rash, and a positive ANA would most likely be diagnosed as:

    1. Rheumatoid arthritis.
    2. Fibromyalgia.
    3. Scleroderma.
    4. Systemic lupus erythematosus.

15. An elderly female client presents to the nurse practitioner with a low-grade temperature and a unilateral throbbing headache. She also reports scalp sensitivity and some visual disturbances. Lab results show a markedly elevated ESR and anemia. She has been relatively healthy except for a recent history of polymyalgia rheumatica (PMR). Symptoms indicate a clinical presentation of:

    1. Bacterial meningitis.
    2. Acute migraine headache.
    3. Temporal (giant cell) arteritis.
    4. Subdural hematoma.

16. A middle-aged female client presents with weight loss, heartburn, dysphagia, dry cough, pain, stiffness of the fingers and knees, and Raynaud's phenomenon. The nurse practitioner recognizes these as the symptoms of:

    1. Rheumatoid arthritis.
    2. Lupus erythematosus.
    3. Graft-versus-host disease.
    4. Scleroderma.

17. The erythematous confluent macular eruption of the face known as the butterfly rash is characteristic of:

    1. Allergic drug eruption.
    2. Systemic lupus erythematosus.
    3. Rosacea.
    4. Seborrheic dermatitis.

18. The nurse practitioner is discussing general health care with a female client who is in remission for SLE. Important points to include are:

    1. Avoid getting pregnant.
    2. Decrease physical and psychological stress.
    3. Avoid isometric and aerobic exercise.
    4. Maintain diet low in fat and carbohydrates.

19. A client presents with sneezing, watery eyes, postnasal drip, full head, and sore throat. The best diagnosis for this client is:

    1. Acute bronchitis.
    2. Allergic rhinitis.
    3. Asthma exacerbation.
    4. Influenza.

20. A 70-year-old woman presents with complaints of morning headache, malaise, and anorexia. The nurse practitioner suspects:

    1. Penumonia.
    2. Temporal arteritis.
    3. Herpes zoster.
    4. Postmenopausal symptoms.

21. When teaching a client about risk factors and prevention of transmission of HIV, which statement is most appropriate?

    1. HIV can be transmitted by casual kissing.
    2. Unprotected oral sex with an infected partner is not advised.
    3. Sharing an office with an HIV-positive person increases the risk of exposure to HIV.
    4. Using the same bathroom as an infected family member puts you at risk of exposure to HIV.

22. Signs and symptoms that alert the nurse practitioner to identify a client who is at an increased risk for HIV infection include:

    1. Night sweats.
    2. Malaise and fatigue.
    3. Frequent sexually transmitted diseases.
    4. Swollen glands and diarrhea.

23. The human immunodeficiency virus is classified as a:

    1. Cytomegalovirus.

    2. Herpetic virus.

    3. Papillomavirus.

    4. Retrovirus.

24. A systemic IgE-mediated antigen–antibody response resulting in a life-threatening massive release of mediators is:

    1. Generalized seizures.

    2. Allergic rhinitis.

    3. Anaphylaxis.

    4. Status asthmaticus.

25. The release of histamine results in:

    1. Bronchospasm, vasodilatation, and vascular permeability.

    2. Bronchodilatation, vasodilatation, and vascular permeability.

    3. Smooth muscle contraction, decreased vascular permeability, and vasoconstriction.

    4. Pain, increased vascular permeability, and bronchodilatation.

26. A 22-year-old female presents with breathlessness, weight loss, nonproductive cough, temperature 38°C (100.4°F), pulse 124, respirations 36, blood pressure 120/78, and a history of a positive HIV serum test. Based on this information, what is the most accurate diagnosis?

    1. *Klebsiella pneumoniae.*

    2. Kaposi's sarcoma.

    3. *Pneumocystis carinii* pneumonia.

    4. Lymphoma.

27. An adult is brought into the clinic and the family states she has a history of anaphylactic reactions. What signs and symptoms indicate to the nurse practitioner the client is experiencing another reaction?

    1. Cough, wheezing, and hives.

    2. Severe malaise, pallor, stridor, and dyspnea.

    3. Anxiety, nasal congestion, and tachycardia.

    4. Rhinorrhea, nausea, and gastrointestinal (GI) cramping.

28. A nurse at the clinic experiences a needle stick from a client with known hepatitis. What should be administered to provide passive immunity?

    1. IgE.

    2. IgA.

    3. IgG.

    4. IgC.

29. Which sign and/or symptom is indicative of a type I hypersensitivity reaction?

    1. Contact dermatitis.

    2. Immediate wheal-and-flare reaction.

    3. Hematuria.

    4. High fever.

30. Which clients are at risk for developing HIV infection/acquired immunodeficiency syndrome (AIDS)?

    1. Immunocompromised clients.

    2. Sexually active teenagers.

    3. Elderly adults.

    4. Marijuana users.

31. Which statement is true regarding latex allergy?

    1. It usually only produces symptoms of contact dermatitis and allergic rhinorrhea.

    2. It is a progressive disease that worsens with continued exposure.

    3. It affects <5% of the health care population.

    4. It is an autoimmune response.

Pharmacology

32. A client newly presenting with signs and symptoms of SLE would have their

medication profile reviewed to determine if they are on any medication that may have caused a drug-induced lupus. Which drug would be most suspect?

1. Digoxin (Lanoxin)

2. Procainamide (Pronestyl).

3. Trimethoprim-sulfamethoxazole (Bactrim).

4. Cimetidine (Tagamet).

33. A client is diagnosed with temporal (giant cell) arteritis. The medication of choice is:

1. Prednisone (Deltasone).

2. Ibuprofen (Motrin).

3. Indomethacin (Indocin).

4. Azathioprine (Imuran).

34. The clinic is notified that a young adult is being brought in with a bee sting and that the individual is having difficulty breathing. Which medication should the nurse practitioner have available for the client's initial care?

1. Lidocaine topical ointment.

2. Epinephrine.

3. Prednisone.

4. Benadryl elixir.

35. The standard drug used for malaria prophylaxis is:

1. Ampicillin (Polycillin, Omnipen).

2. Doxycycline (Vibramycin).

3. Ceftriaxone (Rocephin).

4. Chloroquine phosphate (Aralen).

36. Treatment for allergic rhinitis includes:

1. Antihistamines, corticosteroids, and environmental control.

2. Antibiotics, antihistamines, analgesics, and allergen control.

3. Cholinergic agents, antibiotics, and analgesics.

4. Nasal saline, corticosteroids, and antibiotics.

37. Development of an adverse drug reaction is dependent on which factors?

1. Client age, prior drug reactions, genetic factors, and degree of exposure.

2. Client gender, oral route of administration, and history of atrophic disease.

3. Client age, client gender, and genetic factors.

4. Genetic factors, prior drug reactions, and client gender.

38. A medication frequently used for the prophylaxis as well as initial treatment of *Pneumocystis carinii* pneumonia (PCP) is:

1. Fluconazole (Diflucan).

2. Amphotericin B (Fungizone).

3. Trimethoprim-sulfamethoxazole (Septra, Bactrim).

4. Acyclovir (Zovirax).

39. When instructing the client with allergic rhinitis about the use of nasal decongestants, it is important for them to understand:

1. The condition is self-limiting and will resolve in a matter of weeks whether or not the client is re-exposed to the allergen.

2. Nasal decongestant used continuously for greater than 3 days can result in a worsening of the symptoms.

3. It is not necessary to avoid exposure to the allergen once therapy has been initiated.

4. Allergic rhinitis is only seen in the spring and fall; the condition requires treatment only during these seasons.

40. The major advantage to use of second-generation antihistamines such as astemizole (Hismanal) and loratadine (Claritin) is:

1. Decreased cost.

2. Increased anticholinergic activity.

3. Delayed absorption.

4. Does not cross the blood-brain barrier.

41. What is the desired action of sympathomimetics (adrenergics) when used in the treatment of allergic rhinitis?

    1. Promote vasoconstriction in nasal mucosa.

    2. Block mast cell degranulation.

    3. Decrease the effect of histamines.

    4. Increase degranulation and end-organ response.

42. The nurse practitioner is prescribing astemizole (Hismanal) for a geriatric client's allergy problems. When considering the client's current medications, which medication would be a contraindication to the administration of astemizole?

    1. Erythromycin ethylsuccinate (E.E.S.).

    2. Verapamil (Calan).

    3. Propranolol (Inderal)

    4. Captopril (Capoten).

43. What information is important for the nurse practitioner to include when teaching a client about the use of antihistamines?

    1. Use of topical antihistamines is safe and has relatively few side effects.

    2. Do not use over-the-counter (OTC) medications without consulting the health care provider.

    3. Constipation and urinary retention are expected side effects and do not need to be reported.

    4. Once the antihistamine therapy has been taken for 3 days, avoidance of allergens is not necessary.

44. A primary advantage of using loratadine (Claritin) in treating a client with seasonal allergies is that it:

    1. Is supplied as an enteric-coated pill.

    2. May be prescribed on once-a-day dosing.

    3. Costs considerably less than other medications.

    4. Effectively decreases nasal secretions.

45. What medications are the choice of treatment in the secondary therapy for the client with an anaphylactic reaction?

    1. Antibiotics and anticholinergics.

    2. Nonsteroidal anti-inflammatory drugs (NSAIDs).

    3. Decongestants and expectorants.

    4. Antihistamines and corticosteroids.

6   Answers & Rationales

Physical Examination & Diagnostic Tests

1. **(1)** The reaction to each allergen is important to know. Often clients will indicate they have an adverse reaction to a particular food or medication, such as nausea, stomach pain, or diarrhea, and consider it an allergy. The signs and symptoms of the reaction, speed of onset, how long it lasts, and what successful treatment has been used in the past are important information. Both drug and food allergies should be explored.

2. **(3)** Although all of the tests included in the question may be included in a complete physical examination, laboratory tests specific to the diagnosis of SLE include the ANA, ESR, and C-reactive protein. During flares the ESR and C-reactive protein are elevated. The ANA titer in a client with SLE is positive at a 1:80 ratio.

3. **(3)** The initial screening test for HIV is the ELISA. If the test is positive, confirmation of antibodies is done with a Western blot. Although serology and hepatitis screening along with a CBC and tuberculosis (TB) test are routinely performed, the initial work-up starts with an ELISA test. The CD4 count is performed during the active disease process.

4. **(1)** The majority of clients with SLE have antinuclear antibodies in their blood. There is leukopenia, thrombocytopenia, lymphopenia, and a positive LE cell prep.

Proteinuria with cellular casts is often noted.

5. **(4)** Angioedema is most easily seen in the eyes and mouth, and is edema of the mucous membrane tissue. It can also be observed on the tongue, feet, hands, and genitalia. Diffuse erythema may be seen in the upper body parts. Gastrointestinal symptoms, vomiting, cramping, and diarrhea may also be seen.

6. **(3)** The HIV antibody develops between 6 and 12 weeks after exposure. Because of the variability of antibody development, it is recommended that the test be repeated in 6 months to confirm the findings.

7. **(1)** The most reliable test for the presence of the specific IgE antibody is the skin test. RAST is less sensitive than skin testing and is difficult to standardize and reproduce results. The smear for eosinophils and the CBC are not specific for IgE antibody testing.

8. **(1)** A nasal smear for eosinophils is a simple office procedure. Many clients who have uncomplicated allergic rhinitis have a normal serum IgE. Skin testing should be performed by allergy-trained providers only. RAST testing is higher in cost and lower in sensitivity.

Disorders

9. **(2)** Egg albumin is just one of many identified common antigens that may result in anaphylactic reaction. Others include vaccines, allergen extracts, sulfonamides, penicillins, hormones, legumes (especially peanuts), berries, nuts, seafoods, and venomous bites (bee, wasp, yellow jacket bites). Changes in weather, strong scents, and odors are triggers that may precipitate an asthma attack resulting in bronchospasm and wheezing.

10. **(1)** There is a severe, life-threatening reduction of helper T cells, along with an increase in suppressor T cells. The helper T cells help amplify or increase the production of antibody-forming cells from the B lymphocytes after an encounter with an antigen. Killer T cells are produced after mature helper T cells interact with an antigen. Suppressor T cells suppress the formation of antibody-forming cells from the B lymphocytes which, when their numbers are increased, have a detrimental effect on the immunity and ability of the HIV client to make antibody-forming cells.

11. **(3)** The symptoms most commonly experienced are joint pain, fatigue, Raynaud's phenomenon, chronic or low-grade or recurrent fever, sun sensitivity, hair loss, weakness, butterfly (malar) facial rash, and weight loss. Typically, the pulmonary, cardiac, renal, and central nervous systems are involved.

12. **(2)** HIV infection creates a chronic infectious state in the body that is transmitted via blood and body fluids, and transplacentally.

13. **(3)** Ethical response includes notification of all persons at risk.

14. **(4)** This client is presenting with 4 of the 11 criteria necessary for diagnosing SLE. There is no singular test for SLE, but with the presence of these characteristics plus lab results the diagnosis can be differentiated.

15. **(3)** About 40% of temporal (giant cell) arteritis clients have a history of PMR. The other diagnoses may have some of these symptoms but only arteritis has all the symptoms of those listed in the situation. It is especially critical to note visual disturbances, as these clients can develop sudden blindness.

16. **(4)** The symptom of Raynaud's phenomenon differentiates this as scleroderma. The esophageal dysfunction is often an initial complaint in this disease, which is four times more common in females.

17. **(2)** The butterfly rash is one of the characteristic symptoms of SLE.

18. **(2)** Psychological and physical stress can exacerbate SLE. A balanced diet helps to limit the side effects of some of the medications, while regular exercise helps to reduce arthralgia and myalgia. Barrier contraception is recommended for the female with SLE. Pregnancy is usually allowed during periods of remission.

19. **(2)** The signs and symptoms presented are classic for allergic rhinitis. Acute bronchitis would present with cough and yellow or green sputum production. An asthma exacerbation would present with wheezing, chest tightness, decreased forced vital capacity, and history of exposure to an allergen. Influenza presents with fever, chills, and general malaise.

20. **(2)** The nurse practitioner should rule out temporal arteritis, an inflammatory disorder of unknown etiology affecting large- and medium-sized arteries. It occurs two times more frequently in women, occurs most frequently in the elderly, and occurs rarely in the African-American population.

21. **(2)** Unprotected oral sex with an HIV-positive person puts you at risk for exposure to the virus. Contact such as casual kissing, or sharing an office or bathroom, does not transmit the virus. The virus is transmitted in bodily fluids and secretions.

22. **(3)** The client with frequent sexually transmitted diseases would alert the nurse practitioner to the client's lack of use of protection during sex and the possibility of multiple partners. Night sweats, malaise, fatigue, swollen glands, and diarrhea can be associated with many other illnesses.

23. **(4)** The HIV virus is a retrovirus. It contains an enzyme, reverse transcriptase, that copies RNA into DNA. When the virus binds to a CD4 receptor, it inserts its RNA and enzymes into the cell, where a copy of the virsus's RNA is made and enters the nucleus of the cell. As the infected host cell reproduces, the HIV DNA is duplicated and passed on.

24. **(3)** The massive release of mediators triggers a series of events in target organs. Prior sensitization to the antigen must have occurred to trigger an anaphylactic reaction. Anaphylaxis may result from injection of an antigen, ingested food or drugs, or inhaled antigens.

25. **(1)** The release of histamine results in bronchospasm, vasodilatation, and vascular permeability, leading to wheezing, increased mucous production in the lung, and edema of the airway.

26. **(3)** Based on the history of an HIV-positive test and the symptoms presented, the client is at risk for development of *Pneumocystis carinii* pneumonia. Further examination would include obtaining a chest radiograph, and pulse oximetry to determine oxygen saturation. The lack of purplish lesions is considered in ruling out Kaposi's sarcoma. *Klebsiella pneumoniae* is a nosocomial infection, not community acquired. Lymphoma in HIV usually occurs as non-Hodgkin's as a primary site in the brain.

27. **(2)** Severe malaise, pallor, stridor, and dyspnea are signs and symptoms associated with a severe anaphylactic reaction. Symptoms may occur immediately or up to 2 hours after exposure. Severe reactions require immediate intervention.

28. **(3)** IgG is the major antibody against viruses and bacterias and is the principal mediator of the secondary immune response requiring repeated response to the same antigen. There is no IgC antibody. IgA is the secretory immunoglobulin found in tears, saliva, and mucous secretions of the lung and GI tract. IgE mediates allergic reactions.

29. **(2)** A type I hypersensitivity reaction causes an immediate wheal-and-flare reaction. Contact dermatitis is seen in a type IV (delayed) reaction. Hematuria is seen in a type II reaction caused by the presence of preformed circulating cytotoxic antibodies, such as in a blood transfusion reaction or autoimmune hemolytic anemia. High fever can be seen in the type III hypersensitivity reaction when large quantities of antigen–antibody complexes are released in the body.

30. **(2)** Sexually active teenagers constitute the fastest growing group of HIV-positive clients, due to unprotected sexual activity. Immunocompromised clients and elderly adults are at no greater risk for developing HIV than any other group. Risk factors for the development of HIV include unprotected sexual contact with someone of unknown HIV status, multiple sexual partners, intravenous drug use, hemophiliacs, and clients receiving blood transfusions prior to 1985.

31. **(2)** Latex allergy is a progressive disease that worsens with continual exposure. The symptoms range from contact dermatitis to anaphylaxis. Currently, latex allergy affects 17% of health care workers and 39% of dental professionals. Latex allergy is an acquired immune response to the latex protein allergen. There is no vaccine and the only defense is to avoid contact with latex.

Pharmacology

32. **(2)** Procainamide (Pronestyl) is one of the most common offenders. Twenty per cent of clients receiving this drug develop clinical drug-induced SLE. The other drugs listed have not been associated with SLE.

33. **(1)** This condition, seen primarily in the elderly, can lead to blindness if not treated immediately with corticosteroids. The usual daily dose of prednisone is 60 mg; divided dose initially, then single morning dose (never use every-other-day steroids). Begin a *slow taper* after 4 weeks if asymptomatic and ESR is decreased. Tapering dose is very individualized and the client may be on medications for several months to years. The average time for disease remission is 3–4 years (range 1–10 years).

34. **(2)** Epinephrine would be the first-line drug to be injected for the treatment of the respiratory distress associated with an anaphylactic reaction. The dosage for epinephrine (1:1000 SC) is 0.3–0.5 ml/kg for an adult. Benadryl's onset of action is not fast enough. Lidocaine would only topically treat the pain and not the respiratory problem. Anti-inflammatory medications would not be given initially, but possibly later if needed.

35. **(4)** Chloroquine phosphate is the standard drug used for malaria prophylaxis. The dosage is 5 mg/kg of body weight up to 300 mg for an adult. Doxycycline (Vibramycin) is often used to treat diarrhea associated with traveling to areas where diarrhea is common from drinking the water; it is also used to treat chlamydia and pelvic inflammatory disease. Ceftriaxone (Rocephin) is used in bacterial septicemia or problems of the respiratory and urinary tract. Ampicillin (Polycillin, Omnipen) is used to treat a variety of organisms and as prophylaxis for bacterial endocarditis.

36. **(1)** Unless there is a secondary bacterial infection, antibiotics are not indicated. Antihistamines and reduction of exposure to the allergen will help to reduce the symptoms. For continued control and stabilization of the mast cell, corticosteroids are indicated.

37. **(1)** Adults are at greater risk for development of adverse drug reactions, probably due to the increased number of medications used and the amount of exposures. Clients with prior drug reactions are more likely to develop reactions to new drugs. The risk of an adverse drug reaction occurs in the first 2–3 weeks of therapy. Prolonged course of drug use, high dosage, and intermittent therapy increase the risk of an adverse reaction. Genetic factors may contribute to increased mediators and influencing metabolic pathways. Gender has no effect except with muscle relaxants and chymopapain, where women are at greater risk of developing an adverse drug reaction. Route of drug administration contributes to the risk, with IV, IM, SC, PO, and topical in the order of greatest to least risk.

38. **(3)** Trimethoprim-sulfamethoxazole (Septra, Bactrim) is used to treat as well as prevent *Pneumocystis carinii* pneumonia. Usually, a 21-day course of the drug is indicated. It may take 7–10 days to see a clinical response. Fluconazole (Diflucan) and amphotericin B are antifungal drugs. Acyclovir (Zovirax) is an antiviral used primarily to treat herpes simplex virus types 1 and 2 and herpes zoster (shingles).

39. **(2)** The chronic use of nasal decongestants for greater than 3 days can result in a rebound effect when discontinued. This will lead to increased nasal congestion, which is the result of reflex vasodilatation. The condition may take as long as 2–3 weeks to resolve. Allergic rhinitis is not a self-limiting illness associated only with the spring and fall. Even though therapy is initiated, the client should be instructed to avoid exposure to the allergen as much as possible.

40. **(4)** The second-generation antihistamines do not cross the blood-brain barrier; therefore, they do not cause sedation and/or psychomotor dysfunction. There is little anticholinergic activity and less dry mouth and constipation. The cost of these antihistamines is 15–30 times greater than the first-generation antihistamines. The medications are rapidly absorbed, within 1–2 hours of oral administration on an empty stomach.

41. **(1)** Sympathomimetics (adrenergics) cause vasoconstriction, reducing edema and secretions. Inhaled corticosteroids stabilize mast cells and block degranulation.

42. **(2)** Macrolides (erythromycin) and Hismanal should not be administered concurrently. Fatal dysrhythmias may be precipitated by this combination.

43. **(2)** The client should be instructed not to use OTC medications without consulting the nurse practitioner or pharmacist. The client should be cautioned on the extended use of topical antihistamines. Antihistamines do not affect circulating histamine; therefore, it is important for the client to avoid exposure to a known allergen. Constipation and urinary retention are adverse effects that should be reported to the nurse practitioner.

44. **(2)** An advantage of using loratadine (Claritin) is the once-a-day dosing, which

helps with client compliance. The cost is greater than some of the other first-generation antihistamines. Loratadine/pseudoephedrine (Claritin D) is available as an antihistamine/decongestant with either twice-a-day dosing or (Claritin D 24 Hour) loratadine/pseudoephedrine extended release for once-a-day dosing.

45. **(4)** Medications such as antihistamines and corticosteroids are used to counter mediator release and block release of additional mediators. NSAIDs, antibiotics, and decongestants are not indicated in the treatment of anaphylaxis.

Head, Eyes, Ears, Nose, & Throat (HEENT)

Physical Examination & Diagnostic Tests

Head

1. The nurse practitioner is examining lymph nodes in the neck. What is palpated in the anterior triangle of the neck?

   1. Posterior cervical chain.

   2. Anterior superficial chain.

   3. Periauricular lymph nodes.

   4. Supraclavicular lymph nodes.

Eyes

2. When using an ophthalmoscope, the nurse practitioner:

   1. Holds the ophthalmoscope in the right hand (uses right eye) while examining the client's left eye.

   2. Starts the examination with the lens set at zero.

   3. Begins in a position 1 inch from the eye to check the red light reflex.

   4. Examines the anterior chamber in a well-lighted room and asks the client to focus on an object.

3. The nurse practitioner observes lid lag in a client with:

   1. Myasthenia gravis.

   2. Hyperthyroidism.

   3. Hordeolum.

   4. Chalazion.

4. The nurse practitioner is examining an elderly woman. There is a glossy white circle around the pupils of her eyes, and the pupil has a decreased reaction to the direct light reflex. There is a history of presbyopia. Correct interpretation of these findings is:

   1. Beginning development of cataracts with a significant decrease in visual acuity.

   2. Normal changes in the eyes as a result of the aging process.

   3. A decrease in depth perception and the early eye changes associated with glaucoma.

   4. Visual changes secondary to long-term treatment with digitoxin and corticosteroids.

5. The nurse practitioner is preparing to examine the eyes of an adult client. In order to examine the optic disc and retinal vessels, the practitioner uses what aperture on the ophthalmoscope?

   1. Small aperture.

   2. Red-free filter.

   3. Slit.

   4. Grid.

6. When testing the eyes for the presence of a normal consensual response, the nurse practitioner will:

   1. Shine the light into the client's pupil and observe the rate of pupillary constriction.

   2. Direct the light into one pupil, and observe for the constriction or response of the other pupil.

   3. Hold a card in front of one eye, and have the client focus on a fixed object; remove the card and observe movement of the newly uncovered eye.

   4. Ask the client to focus on an object, then direct a light source to the bridge of the nose while observing for symmetrical reflection in both eyes.

7. On ophthalmic examination, there appears to be a narrowing or blocking of the vein at the point where an arteriole crosses over it. The significance of this finding is:

   1. The client needs to be evaluated for chronic hypertension.

   2. This may be indicative of increased ocular pressure associated with glaucoma.

   3. The finding is associated with papilledema causing decreased venous drainage.

   4. This may represent a small embolus in the retinal vessels.

8. When examining the eyes, the nurse practitioner determines that the pupils change in size when the client focuses from a close object to a distant object. This is interpreted as:

   1. Normal visual accommodation.

   2. Extraocular motor nerves are intact.

   3. Consensual response is appropriate.

   4. Visual acuity is within normal limits.

Ears

9. When examining the ears of an adult client, the nurse practitioner determines the tympanic membrane is gray and translucent. This is interpreted as:

   1. Scarring from previous infections.

   2. Decreased circulation to the membrane.

   3. Presence of serous fluid behind the membrane.

   4. Normal characteristics of the adult ear.

10. The purpose of conducting the Rinne's test is to determine conduction of sound through the bone and through the auditory canal. A normal Rinne's test is described as:

    1. Equal conduction through the mastoid bone and the ear canal.

    2. Air conduction twice as long as bone conduction.

    3. Bone conduction twice as long as air conduction.

    4. Sound is clearer with bone conduction than air conduction.

11. When assessing the tympanic membrane, specific landmarks are determined and

described according to the face of a clock. Normal landmarks for the right tympanic membrane are located:

1. Direct light reflex at the 5- to 6-o'clock position, malleus at the 1- to 2-o'clock position with umbo in center.

2. Manubrium slanted to the left with malleus at the 10-o'clock position.

3. Direct light reflex in center of membrane with malleus at the 9-o'clock position.

4. Umbo to the left with anterior malleolar folds at the 10-o'clock position.

Nose

12. The nurse practitioner understands that nasal mucosa:

1. Is redder than oral mucosa.

2. Is pale and translucent in appearance.

3. Appears pink and boggy, without exudate.

4. Appears dark pink with watery secretion.

Throat

13. Throat cultures are indicated for the following suspects of pharyngitis:

1. Rhinovirus and coronavirus infection.

2. Group A β-hemolytic streptococci.

3. Mononucleosis.

4. *Candida albicans.*

14. A young adult client arrives at the nurse practitioner's clinic with a complaint of low-grade fever, sore throat, a slight headache, and fatigue. On physical examination, the nurse practitioner found exudative tonsils bilaterally, red pharynx with white patches, and enlarged posterior cervical neck nodes. Upon testing, the nurse practitioner would expect to find:

1. Positive rapid strep test.

2. Positive monospot test.

3. Decreased white blood cell (WBC) count.

4. Positive viral throat cultures.

Disorders

Head

15. An adult client presents to the nurse practitioner's office with a white plaque near the base of the tongue. The nurse practitioner notes that the plaque does not wipe off and assesses it as:

1. Hemangioma.

2. Leukoplakia.

3. Papilloma.

4. Erythroplasia.

16. Which of the following are predominant risk factors for oral carcinoma?

1. History of dental infections, age <40.

2. Tobacco use, alcohol use.

3. Herpes simplex virus type 1, tobacco use.

4. Alcohol use, history of dental abscess.

17. The hallmark of early oral cancer is:

1. Tissue retraction.

2. Thickening oral tissues.

3. Persistent (>14 days) local inflammation.

4. Halitosis and cough.

18. An adult female client is being evaluated for a complaint of a sore throat. She states that she has difficulty swallowing and has some mouth pain. On exam, the nurse practitioner finds that the client's mouth, tongue, and pharynx are coated with white curd-like plaques that are difficult to remove with a tongue blade. The course of treatment for this client should include:

1. Referral for evaluation.

2. Amoxicillin 500 mg PO tid × 10 days.

3. Encourage the client to have human immunodeficiency virus (HIV) screening.

4. Clear liquids only for the next few days.

19. The nurse practitioner knows that the most common site for head and neck cancer to occur is the:

    1. Sinuses.

    2. Oral cavity.

    3. Larynx.

    4. Nasal cavity.

Eyes

20. An adult reports awakening with redness and a swollen eyelid. The nurse practitioner notes that the adult is afebrile and the eyelid is nontender and uniformly swollen. The most likely diagnosis is:

    1. Blepharitis.

    2. Hordeolum.

    3. Insect bite.

    4. Dacryocystitis.

21. A client is being prepared for cataract surgery. What information is important for the nurse practitioner to explain to the client?

    1. The procedure is short and the client usually goes home the morning after the surgery.

    2. Both eyes will be patched for the first 24 hours and it is important for the client to stay in bed.

    3. There may be problems with headache and eye pain for the first 24 hours; take the pain medication provided.

    4. Clients usually go home 2–3 hours after the surgery; there will be increased tearing, but it should not be painful.

22. A geriatric client presents at the clinic with complaints of blurred vision that has been getting increasingly worse over the past 2 years. There is also a problem with glare, but no problems with pain. The nurse practitioner would first evaluate for presence of:

    1. Glaucoma.

    2. Retinal detachment.

    3. Degeneration of macula.

    4. Cataracts.

23. An adult client presents to the nurse practitioner for evaluation of a red, itchy eye for 1 day. The client states that when she awoke the eye was matted shut. The client can recall no trauma to the eye. The pupils are equal and reactive and the client denies any pain to the eye. The nurse practitioner treats this client for:

    1. Conjunctivitis.

    2. Corneal abrasion.

    3. Glaucoma.

    4. Iritis.

24. Which assessment of the eye is a deviation from the commonly occurring age-related changes?

    1. Arcus senilis.

    2. Presbyopia.

    3. Sensitivity to glare.

    4. Sustained nystagmus.

25. During a routine physical examination on a 30-year-old client, the nurse practitioner identifies arcus cornealis. The significance of this disorder is:

    1. High potential for future blindness.

    2. None, normal variant of aging process.

    3. Abnormal lipid metabolism requiring medical management.

    4. Hereditary variant of no consequence.

26. A 70-year-old client comes to the clinic complaining of an increased sensitivity to glare, difficulty adapting to darkness, and altered depth perception. The nurse practitioner should suspect.

    1. Cataract.

    2. Macular degeneration.

    3. Glaucoma.

    4. Normal age-related changes.

27. In assessing an adult with bacterial conjunctivitis, the nurse practitioner finds:

    1. Minimal tearing, moderate itching, and profuse exudate.

2. Severe itching, moderate tearing, and minimal discharge.

3. Minimal itching, moderate tearing, and mucoid exudate.

4. Minimal itching, moderate tearing, and profuse exudate.

Ears

28. In teaching clients how to avoid acoustic trauma due to noise in the very loud range, the nurse practitioner knows that noise is loudest from:

    1. Vacuum cleaner.

    2. Power mower.

    3. Clothes washer.

    4. Food blender.

29. A geriatric client is complaining of difficulty hearing. She relates that the problem seems to be getting worse over the past few years. What finding would support a diagnosis of presbycusis?

    1. Unable to hear a watch tick at 1–2 inches from the ear.

    2. Rinne's test indicates air conduction is greater than bone conduction.

    3. History of long-term tetracycline antibiotics for chronic infections.

    4. Long-term family history of chronic hearing loss.

30. An adult is seen by the nurse practitioner for ear pain. The adult is afebrile and reports that she swims frequently for daily exercise. The left ear canal is markedly edematous and moderately inflamed with thick, yellowish drainage at the external meatus. The most likely diagnosis is:

    1. Acute otitis media.

    2. Serous otitis media.

    3. Sinusitis.

    4. Otitis externa.

31. Which of the following organisms is least likely to cause otitis media?

    1. *Moraxella catarrhalis.*

    2. *Streptococcus pneumoniae.*

    3. *Chlamydia trachomatis.*

    4. *Haemophilus influenzae.*

32. Which assessment of the ear would indicate a deviation from the normal aging process?

    1. Dull, retracted, white tympanic membrane.

    2. An elongated lobule.

    3. A sensorineural hearing loss.

    4. Bulging tympanic membrane with a distorted cone of light.

33. The nurse practitioner indicates an understanding of conductive hearing loss in the older client with which statement?

    1. "This has occurred due to damage of the eighth cranial nerve from gentamycin."

    2. "This is a result of an inner ear infection."

    3. "This is a normal part of aging and is referred to as presbycusis."

    4. "This may be reversible after the cerumen is removed from the ear canal."

34. Sensory hearing loss is common in industrial settings and preventable with the use of adequate hearing protection. This type of hearing loss is usually first noted with changes at what level?

    1. 500 Hz.

    2. 200 Hz.

    3. 3000–4000 Hz.

    4. Above 4000 Hz.

Nose

35. An adult client presents to the nurse practitioner's office with fever and complaints of right facial pain, copious yellow nasal discharge, and acute pain and headache when bending over for 5 days. There is no transillumination of the right maxillary sinus and that area is very tender to palpation. The client's diagnosis is:

    1. Chronic sinusitis.

    2. Acute sinusitis.

    3. Dental abscess.

    4. Temporal arteritis.

36. The nurse practitioner is doing health teaching for a group of geriatric women. She would advise them that the most effective preventive measure against the common cold is:

    1. Judicious use of vitamin C during cold season.

    2. Ensuring adequate sleep and fluids.

    3. Meticulous handwashing, preferably with an antibacterial soap.

    4. Avoiding contact with any people who have a runny nose, cough, and sore throat.

Throat

37. A 20-year-old client presents to the nurse practitioner's office with a chief complaint of "severe sore throat" for 3 days. The client states he also ran a fever, but does not know how high it got, and he has been very tired with the sore throat. The physical exam revealed enlarged tonsils with large patchy exudate, inflamed pharynx, and nontender posterior cervical lymphadenopathy. The rest of the exam was nonremarkable. The nurse practitioner would make the diagnosis of:

    1. Infectious mononucleosis.

    2. Leukemia.

    3. Scarlet fever.

    4. Oral candidiasis.

38. Which of the following clinical findings are associated with bacterial streptococcal pharyngitis?

    1. Rhinorrhea.

    2. Cough.

    3. Enlarged tonsils with exudate.

    4. Small oral vesicles.

Pharmacology

39. The antibiotic(s) of choice for acute sinusitis in the adult is (are):

    1. Amoxicillin (Amoxil) 500 mg PO tid × 14 days; trimethoprim-sulfamethoxazole

(TMP-SMX; Bactrim DS) 1 tab q12h PO × 14 days, penicillin V-potassium (Pen-Vee K) 500 mg PO bid × 14 days.

    2. TMP-SMX (Bactrim DS) 1 tab q12h PO × 14 days, Pen-Vee K 500 mg PO bid × 14 days.

    3. Penicillin G 150,000 units IM × 1; amoxicillin 500 mg PO tid × 14 days.

    4. Amoxicillin 500 mg PO tid × 14 days; TMP-SMX (Bactrim DS) 1 tab q12h PO × 14 days.

40. A geriatric client is diagnosed with chronic open-angle glaucoma. She has a past history of bradycardia and first-degree atrioventricular (AV) block. In consideration of her treatment, what medication is to be avoided?

    1. Pilocarpine (Isopto Carpine).

    2. Timolol (Timoptic).

    3. Hydrochlorothiazide (Diuril).

    4. Acetazolamide (Diamox).

41. Which antibiotic would be appropriate for the nurse practitioner to prescribe for β-lactamase production by strains of *Haemophilus influenzae* and *Moraxella catarrhalis* in an adult with acute otitis media?

    1. Amoxicillin (Amoxil).

    2. Trimethoprim-sulfamethoxazole (Bactrim).

    3. Penicillin V potassium (Pen-Vee K).

    4. Metronidazole (Flagyl).

42. The treatment plan for a client diagnosed with infectious mononucleosis includes which of the following?

    1. Rest during acute phase.

    2. Avoid exercise during acute phase.

    3. Corticosteroids during acute phase.

    4. Ampicillin orally for 10 days.

43. A client has had yellowish green nasal drainage and frontal headache for a week. The client's temperature has gone up to 101.2°F on most afternoons and she has a

cough that worsens when she lies down. The physical exam is within normal limits except for the drainage and a slightly erythematous pharynx. She does not have any drug allergies and has not been on any medications in the last few months. Which medication would be best to prescribe for her?

1. Diphenhydramine hydrochloride (Benadryl).

2. Erythromycin (E-Mycin).

3. Pseudoephedrine hydrochloride (Sudafed).

4. Amoxicillin (Amoxil).

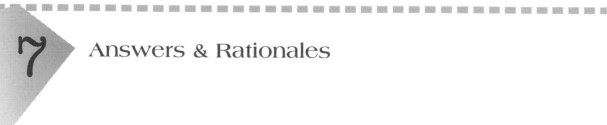

Answers & Rationales

Physical Examination & Diagnostic Tests

Head

1. **(2)** The conceptualization of triangles is useful in determining the location of palpable lymph nodes in the neck. The sternocleidomastoid muscle is the division between the anterior (containing the anterior superficial cervical chain) and the posterior (containing the posterior cervical chain) triangles. The trapezius muscle marks the posterior border of the posterior triangle. The supraclavicular or scale nodes are palpated in the angle formed by the clavicle and the sternocleidomastoid muscle.

Eyes

2. **(2)** The correct use of the ophthalmoscope involves using the right hand and right eye to examine the client's right eye. The room should be semidarkened for best visualization. The examiner initially inspects the lens and vitreous body from a distance of about 12 inches (at zero setting) and moves closer to the eye, usually rotating the lenses to the positive numbers (+15 to +20), which assists in focusing on near objects.

3. **(2)** If the lid margin falls above the limbus (junction line where the sclera and cornea meet) so that some sclera is visible, hyperthyroidism may be present. The lid may lag behind the limbus as the gaze moves from an upward to a downward position. Ptosis is a drooping lid margin that falls at the pupil or below and may

indicate an oculomotor lesion or myasthenia gravis. A chalazion is an inflammation or cyst of the meibomian glands that lie within the posterior portion of the eyelid. A localized infection of the small glands around the eyelashes in the hair follicle at the lid margin is called a hordeolum.

4. **(2)** With cataracts there is a clouding of the lens, not a circle around the pupil. The circle around the pupil is arcus senilis, which is normal in the geriatric client. The visual acuity of the client cannot be determined from the information provided. There are no observable pupillary changes in the beginning stages of glaucoma, which is identified by checking the intraocular pressure.

5. **(2)** The red-free filter is used to examine the optic disc for pallor and vascular changes as well as to assess for retinal hemorrhages. The small aperture is used for small pupils, the slit is for the anterior eye, and the grid is for estimating the size of lesions found in the fundal area.

6. **(2)** Consensual response is pupillary constriction of one eye when there is a direct light stimulus to the pupil of the other eye.

7. **(1)** AV nicking is associated with longstanding hypertension. Intraocular pressure cannot be determined from an ophthalmic examination. Papilledema is

associated with swelling around the optic disc, and small emboli are represented by an abrupt impediment or severe narrowing of an arteriole not associated with where the retinal veins and arteries cross.

8. **(1)** Changes in pupil size when focusing from near to distant objects is normal accommodation. The term extraocular eye movements refers to the ability to move the eye. Consensual response is constriction of the eye in response to light being shown in the opposite eye. The Snellen eye chart is used to determine the visual acuity.

Ears

9. **(4)** This describes the normal characteristics of the tympanic membrane. There is no evidence of scarring or fluid.

10. **(2)** The normal Rinne's test is air conduction twice as long as bone conduction (AC > BC).

11. **(1)** This describes the correct position for these landmarks on the right ear. In Option #2 the manubrium slants to the right with the malleus at the 1- to 2-o'clock position for the right ear. Option #3 describes the correct position for the left ear. In Option #4, the umbo is in the center with the anterior folds at the 1- to 2-o'clock position for the right ear.

Nose

12. **(1)** The nasal mucosa is redder than oral mucosa. Increased redness of the nasal mucosa usually indicates infection. Pale, boggy turbinates along with watery secretion often occurs with allergic rhinitis. The normal secretion is mucoid. Purulent, crusty, or bloody secretions are abnormal.

Throat

13. **(2)** Rapid screening for strep can be done from throat swab with antigen agglutination kits, but there is a 5–10% false-negative rate; therefore, it is suggested that culture should be performed. The heterophile antibody test, or monospot test, which rapidly detects heterophile antibodies, compares with the sensitivity and specificity (95% specific and 90% sensitive) of older

heterophile antibody tests to diagnose mononucleosis. *Candida albicans* and rhinovirus are not diagnosed by bacterial cultures. Oral candidiasis can be diagnosed with a potassium hydroxide (KOH) smear.

14. **(2)** The client in this situation had risk factors (age) and symptoms of mononucleosis; therefore, the monospot (heterophile antibody) test should be conducted. The classical triad of mononucleosis symptoms includes sore throat, fever, and posterior cervical lymphadenopathy with or without mild tenderness. Rapid screening for strep can be done from throat swab with antigen agglutination kits. A WBC count would be ordered for bacterial pharyngitis, in that WBC elevation is found with bacterial infection and a decrease is associated with viral agents.

Disorders

Head

15. **(2)** Leukoplakia is a white patch present on the oral mucosa that cannot be rubbed off. Hemangiomas are benign blood vessel proliferation of the lips, tongue, or buccal mucosa. Erythroplasia is an asymptomatic red, velvety lesion of the mouth. Papillomas are benign verrucous lesions, which are manifestations of human papillomavirus infection.

16. **(2)** The high risk factors for oral cancer are tobacco and alcohol use. The risk increases with the number of cigarettes smoked per day. The disease is age related, occurring in those over 40 years of age, and increasing with age. The male/female ratio is 3:1. Other risk factors are use of cigars, pipes, and smokeless tobacco. Human papillomavirus has been considered in the etiology for squamous cell carcinoma in the upper head and neck.

17. **(3)** Erythroplasia is accompanied by an inflammatory reaction in a client with suspected oral cancer. If the erythematous lesion persists over 14 days, a high suspicion of early oral cancer exists. Tissue retraction and thickening of the oral tissues are later signs of oral cancer. Halitosis (odor) may be associated with dysfunction within the oral cavity, nasal cavity, sinuses, or esophageal disorders. Cough is the primary symptom of respiratory disorders such as acute bronchitis and pneumonia.

18. **(3)** Adults who present with thrush (oral candidiasis) may be immunologically impaired. It is important to make the diagnosis of HIV early to start treatment modalities. Treatment with amoxicillin may actually worsen the condition.

19. **(2)** The nurse practitioner knows the risk factors for head and neck cancer include tobacco and alcohol use; poor oral hygiene; and occupational exposure to asbestos, coke, nickel, wood, or leather. The most common site is in the oral cavity, accounting for 48% of the head and neck cancer diagnoses.

Eyes

20. **(3)** Generalized, diffuse swelling and erythema of the eyelid is associated with an insect bite. Blepharitis is a chronic inflammatory condition characterized by erythema and scaling of the lid margins. Hordeolum or stye is an acute, purulent inflammation of the sebaceous glands (usually the meibomian or zeisian) of the eyelids and usually does not involve the entire eyelid. It may be painful, especially over the gland. Dacryocystitis is an inflammation of the lacrimal sac characterized by erythema and swelling over the lacrimal duct.

21. **(4)** Clients go home almost immediately after the procedure. Eye patches may be worn for the first 24 hours. Care should be taken to protect the operative eye from injury. There is some discomfort, but pain should not be a problem. The client can be up and around as tolerated.

22. **(4)** Cataracts are characterized by painless loss of visual acuity over a period of time. Retinal detachment most often occurs suddenly, with partial loss of the field of vision. Glaucoma results in the loss of peripheral vision and macular degeneration primarily involves the central vision field.

23. **(1)** In corneal abrasion, glaucoma, and iritis the chief complaint is pain. Conjunctivitis presents with no pain and with a history of purulent discharge.

24. **(4)** Sustained nystagmus is indicative of a neurologic complication. The other options include normal age-related changes.

25. **(3)** Arcus cornealis is the deposit of lipids at the junction of the cornea and sclera that is present in many people over age 50. When identified in younger individuals, it points to a disorder of lipid metabolism.

26. **(4)** These assessments are normal age-related changes. Signs and symptoms of cataracts include reduced visual acuity; painless, progressive loss of vision; and sensitivity to light, especially on night driving. Reduced color discrimination and double vision may also be seen. Macular degeneration will present with a loss of the central vision. Primary open-angle glaucoma will present with occasional headaches, occasionally halos around lights, and it may be asymptomatic in the early stages. Primary angle-closure glaucoma will present with episodes of blurred vision, halos around lights at night, and redness with congestion.

27. **(4)** Classic signs of bacterial conjunctivitis include those symptoms listed along with complaints of eyelids being "glued shut" upon arising in the morning. Option #2 is indicative of allergic conjunctivitis. Option #3 is indicative of viral conjunctivitis.

Ears

28. **(2)** Although all of these household appliances are noisy, the client should wear ear plugs or muffs when using a power lawnmower regularly for long periods of time.

29. **(1)** Inability to hear a watch tick at 1–2 inches from the ear is a classic sign of hearing loss characteristic of advancing age. The Rinne's test will indicate bone conduction is two times greater than air

conduction. Tetracyclines are not ototoxic and the family history may or may not contribute to the problem.

30. **(4)** The adult has the clinical findings of otitis externa. Otitis externa is an inflammation and/or infection of the external ear canal predisposed by excessive wetness such as swimming. Common organisms responsible for otitis externa include *Pseudomonas aeruginosa*, *Proteus mirabilis*, and *Enterobacter aerogenes*. Sinusitis clinical findings focus on sinus tenderness, and a purulent nasal discharge. Clinical findings of otitis media include ear pain, full or bulging tympanic membrane, decreased or negative mobility, and possible erythema. Findings associated with serous otitis media include opaque or translucent tympanic membrane with presence of air bubbles; landmarks may be absent and the light reflex may be diffuse or absent.

31. **(3)** The most frequent bacterial organisms that infect the middle ear are similar to those of the nasopharynx: *Streptococcus pneumoniae*, *Haemophilus influenzae*, and *Moraxella catarrhalis*. Viruses may also cause acute otitis media. *Chlamydia trachomatis* is not a frequent causative agent.

32. **(4)** This would be indicative of an inflammation of the middle ear (acute otitis media). The other options include normal changes that occur with aging.

33. **(4)** Conductive hearing loss may result from acute otitis media, perforation of the eardrum, and obstruction of the ear canal, as by cerumen. The other distractors result in sensorineural hearing loss.

34. **(4)** This type of hearing loss presents with high-frequency loss, above the 4000-Hz level and then progresses into voice frequencies at 2000–3000 Hz.

Nose

35. **(2)** The client is experiencing the classic characteristics of acute sinusitis. Chronic sinusitis has nasal discharge, congestion, headache, or cough for over 30 days. A dental abscess has a severe tooth-associated pain, and jaw tenderness. Temporal arteritis causes pain in the jaw, tongue, and face but no nasal discharge.

36. **(3)** Transmission of cold viruses is spread indirectly (e.g. self-innoculation from virus being on surfaces of inanimate objects, to mucous membranes of the nose and mouth). It is less likely to be spread by the aerosol route. So, one should avoid touching the nose and mouth unless the hands have been thoroughly washed. It is impractical to avoid contact, as cold viruses are found everywhere. Although many individuals believe vitamin C prevents colds, there is little research to support the claim.

Throat

37. **(1)** Mononucleosis is commonly seen in adolescents and young adults. It often presents with fever, exudate on the tonsils, generalized lymphadenopathy, malaise, posterior cervical adenopathy, and palatine petechiae. Leukemia presents with anorexia, irritability, lethargy, and bone pain. The peak incidence is is 3- to 5-year-olds. Scarlet fever presents in children 2–10 years old, with fever, abdominal pain, headache, sore throat, and strawberry tongue. Oral candidiasis presents with white curd-like plaques on an erythematous mucosa. The tongue is red with a white coat.

38. **(3)** Characteristics of bacterial pharyngitis include headache, mild to severe erythema of tonsils with white or yellow exudate, dysphagia, positive anterior cervical nodes, sore throat with dysphagia, fever over 101°–102.5°F, and nausea. Viral organisms as Herpangina present with small oral vesicles. Cough is the primary symptom of acute bronchitis. Rhinorrhea is associated with allergic rhinitis.

Pharmacology

39. **(4)** Amoxicillin (Amoxil) is the first-line antibiotic for acute uncomplicated sinusitis in the adult because of cost-effectiveness, efficacy, and cure rates ranging from 67%–100%. Even though 35% of *H. influenzae* and 75% of *M. catarrhalis* produce β-lactamase, cure rates when using amoxicillin have not been significantly different. Therefore, several other drugs may be utilized with similar clinical response to amoxicillin. These include ampicillin, TMP-SMX (Bactrim), cefaclor (Ceclor), cefuroxime axetil (Ceftin), loracarbef (Lorabid), and amoxicillin-clavulanate potassium (Augmentin).

40. **(2)** β-Adrenergic blockers cause problems with bradycardia; the timolol (Timoptic) can be absorbed systemically from the eye and should not be used.

41. **(2)** Amoxicillin is ineffective against β-lactamase production. Erythromycin/sulfa, trimethoprim/sulfa, and cephalosporins are effective against β-lactamase production by strains of *H. influenzae* and *M. catarrhalis*. Pen-Vee K and metronidazole are not effective in this group. Cephalexin, cefuroxime, or cefixime can be used as alternatives.

42. **(1)** The treatment of mononucleosis includes bed rest while the client has fever and myalgia (10–14 days), supportive acetaminophen or ibuprofen, warm saline gargles, and throat lozenges or spray. The client must avoid strenuous exercise and contact sports the first 2–3 weeks. Corticosteroids are recommended only in clients with impending airway obstruction. Ampicillin is not recommended due to allergic reaction and rash reaction. About 95% of clients with mononucleosis recover uneventfully with supportive treatment.

43. **(4)** The client is experiencing symptoms of acute sinusitis. The first-line antibiotic to prescribe for this condition is amoxicillin due to safety and efficacy. Oral antihistamines such as diphenhydramine should not be used unless the client has allergies. Oral decongestants (pseudoephedrine hydrochloride) are not as effective as topical agents in clients with sinusitis. Erythromycin is not a first-line antibiotic for sinusitis.

8 Integumentary

Physical Examination & Diagnostic Tests

1. The nurse practitioner describes an annular skin lesion as usually arranged in:

   1. Groups of vesicles erupting unilaterally.

   2. A line.

   3. A pattern of merging together, not discrete.

   4. A circle or ring-shaped.

2. A client has pitting of the nails. The nurse practitioner understands this is associated with:

   1. Psoriasis.

   2. Iron deficiency anemia.

   3. Malnutrition.

   4. Hyperthyroidism.

3. The nurse practitioner is inspecting a dark-skinned individual for signs of jaundice. The best place to observe is:

   1. Sclera of the opened eye.

   2. Palms and soles of the hands and feet.

   3. Oral mucosa.

   4. Nail beds.

4. When assessing the hydration status of a client, the best place to evaluate skin turgor on an adult is:

   1. Just below the clavicle.

   2. Below the scapula on the back.

   3. On the inside of the forearm.

   4. Back of the hand.

5. The Wood's lamp is used to evaluate skin lesions. When the light is shown on the client's skin, a green-yellow fluorescence indicates:

   1. Presence of fungi.

   2. Lichenification.

   3. Keratinized cells.

   4. Bacterial colonies.

6. On examination of a client's skin, the nurse practitioner finds a lesion that is about 0.75 cm in diameter, brown, circumscribed, flat, and nonpalpable. The correct term for this lesion is:

   1. Macule.

   2. Papule.

   3. Nodule.

   4. Wheal.

7. The history and physical of a client indicates past occurrences of lichenification. The nurse practitioner identifies the characteristics of this lesion as:

   1. Dried, crusty exudate, slightly elevated.

   2. Rough thickened epidermis, accentuated skin markings.

   3. Keratinized cells shaped in an irregular pattern with exfoliation.

   4. Loss of epidermis with hollowed-out area and dermis exposed.

8. Clubbing of the nails occurs in clients with chronic respiratory conditions. The nurse practitioner assesses for this condition by:

   1. Evaluating the nail for transverse depressions and ridges.

   2. Placing both of the client's hands together with palms inward and index fingers aligned.

   3. Placing nail beds of each index finger together to determine angle of nail plate.

   4. Determining if there is diffuse discoloration of the nail bed from decreased oxygenation.

9. A circumscribed, elevated lesion >1 cm in diameter and containing clear serous fluid is best described as a:

   1. Papule.

   2. Vesicle.

   3. Bulla.

   4. Pustule.

10. In performing a skin assessment, the nurse practitioner understands that the following characteristic of a mole would necessitate immediate intervention:

    1. A 5-mm, symmetrical, uniformly brown mole on the thigh that has been present and has not changed in appearance for over 5 years.

    2. Multiple small (1- to 3-mm) flat moles across the upper back that are dark brown in color, round, and have smooth edges.

    3. A 3-cm waxy papule, with a "stuck-on" appearance, noted on the face.

    4. A new 2-mm mole that is brown with a red, irregular border, and is occasionally pruritic.

11. Dermatophyte skin infections can be diagnosed from skin scrapings and prepped with which solution for microscopic exam?

    1. Hydrochloric acid.

    2. 20% potassium hydroxide (KOH) solution.

    3. Gram's stain.

    4. Distilled water.

Skin Disorders

12. A client complains of intolerable itching in the pubic hair. On examination the nurse practitioner notes erythematous papules and tiny white specks in the pubic hair. The differential diagnosis includes all **except**:

    1. Pediculosis pubis.

    2. Scabies.

    3. Impetigo.

    4. Atopic dermatitis.

13. An elderly lady has an area of vesicles in clusters with an erythematous base that extend from her spine, around and under her arm and breast, to the sternum on her left side. She says the area was very tender last week and the vesicles started erupting yesterday. She is complaining of severe pain in the area. The diagnosis for this condition is:

1. Psoriasis.

2. Herpes zoster.

3. Contact dermatitis.

4. Cellulitis.

14. Which is a true statement about psoriasis?

   1. It usually is worse in the summer.

   2. It is highly contagious.

   3. It can be aggravated by stress.

   4. All clients have accompanying pruritis.

15. A client with actinic keratosis should be told:

   1. These are a normal part of aging and are benign.

   2. These lesions can develop into squamous cell carcinomas.

   3. This is part of an allergic reaction and the offending allergen needs to be identified.

   4. This skin condition responds well to sunlight, which will help alleviate the symptoms.

16. The following are all true statements regarding urticaria **except**:

   1. Most cases of acute urticaria are mediated by immunoglobulin E (IgE) mast cell degranulation after exposure to certain substances.

   2. Chronic urticaria may be related to occult infections.

   3. Urticaria is characterized by itchy red swellings of a few millimeters to a few centimeters in size.

   4. Laboratory studies are necessary to identify the causative agent.

17. A client who is known to be human immunodeficiency virus (HIV)-positive presents with several painless, persistent, raised purple lesions on the face. The most likely cause is:

   1. Seborrheic dermatitis.

   2. Molluscum contagiosum.

3. Kaposi's sarcoma.

4. Fungal infection.

18. During the physical examination, the nurse practitioner assesses a macular-papular skin lesion on a client's back that is warty, scaly, greasy in appearance, and light tan in color. The nurse practitioner would make the diagnosis of:

   1. Actinic keratosis.

   2. Basal cell carcinoma.

   3. Seborrheic keratosis.

   4. Senile lentigo.

19. The nurse practitioner would expect to make which assessment with an older client diagnosed with herpes zoster (shingles) during the prodromal stage?

   1. Erythematous lesions present over four different parts of the body.

   2. A red, pinpoint, painless rash.

   3. A burning pain in a line on only half of the client's chest that does not cross the midline.

   4. Painless purulent lesions for 2 days followed by complaints of itching, burning, and nausea.

20. What would be the appropriate management for a client with herpes zoster (shingles)?

   1. Acyclovir (Zovirax).

   2. Miconazole (Monistat-Derm).

   3. Clotrimazole (Lotrimin).

   4. Corticosteroid (prednisone).

21. An elderly retired farmer's wife presents with a dome-shaped pearly firm nodule with telangiectasia on her nose. In making a differential diagnosis, the nurse practitioner recognizes this to be:

   1. Compound nevus.

   2. Melanoma.

   3. Bullous pemphigoid.

   4. Basal cell carcinoma.

22. An adult female presents with an irregular variegated nevus on her lower left back that has doubled in size in the past 3 months. The nurse practitioner should:

    1. Do a punch biopsy to confirm the diagnosis.

    2. Take a photograph of the lesion and recheck it in 1 month.

    3. Refer immediately to a dermatologist.

    4. Reassure the client that these are normal changes related to hormone variations.

23. A client presents with pain in her right chest wall for the past 48 hours. Upon examination, the nurse practitioner notices a vesicular eruption along the dermatome and identifies this as herpes zoster. The nurse practitioner informs the client:

    1. All symptoms will disappear in 3 days.

    2. Oral medication can dramatically reduce the duration and intensity of symptoms.

    3. She has chickenpox and can be contagious to his grandchildren.

    4. The eruptions will recur at regular intervals.

24. A young adult female presents to the nurse practitioner's office stating that she has a red rash over her trunk that itches, and has been present for 2 weeks. She has tried over-the-counter lotions and creams, with no relief of symptoms. She states that it started as a small, round red patch on her chest, and has since spread across her chest, back, arms, and legs. Physical exam reveals a generalized distribution of erythematous, scaly macular lesions that run parallel to each other, creating a "Christmas tree" pattern. The nurse practitioner should:

    1. Do a thorough medication history, investigate any potential allergens, and send client to an allergy specialist.

    2. Prescribe triamcinolone acetonide 0.025% (Aristocort A) cream bid for 2 weeks.

    3. Teach client to expose self to modest amounts of sunlight without burning, and use calamine lotion or oatmeal baths for symptom relief.

    4. Refer client to a dermatologist for a biopsy.

25. An adult female client presents to the nurse practitioner's office complaining of flu-like symptoms, a large red spot in the right groin, headaches, and generalized muscle pain. These symptoms have persisted for approximately 4–5 weeks. In taking the client's history, it would be most important to determine whether the client:

    1. Was using new skin care products, detergents, and so forth.

    2. Was taking any new medications, vitamins, herbal therapies, and the like.

    3. Has had a recent insect bite or potentially been exposed to insects, such as ticks (e.g., camping trips, travel to heavily wooded areas).

    4. Has been exposed to anyone who has tuberculosis.

Pharmacology

26. An obese woman presents to the clinic with complaints of tenderness and irritation under both of her breasts. The examination reveals a very irritated, moist, inflamed area with macules and papules present. The best treatment for this woman is:

    1. Nystatin cream two or three times a day for 10 days; encourage thorough drying of the area and exposure to light and air.

    2. Systemic anti-staphylococcal antibiotics (dicloxacillin) and soaking with moist pads of normal saline three times a day.

    3. Gentle washing of the area and removal of crusts, then application of antibiotic ointment.

    4. Antiviral treatment (acyclovir) and topical ointment to prevent secondary infection.

27. Which classification of drugs have the potential to aggravate psoriasis?

    1. β-Blockers.

    2. Thiazide diuretics.

    3. Vasodilators.

    4. Monoamine oxidase (MAO) inhibitors.

28. In treatment of severe inflammatory acne for a female adolescent, the nurse practitioner understands:

    1. Isotretinoin (Accutane) provides an effective first-line therapy.

    2. The benefits of treatment will be noted in 5–7 days.

    3. The importance of counseling on stringent dietary changes.

    4. Systemic antibiotics are effective treatments.

29. A young mother brings her infant to the family nurse practitioner with complaint of difficulty with diaper rash. She reports the infant has had it for about a week. Upon exam the diaper area appears beefy red with sharply marginated dermatitis. Satellite lesions are also noted. The family nurse practitioner recommends:

    1. Change from disposable diapers to cloth diapers with plastic pants.

    2. Application of nystatin (Mycostatin) after each diaper change.

    3. Apply wet soaks three times daily.

    4. Apply oil liberally after bathing.

30. All of the following are true of postherpetic neuralgia **except**:

    1. Capsaicin (Zostrix) cream may alleviate some of the discomfort.

    2. The majority of clients who have postherpetic pain lose it gradually, day by day, week by week.

    3. Acyclovir (Zovirax) 200 mg, 5 capsules a day PO in divided doses, is an effective therapy.

    4. It is more common in clients over age 60.

31. When treating genital warts with topical podophyllin, it is important for the family nurse practitioner to:

    1. Apply preparation directly to the wart and approximately 5 mm around the base of the wart.

    2. Cover with a dressing so the solution remains moist and caution the client not to remove for 24 hours.

    3. Instruct the client to wash off medication in 4–6 hours.

    4. Treat with liquid nitrogen before applying podophyllin.

32. What is the recommended treatment of rosacea?

    1. Oral hydrocortisone.

    2. Oral ketoconazole.

    3. Low-dose tetracycline.

    4. Topical 5-fluorouracil.

33. When using lidocaine with epinephrine 1–2% as a local anesthetic in the repair of an injury, it is essential to keep in mind that the maximum allowable dose is:

    1. 7 mg/kg.

    2. 2 mg/kg.

    3. 10 mg/kg.

    4. 5 mg/kg.

34. On a return visit to the clinic, a woman who is receiving sulfonamide therapy exhibits the following symptoms: generalized rash, mucous membrane lesions, sloughing of the skin of the palms and feet, high fever, and generalized malaise. These findings would alert the nurse practitioner to consider:

    1. Hepatitis B.

    2. Stevens-Johnson syndrome.

    3. HIV infection/acquired immunodeficiency syndrome (AIDS).

    4. *Pneumocystis carinii* pneumonia.

35. An adolescent female presents to the nurse practitioner's office with a prolonged history of facial acne. She has been seen by several dermatologists, and has been treated over the past 3 years with multiple therapies, including topical antibiotics, drying agents, intralesional injections of corticosteroids, and multiple systemic antibiotics, without success. After consulting with the collaborating physician, the nurse practitioner prescribes isotretinoin (Accutane). Teaching/counseling related to the use of this medication includes:

    1. No dietary/alcohol restrictions are necessary.

    2. Exposure to sunlight without burning can be helpful in hastening the healing process.

    3. Eliminate all fat from the client's diet.

    4. Emphasize the importance of using effective contraception if the client is sexually active, due to the teratogenicity of the drug.

36. A female client presents for an office visit with complaints of a measles-like rash on her trunk and spreading to extremities. She was seen several days ago for a urinary tract infection and started on trimethoprim-sulfamethoxazole (TMP-SMX; Bactrim DS) 1 tab PO bid. The recommended action for the nurse practitioner is to:

    1. Instruct the client to continue Bactrim and see if any change occurs in the rash.

    2. Discontinue Bactrim.

    3. Take client off Bactrim for 3 days and restart the medication.

    4. Decrease Bactrim to half dose.

Answers & Rationales

Physical Examination & Diagnostic Tests

1. **(4)** Annular skin lesions may be arranged in a circular manner or in an arciform (arc-shaped) pattern (i.e., tinea corporis). Multiple groups of vesicles erupting unilaterally following the course of cutaneous nerves is herpetiform or zosteriform (i.e., herpes zoster). Linear lesions are arranged in a line (i.e., allergic contact dermatitis to poison ivy). Confluent lesions become merged together and are not discrete (i.e., scarlet fever rash).

2. **(1)** Psoriasis, peripheral vascular disease, diabetes, tuberculosis, and other infectious diseases such as syphilis are associated with pitting deformities of the nail that may vary from pinpoint size to pinhead size and may be linear or irregular in distribution. Iron deficiency anemia, eczema, malnutrition, and pellagra are associated with koilonychia (spoon nails). Hyperthyroidism and hypothyroidism are associated with onycholysis, which is a separation of the nail from the nail bed, originating at the free edge and progressing proximally.

3. **(1)** The place to inspect is in that portion of the sclera that is observed when the eye is open. If jaundice is suspected, the posterior portion of the hard palate should be examined for a yellowish cast. Pallor and cyanosis can be noted in the nail bed, palms, and soles.

4. **(1)** Just below the clavicle or on the abdomen for an adult and on the abdomen for infants and children are the most reliable areas for indication of hydration status.

5. **(1)** Fungal lesions will be visualized as a green-yellow fluorescence when viewed with the Wood's lamp in a dim room.

6. **(1)** A macule is <1 cm in diameter; nonpalpable; and brown, red, purple, or tan (freckles, flat moles, rubella). A papule is elevated and palpable (warts, pigmented nevi). A nodule is 1–2 cm in diameter, elevated, and deeper (lipoma). A wheal is elevated, irregular, and has a variable diameter (insect bites, urticaria).

7. **(2)** Lichenification occurs with chronic irritation, often of an exposed extremity (chronic dermatitis). Crusts are dried exudate, scales are heaps of keratinized cells from exfoliation (psoriasis), and loss of epidermis is excoriation as seen in an abrasion.

8. **(3)** The angle of the nail beds should form a diamond when the nail beds are approximated. Transverse ridges and grooves may occur from trauma. Placing the palms together provides no assessment data, and diffuse discoloration may be from a fungal infection or an injury.

9. **(3)** Bulla is the correct term. A papule is solid, a vesicle is <1 cm in diameter, and a pustule contains a purulent exudate.

10. **(4)** The appearance of a new mole with high-risk features including irregular border, color changes, and changes in sensation (i.e., pruritis) would necessitate immediate biopsy to rule out melanoma, and/or referral to a dermatologist. Uniform moles, those that are symmetrical and have smooth borders, and those that are not showing signs of change are those that can be followed with annual skin assessments. Seborrheic keratosis is a benign skin growth that usually presents on sun-exposed areas, and appears waxy or "stuck-on," requiring no treatment.

11. **(2)** Under microscope exam, fungal scrapings in KOH solution will appear as thread-like hyphae crossing cell walls. The other solutions are not indicated for use to identify dermatophytes.

Skin Disorders

12. **(3)** Intense itching is characteristic of pediculosis pubis, scabies, and atopic dermatitis. Impetigo starts out as a tender erythematous papule and progresses through a vesicular to a honey-crusted stage with no itching.

13. **(2)** Herpes zoster typically presents with a history of tenderness followed by eruptions and vesicles that follow a dermatome on one side of the body. This is very painful. Other symptoms may include fever, headaches, and malaise.

14. **(3)** Stress can aggravate psoriasis. Sunlight helps psoriasis, so it is usually better in the summer. It is not contagious and only about 30% of clients with psoriasis itch.

15. **(2)** Actinic keratoses are potentially precancerous lesions, and are found in areas of skin exposed to sunlight. Due to the increasing popularity of sunbathing, they can even be seen in persons in the 30- to 50-year-old age group.

16. **(4)** Laboratory studies are not likely to be helpful in evaluation of urticaria. Identification of causes is usually based on history and physical findings. The other statements are true of urticaria.

17. **(3)** Although any one of these skin conditions can affect the skin, particularly of an HIV-positive client, the description relates most closely to Kaposi's sarcoma and warrants a biopsy.

18. **(3)** The assessment describes a seborrheic keratosis. The actinic keratosis is an irregular, rough, scaly, white to erythematous macular lesion found most commonly on the dorsal surface of the hands, arms, neck, and face. It has malignant potential. The basal cell carcinoma is a smooth, round nodule with a pearly gray border and central induration. The senile lentigo are gray-brown, irregular, macular lesions on sun-exposed areas of the face, arms, and hands.

19. **(3)** Herpes zoster (shingles) is a vesicular dermatomal eruption related to a reactivation of latent varicella virus. It increases with advanced age and is characterized by burning pain and paresthesia along one or two dermatomes. This will not cross the midline. This discomfort may be accompanied by fever, malaise, or headache. The vesicular stage lasts 2–3 weeks. The vesicles are very painful and grouped along one or two dermatomes. They are initially clear or blood-filled and become purulent. The area along the dermatome is erythematous, and the vesicles crust and then scab, which may leave hypopigmented scars. The other options discuss painless lesions and are not specific to this prodromal stage.

20. **(1)** Antiviral therapy with acyclovir 800 mg five times per day for 7 days may speed healing if started within 2–3 days of onset, especially in immunocompromised individuals. Miconazole and clotrimazole are antifungal creams, and the prednisone would only be used to decrease the incidence of postherpetic neuralgia. Prednisone may increase the incidence of disseminated infection.

21. **(4)** These are classic signs of a basal cell carcinoma, a diagnosis also supported by the employment history of the client. Melanoma would be pigmented, compound nevus would not be firm or have telangiectasia, and bullous pemphigoid results in bullous lesions.

22. **(3)** Refer the client immediately to a dermatologist, since these are highly suspicious findings of a melanoma. Biopsy should never be done on a melanoma, and any delay in time could be detrimental to the outcome.

23. **(2)** Oral acyclovir is very effective in reducing the intensity and duration of symptoms if started early in the course of the disease. Herpes zoster does not usually recur at regular intervals, but it frequently lasts for several weeks.

24. **(3)** This client presents with a classic case of pityriasis rosea, a benign, self-limiting skin eruption of unknown etiology. Although a medication/allergen history would be warranted, referral to an allergy specialist or dermatologist would not be necessary. Triamcinolone would not be indicated, as the treatment is mainly symptomatic. Sunlight in moderate amounts has been shown to hasten healing in some cases.

25. **(3)** The signs and symptoms presented are classic for Lyme disease, which is transmitted by ticks. Therefore, it would be important to inquire about potential exposure to ticks in the time period prior to the development of signs and symptoms. Exposure to new skin care products would be important if the nurse practitioner suspected an allergic reaction, which is not consistent with the signs and symptoms presented. While a thorough medication history should always be done, it is most likely not going to reveal the cause of the signs and symptoms in this case. Tuberculosis does not present in this manner.

Pharmacology

26. **(1)** The description is consistent with intertriginous candidiasis, which is treated with an antifungal ointment or oral medication. It is not a staphylococcal infection; the area does not need to be kept moist but needs to be kept dry. An antibiotic ointment will not relieve the problem. Herpes zoster is treated with antiviral medications; this is not described as particularly painful, and it is bilateral.

27. **(1)** β-Blockers can exacerbate psoriasis. They are believed to decrease cyclic-AMP–dependent protein kinase (an inhibitor of cell proliferation). There is no known effect with the other stated classifications.

28. **(4)** Systemic antibiotics (such as tetracycline) offer the most effective treatment in inflammatory acne. Accutane is also very effective but, because of serious teratogenic side effects, it is not first-line treatment. Improvement in acne will not be noted for 4−8 weeks, and dietary changes have not been demonstrated to have any beneficial effect.

29. **(2)** Appearance is indicative of *Candida albicans*, which is best treated with nystatin. The other choices would aggravate the diaper rash due to promotion of overhydration.

31. **(3)** Acyclovir offers no benefit for postherpetic pain, since this is a treatment for the acute phase during initial eruption of vesicular lesions.

31. **(3)** Clients need to be instructed to wash off podophyllin. It is to be applied sparingly, to only the wart, while avoiding normal skin and allowed to dry thoroughly before the client dresses. There is no rationale to treat with both liquid nitrogen and podophyllin.

32. **(3)** Systemic treatment with low-dose tetracycline is very effective for rosacea. Topical treatment with metronidazole or low-dose hydrocortisone may also be useful. Oral cortisone and antifungal agents are not known to be effective. Topical 5-fluorouracil is used in the treatment of actinic keratosis, a precancerous skin condition.

33. **(1)** The correct answer is 7 mg/kg lidocaine with epinephrine for adults and 5 mg/kg for lidocaine without epinephrine. Although local anesthetics are commonly used, the maximum allowable doses are rarely emphasized, and overdose can result in anaphylactic shock.

34. **(2)** Stevens-Johnson syndrome is a severe form of erethema multiforme that can be fatal. The clinical picture of this syndrome is mucous membrane lesions, conjunctival and corneal lesions, fever, malaise, arthralgia, and sloughing of the skin of the hands and feet. The characteristics that differentiate this condition are the eruption of vesicles and ulcerations of the mucosa and the sloughing skin.

35. **(4)** Isotretinoin is extremely teratogenic; therefore, a sexual assessment along with a pregnancy test in women with child-bearing capacity, and contraceptive counseling should be done for all clients. The combination of alcohol and isotretinoin can cause a disulfiram-like reaction; therefore, the use of alcohol should be avoided. Isotretinoin can cause photosensitivity, so the nurse practitioner should counsel the client to avoid sunlight, wear protective clothing and sunglasses, and apply sunscreen to all sun-exposed areas without acne. No conclusive relationship between diet and acne has been established.

36. **(2)** In case of suspected drug reactions, it is recommended the drug be eliminated and documented in the client's record so it is not reintroduced.

Endocrine

9

Physical Examination & Diagnostic Tests

1. What is the correct procedure for palpation of a client's thyroid gland?

   1. Stand behind the client, hyperextend the head, and palpate both sides simultaneously.

   2. Have the client lower her chin and lean her head slightly toward the side being evaluated.

   3. Hyperextend the head and have the client lean away from the side being evaluated.

   4. Have the client lean away from the side being examined and take a swallow of water.

2. When a client sips water and swallows, the thyroid gland:

   1. Moves downward and slightly posterior and feels smooth on palpation.

   2. Elongates and enlarges during the swallow and immediately returns to a resting position at the end of palpation.

   3. Moves slightly out during the sipping and backward during the swallowing.

   4. Moves upward during the swallow and feels symmetrical and smooth to palpation.

3. Which question is **not** part of the Carville Diabetic Foot Screen?

   1. Has there been a change in the foot since the last evaluation?

   2. What was the last fasting blood glucose and glycosylated hemoglobin (HgbA$_{1c}$)?

   3. Does the foot have an abnormal shape?

   4. Are the nails thick, too long, or overgrown?

4. While conducting the interview for a physical examination, the nurse practitioner identifies what finding in the client's history as being commonly associated with thyroid carcinoma?

   1. Family history of thyroid cancer.

   2. History of hyperthyroidism.

   3. Irradiation of the neck.

   4. Smoking for 15 years.

5. When doing a physical examination on a client with hyperthyroidism, a common neurologic finding is:

   1. Memory, attention, and problem-solving deficits.

   2. Diminished deep tendon reflexes.

   3. Severe cognitive impairment.

   4. Delusions and psychosis.

6. The treatment goal for glycemic control in a type II diabetic is to achieve and maintain an $HgbA_{1c}$ of:

   1. <10%.

   2. Between 6% and 9%.

   3. <7%.

   4. >8%.

7. Which finding would alert the nurse practitioner that a client might be experiencing a problem with the endocrine system?

   1. Coagulation abnormalities and fatigue.

   2. Growth abnormalities and glucose intolerance.

   3. Hypoxia and jaundice.

   4. Steatorrhea and abdominal distention.

8. The nurse practitioner notes a solitary thyroid nodule on a client during a routine physical examination. The diagnostic test of choice is:

   1. Thyroid scan and antibody level.

   2. Thyroid-stimulating hormone (TSH) and ultrasound.

   3. X-ray of the thyroid.

   4. Fine-needle aspiration (FNA) biopsy.

9. An adult female client presents to the nurse practitioner's office complaining of fatigue, weakness, and weight gain over the past 4 months. Physical examination reveals an elevated blood pressure, facial and supraclavicular fullness, hirsutism noted on the face, proximal muscle weakness, and

facial and truncal distribution of acne. Appropriate laboratory tests the nurse practitioner should order include:

   1. Antinuclear antibody test (ANA) and rheumatoid factor (RF).

   2. 3-hour glucose tolerance test and lipid profile.

   3. Red blood cell (RBC) count and a calcium level.

   4. Dexamethasone suppression test, a urine free cortisol level, and TSH and thyroxine (T_4) level.

10. In evaluating the laboratory values taken from a client with Graves' disease, one should expect:

    1. TSH levels to be increased.

    2. TSH levels to be decreased.

    3. TSH levels to be within normal limits.

    4. T_4 levels to be decreased.

11. What information is correct regarding foot screening using a nylon filament (5.07 Semmes-Weinstein)?

    1. Use a 25-gm filament and apply along perimeter of any scar or ulcer tissue.

    2. Apply the filament at a 45-degree angle to the skin surface.

    3. Apply sufficient force for approximately 1.5 seconds to cause the filament to bend.

    4. Slide the filament across the skin and make repetitive contact to each of the ten sites.

Disorders

12. The etiology of type I diabetes can be best described as:

    1. An autosomal dominant genetic disorder.

    2. Autoimmune destruction of the β-cells.

    3. Overnutrition and resulting obesity as the major risk factor.

    4. Prevented by exercise, which increases the concentration of insulin receptors.

13. The nurse practitioner should do an annual referral for the client who has had diabetes for over 5 years to:

    1. A cardiologist.

    2. A dietitian.

    3. A vascular surgeon.

    4. An ophthalmologist.

14. Hirsutism presenting in a young female with normal menstruation and normal plasma androgens is most likely:

    1. An ovarian tumor.

    2. Cushing's syndrome.

    3. Idiopathic.

    4. Polycystic ovary disease.

15. Pathophysiologic reasons for decreased testosterone level develop in the:

    1. Hypothalamus, posterior pituitary, adrenals.

    2. Anterior pituitary, adrenals, testes.

    3. Testes, adrenals, posterior pituitary.

    4. Hypothalamus, anterior pituitary, testes.

16. The most common cause of poor control of type I diabetics during the adolescent period is:

    1. Emotional disturbance.

    2. Noncompliance with dietary restrictions.

    3. Poor adherence to blood testing and insulin injections.

    4. All of the above.

17. When counseling a diabetic client on foot care, it is important to emphasize:

    1. Daily foot soaks in warm, soapy water.

    2. Careful daily foot inspections.

    3. Trim corns and calluses regularly.

    4. Trim toenails as close to the bed of the nail as possible and round nails to avoid scratching other toes.

18. An adult client presents to the nurse practitioner for evaluation of polyuria, polydypsia, and weight loss. Which lab result would require immediate intervention by the nurse practitioner?

    1. An $HgbA_{1c}$ of 14%.

    2. A serum glucose of 150 mg/dl.

    3. An $HgbA_{1c}$ of 6.0%.

    4. A serum glucose of 65 mg/dl.

19. An adult client is being evaluated for hypoglycemia due to a blood sugar of 58 mg/dl on a screening SMAC-20. The nurse practitioner can begin her differential diagnosis by:

    1. Deciding if the hypoglycemia is fasting or postprandial.

    2. Ascertaining if it is related to alcohol use.

    3. Deciding if the client has other medical problems.

    4. Reassuring the client that it is a benign problem.

20. A middle-aged normally healthy female presents for evaluation of intermittent palpitations. She originally thought it was related to job stress. She also reports mood variability, tremulousness, difficulty falling asleep, and a 10-lb weight loss despite a normal appetite. She feels warm most of the time and wonders if she is perimenopausal. She has no history of heart disease. The objective data that would yield the most useful information would be:

    1. Electrocardiogram (ECG).

    2. TSH, free T_4.

    3. Electrolytes.

    4. Holter monitor.

21. An adult client presents to the clinic complaining of fatigue, weakness, weight gain in spite of lack of appetite, and feelings of depression. Her physical examination reveals an obese, alert female with thinning hair, bilateral chest puffiness, increased facial hair, supraclavicular fat pad, thin arms and legs, purple striae on abdomen, and multiple ecchymotic areas on extremities. Her vital signs are blood pressure (BP) 158/96, pulse 88, respirations 22. Laboratory studies include fasting blood sugar (FBS) 200 mg/dl, electrolyte panel is within normal limits (WNL) except for potassium 3.0 mEq/L, hemoglobin 11.8 gm, and hematocrit 34%. The nurse practitioner suspects:

    1. Addison's disease.

    2. Pheochromocytoma.

    3. Cushing's syndrome.

    4. Hypoaldosteronism.

22. Which of the following is the best alternative for treating hyperthyroidism diagnosed during the first trimester of pregnancy?

    1. Radioactive iodine in smaller than usual dose during the first trimester.

    2. Propylthiouracil during the first trimester, subtotal thyroidectomy during the midtrimester, no thyroid replacement.

    3. Propylthiouracil during the first trimester, subtotal thyroidectomy during the midtrimester, thyroid replacement.

    4. No treatment until after delivery.

23. Clinical findings in a client with hypothyroidism include:

    1. Hyperactive bowel sounds.

    2. Oily skin and acne.

    3. Postural tremors of the hands.

    4. Edema of the face and eyelids.

24. A young adult female reports anxiety, tremulousness, headaches, palpitations, and sweating 2–4 hours after eating. Physical exam is normal. No labs are currently available. No history of any medical

conditions are noted. The most likely diagnosis is?

    1. Dumping syndrome.

    2. Hypoglycemia.

    3. Alcohol abuse.

    4. Hyperthyroidism.

25. Which of the following is the most likely etiology for hypercalcemia in the medically well asymptomatic adult?

    1. Hyperthyroidism.

    2. Hyperparathyroidism.

    3. Hyperpituitarism.

    4. Hypothyroidism.

26. A middle-aged female with no previous medical history presents with a 30-lb weight gain in 2.5 months. She denies any medication use or allergies. She was currently laid off of a very active job and has been sedentary. Physical exam reveals BP 172/111, central obesity, FBS 200 mg/dl. The most likely cause of the client's weight gain is:

    1. Cushing's disease.

    2. Hypothyroidism.

    3. Depression.

    4. Diabetes.

27. A middle-aged female accompanied by her daughter to the clinic presents with agitation, confusion, fever, tachycardia, and diaphoresis. The daughter states these symptoms were preceded by nausea, vomiting, and abdominal pain. There is no history of cardiac disease, diabetes, or substance abuse. She was started on some "anti drug" 2 weeks ago and scheduled for some kind of throat surgery next week (per daughter). Based upon this history, the nurse practitioner immediately orders:

    1. TSH, T$_4$.

    2. Urinalysis.

    3. Spinal tap.

    4. Computed tomography of head.

28. A 45-year-old female client presents to the nurse practitioner's office complaining of a 6-month history of fatigue, 15-lb weight gain, lethargy, an inability to tolerate cold temperatures, forgetfulness, hair loss, and constipation. Physical findings include dry coarse skin, periorbital edema and puffy face, bradycardia, hyporeflexia and muscle weakness, and a smooth goitrous thyroid. The nurse practitioner would make the diagnosis of:

    1. Congestive heart failure (CHF).
    2. Diabetes mellitus (DM).
    3. Hypothyroidism.
    4. Thyroid cancer.

29. A diabetic client has been taking 6 U of regular insulin and 12 U of Lente insulin in the morning. In the evening she has been taking 3 U of regular insulin and 8 U of Lente insulin. The client has been monitoring her blood glucose levels and she shows the nurse practitioner the following chart.

	7 AM	Noon	5 PM	Bedtime
Monday	100	76	98	109
Tuesday	119	75	88	110
Wednesday	119	66	86	100
Thursday	123	70	111	122
Friday	128	60	99	110

    The nurse practitioner adjusts the client's insulin by:

    1. Increasing the regular insulin.
    2. Decreasing the regular insulin.
    3. Decreasing the Lente insulin.
    4. Increasing both insulins.

30. The role of the nurse practitioner in the initial management of a client with a thyroid nodule involves:

    1. Referring the client to an endocrinologist for further evaluation.
    2. Obtaining a fine-needle aspiration of the nodule and sending to cytology.
    3. Ordering an ultrasound and thyroid scan.
    4. Ordering levothyroxine (Synthroid) to reduce the size of the nodule.

31. When teaching a diabetic client about "sick day" guidelines, the nurse practitioner explains:

    1. Stop measuring blood glucose and only check urine for ketones.
    2. Do not take your usual dose of insulin at the usual time.
    3. Be sure to take metformin (Glucophage) and acarbose (Precose), even if nausea and vomiting are present.
    4. Administer extra doses of regular insulin according to instructions for blood glucose levels above 240 mg/dl.

32. A young adult female client presents to the clinic with complaints of nervousness, tremulousness, palpitations, heat intolerance, fatigue, weight loss, and polyphagia. After a complete history and physical examination, along with thyroid function tests, the nurse practitioner makes the diagnosis of hyperthyroidism, recognizing that the most common cause of this condition is:

    1. Thyroid cancer.
    2. Graves' disease.
    3. Pituitary adenoma.
    4. Postpartum thyroiditis.

33. A young adult female client presents to the nurse practitioner's office, stating that she found a lump in her neck. Physical examination reveals a firm, 2-cm nodule that is fixed and nontender located on the right lobe of the thyroid gland. Right posterior cervical lymphadenopathy is also noted. The nurse practitioner should:

    1. Order a TSH level to determine thyroid function, and refer the client to a surgeon for a fine-needle biopsy of the nodule.
    2. No intervention is necessary at this time; schedule a follow-up visit in 6 months.
    3. Prescribe levothyroxine (Synthroid) 0.1 mg PO daily and schedule a 6-week follow-up visit.
    4. The client's thyroid should immediately be ablated with radioactive iodine, and the patient should be referred to an endocrinologist.

34. A client with Graves' disease is placed on radioactive I^{131} therapy. When teaching about this treatment, it is important for the nurse practitioner to include what information?

    1. Clients are highly radioactive for approximately 7 days following treatment and need to be isolated.

    2. Clients should not become pregnant during or after receiving this therapy because of the teratogenic effects to the fetus (e.g., chromosomal abnormalities).

    3. Clients may become hypothyroid after this treatment, and will therefore need to have regular TSH and T$_4$ levels drawn, with the potential for thyroid hormone replacement therapy.

    4. This therapy is contraindicated in clients with cardiac disease.

Pharmacology

35. Clients started on metformin (Glucophage) need to be monitored closely for the following potential side effect:

    1. Significant increase in weight.

    2. Elevation of low-density lipoprotein (LDL) cholesterol level.

    3. Lactic acidosis.

    4. Increase in insulin requirements.

36. The nurse practitioner has ordered a client with type II diabetes to take glipizide (Glucotrol) 10 mg PO bid. In evaluating the medication's effectiveness, it is thought to reduce blood glucose by:

    1. Delaying the cellular uptake of potassium and insulin.

    2. Stimulating insulin release from the pancreas.

    3. Decreasing the body's need and utilization of insulin at the cellular level.

    4. Interfering with the absorption and metabolism of fats and carbohydrates.

37. The nurse practitioner would expect which symptom to be a side effect of metformin (Glucophage)?

    1. Gastrointestinal upset.

    2. Photophobia.

    3. Hyperglycemia.

    4. Skin eruptions.

38. A client is receiving antithyroid medication. The nurse practitioner understands that:

    1. Lifelong daily treatment is necessary to keep TSH levels within the normal range.

    2. Antithyroid medications do not cross the placenta.

    3. The medications are somewhat expensive and have serious cardiac and hematologic side effects.

    4. Clients remain on the medications for 1–2 years and then the medication is gradually withdrawn.

39. When prescribing an antihypertensive medication for a type II diabetic client with hypertension, the drug classifications that would tend to reduce insulin sensitivity are:

    1. Diuretics and calcium channel blockers.

    2. Diuretics and β-blockers.

    3. Calcium channel blockers and angiotensin converting enzyme (ACE) inhibitors.

    4. α-Blockers and ACE inhibitors.

40. A 35-year-old female sees the nurse practitioner with a complaint of cold intolerance, fatigue, dry skin, weight gain, and heavy menstrual periods. Upon physical exam, she is found to have a pulse of 58 bpm, a "waxy" sallow complexion, and a firm goiter. A TSH is checked and found to be 176 mU/L. The best treatment choice for this client is:

    1. Begin levothyroxine (Synthroid) at 0.025 mg PO qd and repeat TSH in 2 weeks.

    2. Administer a "loading dose" of oral levothyroxine (Synthroid), as well as starting a full replacement dose of levothyroxine (Synthroid).

3. Administer a "loading dose" of IV levothyroxine (Synthroid), and start on a half replacement dose of levothyroxine (Synthroid).

4. Begin levothyroxine (Synthroid) at a dose of 0.1 mg PO qd and recheck TSH in 6 weeks.

41. The nurse practitioner is seeing an obese, middle-aged female client for a follow-up visit. She was diagnosed as a type II diabetic 3 months ago and started on a regimen of diet and exercise. Today her fasting plasma glucose is 200 mg/dl and her HgbA$_{1c}$ is 10%. She has lost 2 lb. She reports her home monitoring glucose has ranged from 180–300 mg/dl. The rest of her chemistry profile is WNL. The best treatment choice for this client is:

   1. Review her diet and exercise plan, increase exercise regimen, and reduce caloric intake. Schedule her for another follow-up in 3 months.

   2. Start her on sliding-scale insulin and instruct her on recording glucose and insulin requirements. Schedule her to return in 1 week to be re-evaluated for long-acting insulin.

   3. Initiate treatment with metformin (Glucophage).

   4. Initiate treatment with an oral sulfonylurea agent (i.e., glyburide).

42. What is associated with chronic overtreatment with levothyroxine (Synthroid)?

   1. Tachycardia.

   2. Severe osteoporosis.

   3. Insomnia.

   4. Sweating.

43. A middle-aged female presents for a diabetes follow-up exam. She has been in good health without identified complications of diabetes. Her FBS is 100 and her personal records indicate that she is taking insulin in the prescribed amounts and at the prescribed times. Her vital signs are BP 142/98, pulse 80, respirations 20. Today's plan would include:

   1. Begin diuretics and a β-blocker.

   2. Begin ACE inhibitor and consider a diuretic.

   3. Get an ECG and chest x-ray.

   4. Return for BP check in 5–7 days.

44. An adult female has recently been started on insulin. Her regimen is two daily injections with two thirds of total daily insulin in the morning and one third in the evening. She is using the 70/30 mixture of intermediate- and short-acting insulin in both injections. She presents for a follow-up visit with her log of blood glucose. The nurse practitioner notes that her recorded glucose levels before the evening meal have been in the 60- to 70-mg/dl range. Other checks during the day are in 100- to 120-mg/dl range. What adjustments need to be made?

   1. Intermediate insulin, change 70/30 combination to self-mix and reduce AM intermediate dose.

   2. Regular insulin, reduce AM dose of 70/30.

   3. Intermediate insulin, reduce AM dose of 70/30.

   4. Regular insulin, change 70/30 to self-mix and reduce AM regular dose.

45. A client on antithyroid drug therapy for hyperthyroidism presents with complaints of palpitations and dry mouth for the past 2 days. She has had a cough and cold symptoms for the past 3 days that she has been treating with over-the-counter medications. Which medication would the nurse practitioner encourage the client to avoid?

   1. Benzocaine (Chloraseptic) lozenge.

   2. Guaifenesin (Robitussin).

   3. Ibuprofen (Advil).

   4. Sudafed (Pseudoephedrine).

46. What is the most frequent complaint of clients who use insulin pumps?

    1. Problems with elevated glucose after changing the catheter type (nonneedle) infusion set.

    2. Skin and site problems related to dressing adhesive not sticking, redness and pain at infusion site, and allergic response to tape.

    3. Mechanical problems with the pump's digital readout.

    4. Understanding "sick day" management modifications.

47. The nurse practitioner understands that troglitazone (Rezulin) is indicated for:

    1. Prenatal clients with gestational diabetes.

    2. Brittle type I clients.

    3. Type II clients who require insulin and who have poor glycemic control and insulin resistance.

    4. Type II clients to prevent the rapid postprandial blood glucose surges by delaying carbohydrate absorption.

48. An older client with a history of hypertension and coronary bypass surgery has been diagnosed with hypothyroidism. Appropriate medication management is:

    1. Levothyroxine (Synthroid) 0.1 mg daily and return in 6 weeks for follow-up.

    2. Desiccated thyroid extract 2 grains daily and return in 6 weeks for follow-up.

    3. Levothyroxine (Synthroid) 0.025 mg daily for 6 weeks with slow gradual increase in dosage every 4–6 weeks until therapeutic level is obtained.

    4. Methimazole (Tapazole) 15 mg daily in three divided doses, gradually increasing

dose every 4 weeks until a therapeutic level is obtained.

49. A client is newly diagnosed as being hypothyroid and is placed on levothyroxine (Synthroid) 0.1 mg PO daily. Follow-up by the nurse practitioner should include:

    1. No follow-up visits are necessary.

    2. The client should return to the clinic in 4–6 weeks to evaluate the response to treatment, including a TSH level, and to determine if there has been symptomatic improvement.

    3. The client should have weekly levothyroxine levels drawn.

    4. The client should have monthly complete blood counts (CBCs) while on levothyroxine (Synthroid), because the medication has been found to be myelosuppressive.

50. Classes of medications commonly used to treat hyperthyroid conditions include:

    1. Antibiotics and corticosteroids.

    2. ACE inhibitors, anxiolytics, and antithyroid medications.

    3. β-Blockers, nonsteroidal anti-inflammatory drugs (NSAIDs), and antithyroid medications.

    4. Calcium channel blockers and corticosteroids.

51. The nurse practitioner understands that lisproinsulin (Humalog):

    1. Can be injected just prior to eating.

    2. Is less costly than regular insulin.

    3. Increases the likelihood of late postprandial hypoglycemia due to its length of action.

    4. Has a long-term safety profile and does not cause any teratogenic effects.

9 Answers & Rationales

Physical Examination & Diagnostic Tests

1. **(2)** When examining the thyroid, it is important to have the client relax the sternocleidomastoid muscles. This can be done by having the client lean toward the side being evaluated.

2. **(4)** The thyroid gland is fixed to the trachea and thus ascends during swallowing. This assists the nurse practitioner in distinguishing thyroid structures from other neck masses. The gland's size, degree of enlargement, consistency, surface characteristics, and presence of nodules or bruits are noted during the examination.

3. **(2)** There are five questions to the Carville Diabetic Foot Screen. They are as follows: Has there been a change in the foot since the last evaluation? Is there a foot ulcer now or history of foot ulcer? Does the foot have an abnormal shape? Is there weakness in the angle or foot? Are the nails thick, too long, or overgrown?

4. **(3)** Papillary carcinoma is the most common form of thyroid cancer. It is associated with a history of exposure to radiation. Family history, history of hyperthyroidism, and smoking are not considered significant risk factors for this malignancy.

5. **(1)** The high level of thyroid hormone affects the nervous system, causing sympathomimetic symptoms such as brisk deep tendon reflexes, fine, rapid tremor of the hands, restlessness, irritability, insomnia, dreams, nightmares, and rarely severe cognitive impairment and psychosis.

6. **(3)** The American Diabetes Association (ADA) recommends <7% as an important treatment goal to decrease risk of long-term complications. A lab result of >8% HgbA$_{1c}$ is an indication that action needs to be taken, either by a change of medication or reinforcement of education.

7. **(2)** Growth abnormalities are associated with anterior pituitary dysfunction, and glucose intolerance is associated with diabetes due to pancreas dysfunction. Coagulation abnormalities and fatigue would be associated with hematologic dysfunction. Hypoxia would be associated with oxygenation problems and jaundice with liver or biliary problems. Steatorrhea is associated with malabsorption syndrome and cystic fibrosis.

8. **(4)** Although the primary care provider may obtain TSH and antibody levels, the preferred diagnostic tool for the endocrinologist is the fine-needle aspiration biopsy. Although scans, sonography, and x-ray tests can be used in initial screening, they do not assist in the determination of whether the nodule is malignant or not. The aspirate is sent for cytology and interpretation.

9. **(4)** The dexamethasone suppression test is the best screening test for Cushing's disease, for which a 24-hour urine for free cortisol is the best confirmatory test. TSH and T_4 levels may also be appropriate to rule out a thyroid condition, as some of the client's signs and symptoms are consistent with thyroid dysfunction. ANA and RF are ordered when rheumatoid arthritis or systemic lupus erythematosus (SLE) is suspected; this client's clinical picture is not consistent with these conditions. An RBC count would be done to rule out anemia, a potential problem for this client based on the history of fatigue, but the rest of the clinical picture points to something more than anemia. There are no clinical findings to support blood for a calcium level being drawn.

10. **(2)** TSH levels should be decreased in a client with Graves' disease, because thyroid-stimulating immunoglobulins bind to TSH receptors, which increase T_4 synthesis and release, subsequently suppressing TSH levels.

11. **(3)** The correct procedure is to use a 10-gm (5.07 Semmes-Weinstein) filament and apply to ten sites on the foot (one on the top of the foot, nine on the heel, sole, and toes). The filament is to be applied perpendicularly (90-degree angle) to the skin surface with sufficient force for 1.5 seconds to cause the filament to bend. The filament should not be allowed to slide across the skin or make repetitive contact to each test site. Randomizing the selection of test sites (start with big toe → heel → instep area → little toe → etc.) and the time between successive tests and having clients close their eyes helps to reduce client guessing.

Disorders

12. **(2)** Type I diabetes is caused by destruction of the β-cells mediated through the immune system. The other three choices refer to type II diabetes.

13. **(4)** An annual eye exam with the pupils dilated should be done by a specialist who can recognize subtle abnormalities. Although the other referrals can offer important contributions to diabetic care, it would be on an as-needed basis rather than annually.

14. **(3)** Because of the normal menstrual periods and androgen plasma level, this would be considered idiopathic. Diseases related to the ovaries would cause changes in the menstrual cycle, and with Cushing's syndrome the client would have adrenal androgen overproduction.

15. **(4)** Testosterone production is regulated by the hypothalamic-pituitary-testicular (HPT) axis. Thus abnormalities in any one of these areas can affect the production of testosterone.

16. **(4)** All of these contribute significantly to difficulty controlling diabetes in the teen years. Hormonal changes and the desire to become independent increase emotional conflicts. Teens have a great desire to be like their peers and do not want to be regimented in following a specific diet and adhering to a treatment plan.

17. **(2)** It is important for diabetics to have their feet inspected daily, either per self-exam or by a family member. Feet should be washed daily but never soaked. Corns and calluses should be cared for by a professional. Nails should be trimmed straight across to avoid injury to the nail beds.

18. **(1)** The normal serum glucose for adults ranges from 70–120 mg/dl. Diabetic acidosis is not of concern until the glucose is >300 mg/dl. An HgbA$_{1c}$ of >8.0% indicates poor glucose control over the past few months.

19. **(1)** True hypoglycemia can be organized around whether it is fasting or postprandial. Postprandial hypoglycemia may be caused by early adult-onset diabetes or postgastrectomy syndrome. Fasting hypoglycemia is most commonly caused by excessive doses of insulin or sulfonylureas.

20. **(2)** This middle-aged female client presents with many of the classic symptoms of early hyperthyroidism. A suppressed TSH with an elevated free T_4 establish the diagnosis of hyperthyroidism.

21. **(3)** The client's physical findings and habitus along with hypertension and hypokalemia are associated with Cushing's syndrome, which is a state of excessive cortisol production caused by a pituitary tumor. A Cushing's-like syndrome is often associated with prolonged glucocorticoid administration. Obesity is the primary finding in Cushing's syndrome, along with the "moon face," "dowager" or "buffalo hump," truncal obesity, hirsutism in women, and impotence and loss of body hair in men. Addison's disease is characterized by hyperkalemia, hyponatremia, hypoglycemia, anemia, and hypercalcemia. Clients with hypoaldosteronism (impaired renin secretion) have hyperkalemia. Pheochromocytoma would be in the differential diagnosis of this client because of the hypertension; the other findings are not consistent with this diagnosis.

22. **(3)** Low-dose antithyroid drugs are considered a good alternative to prevent the ill effects of hyperthyroidism on the mother and developing fetus until surgery can be performed. It is noted that some opt to use an antithyroid drug until after delivery and then have surgery. Removal of the thyroid during the second trimester can be performed safely and is the usual recommendation. Replacement is essential after removal of the gland.

23. **(4)** Accumulation of hyaluronic acid in interstitial tissues increases capillary permeability to albumin and accounts for the interstitial edema that is noted in the face and eyelids of individuals with hypothyroidism.

24. **(2)** While alcohol abuse may be a cause for hypoglycemia, this client is presenting with classic symptoms of postprandial hypoglycemia. It would be a good idea to assess for alcohol abuse as the etiology of the diagnosis of hypoglycemia.

25. **(2)** Hyperparathyroidism accounts for more than 60% of hypercalcemic clients and is likely to be the explanation for elevated serum calcium levels.

26. **(1)** While Option #3 may explain the weight gain, Cushing's disease is correct for the constellation of symptoms of rapid weight gain, hypertension, and elevated blood sugar. These symptoms suggest adrenal dysfunction. Serum cortisol and adrenocorticotropic hormone levels should be checked.

27. **(1)** This woman is likely experiencing the life-threatening syndrome that can occur in decompensated hyperthyroidism. The clues are her symptom presentation and progression, the new "anti drug," and upcoming throat surgery.

28. **(3)** The symptoms describe the classic presentation of a client with hypothyroidism. A client with CHF would exhibit jugular venous distention, has rales, and peripheral edema. The criteria for diagnosing DM are polydipsia, polyphagia, polyuria, and weight loss. Thyroid cancer commonly presents without physical symptoms, and often the only physical finding is a hard, fixed nodule on the thyroid gland.

29. **(2)** The client's blood sugars are low around lunch time, which is when the regular insulin is peaking (3–4 hours), so a reduction in the regular insulin would help this problem.

30. **(1)** The nurse practitioner's role in primary care for a client with a thyroid nodule involves initially the early identification of the thyroid nodule on physical examination, referring the client to an endocrinologist for further evaluation, and possibly obtaining some preliminary TSH and antibody testing. The endocrinologist performs the FNA. Levothyroxine may or may not be used to diminish the size of the nodule based on the findings from the FNA and the endocrinologist's chosen treatment plan.

31. **(4)** It is important for the diabetic client to understand that when they are sick their blood glucose level will probably increase, even when they are not eating. It is most important they monitor blood glucose levels every 2–4 hours and check urine for ketones, if glucose level is >240 mg/dl. In Option #3, these medications *should not* be given until the client's nausea and vomiting have subsided and they have resumed a normal diet (blood glucose monitoring is important during this period of time).

32. **(2)** Graves' disease, an autoimmune condition also known as diffuse toxic goiter, is the most common cause of hyperthyroidism in this age group. Much less common causes include cancer of the thyroid, adenoma of the pituitary gland, and postpartum (or silent) thyroiditis.

33. **(1)** The TSH level should be determined to establish whether the client is euthyroid, hypothyroid, or hyperthyroid. The client should also be sent to an endocrinologist/ surgeon because all nodules of the thyroid should be biopsied to rule out malignancy. Watching and waiting is inappropriate without having a biopsy performed. Thyroid hormone replacement therapy would only be indicated in those clients found to be hypothyroid and in whom thyroid cancer has been ruled out. Thyroid ablation may be indicated in clients whose fine-needle biopsy results are positive for thyroid cancer, but this cannot be determined without a surgeon's intervention.

34. **(3)** Hypothyroidism often follows this treatment, with 50% of clients requiring replacement therapy in the first year, and nearly 100% within 10 years. For this reason, regular monitoring of TSH and T_4 levels should be performed. Clients emit a small amount of radioactivity after receiving the dose used to treat this condition, and do not require isolation for 7 days. Radioactive iodine is very safe, without an increased risk of gonad chromosomal abnormalities; therefore, there is no contraindication to becoming pregnant after therapy, although clients are counseled to avoid pregnancy while on treatment and to avoid children and pregnant women after receiving the oral ablation dose. This therapy is recommended for those clients who have cardiac disease associated with their thyroid condition.

Pharmacology

35. **(3)** Lactic acidosis is a potentially severe and fatal reaction to metformin. Metformin does not contribute to weight gain—it often helps with weight loss, and decreases LDL, triglycerides levels, and insulin requirements.

36. **(2)** The sulfonylureas reduce blood glucose by stimulating insulin release from the pancreas. Also, over a long period of time, they may actually increase insulin effects at the cellular level and decrease glucose production by the liver. This is the reason why sulfonylureas are used in type II diabetics who still have a functioning pancreas.

37. **(1)** Anorexia, nausea, and a metallic taste in the mouth are common side effects. Over time, the gastrointestinal (GI) symptoms subside and can be relieved by taking the medication with food or by starting at a lower dose.

38. **(4)** Antithyroid medications (propylthiouracil or methimazole) are relatively inexpensive and do cross the placenta. The client remains on the medication for 1–2 years with the hope of a permanent remission of symptoms when they are withdrawn.

39. **(2)** Both of these drug classifications tend to reduce insulin sensitivity and can cause hyperglycemia. ACE inhibitors, calcium channel blockers, and selective α-blockers are metabolically neutral; some may actually have a beneficial effect.

40. **(4)** The client's symptoms indicate hypothyroidism along with the elevated TSH; the normal range for TSH is 0.5–4.7 mU/L. A full replacement dose of levothyroxine (Synthroid) should be started based on the client's age and her TSH level should be checked in 6 weeks, since it can take that long for a given dose to become effective. Loading doses should never be

given except for coma, which is treated by IV medication in the hospital.

41. **(3)** Metformin is a better option in an obese client, as metformin is frequently associated with weight loss while sulfonylureas may actually cause a weight gain. Insulin is also not a good choice, as it is an overly aggressive approach with mildly elevated glucose. Clients also tend to be less receptive to treatment requiring injections. Diet and exercise were unsuccessful, and the longer her blood sugar remains elevated, the greater the risk for end-organ damage.

42. **(2)** All but osteoporosis are related to acute overdosage of levothyroxine and can be relieved by omitting the dose for 3 days and then starting on a lower dose.

43. **(4)** In order to initiate treatment for elevated BP it is recommended that three elevated readings be recorded on three separate occasions. There is no evidence to suggest that this woman had an elevated BP on prior visits.

44. **(1)** This is the best answer, as the AM intermediate dose affects the glucose level before dinner. Altering the regular insulin will affect levels before lunch and before bedtime; these levels are OK. In order to reduce the intermediate insulin while maintaining the level of regular insulin, the client will need to self-mix the intermediate and regular insulin using less of the intermediate.

45. **(4)** Sudafed (Pseudoephedrine) and other decongestant medications that contain sympathomimetics lead to adverse reactions of central nervous system (CNS) overstimulation, palpitations, headache, hypertension, nervousness, and the like. Robitussin in combination (i.e., Robitussin-CF [dextromethorphan, phenylpropanolamine, guaifenesin]) or Robitussin-PE [pseudoephedrine, guaifenesin] can also cause palpitations and CNS overstimulation. Robitussin-DM (dextromethorphan, guaifenesin) usually has predominantly GI upset, drowsiness, headache, and rash as adverse effects.

46. **(2)** Infusion site problems and skin irritation are by far the most frequent complaints of a client who uses an insulin pump. Often, they are the major reasons for the client's decision to discontinue using the pump. Clients also find it is more time consuming and costly. However, the Diabetes Control and Complications Trial (DCCT, 1993) reported a reduced risk of microvascular complications when insulin pumps and multiple daily injections were used.

47. **(3)** Prenatal clients are managed with insulin, not an insulin sensitizer. Troglitazone (Rezulin) acts by decreasing peripheral insulin resistance in skeletal muscle and adipose tissue without enhancing insulin secretion. It improves glucose tolerance and decreases insulin resistance in insulin-dependent type II diabetics. Option #4 refers to the action of α-glucosidase inhibitor (e.g., acarbose [Precose] and miglitol [Glyset]).

48. **(3)** Older clients, especially with heart disease, need to be started on the smallest amount of thyroid medication replacement (0.025 mg not 0.1 mg) and gradually increased until a therapeutic level is achieved. If replaced too quickly, the heart may decompensate. Two grains of thyroid extract is too much. Methimazole (Tapazole) is an antithyroid medication and is indicated for treatment of hyperthyroidism.

49. **(2)** The response to therapy is based on clinical symptomatology and a TSH assay approximately 4–6 weeks after initiation of therapy. This is continued until a stable dose is obtained. TSH and a free T_4 level are the two standard tests that can be used to monitor the status of the thyroid; a levothyroxine level cannot be drawn. Levothyroxine (Synthroid) is not a myelosuppressive agent.

50. **(3)** β-Blockers are initially prescribed to reduce the signs and symptoms of the condition and to reduce the peripheral conversion of T_4 to triiodothyronine (T_3); NSAIDs are indicated for reducing inflammation associated with thyroiditis; and antithyroid medications, such as propylthiouracil (PTU) or methimazole (Tapazole), are used to treat severe hyperthyroidism. Corticosteroids are sometimes used in the treatment of thyroiditis, but the remaining classes of medications are not routinely used in the management of hyperthyroidism (namely, antibiotics, ACE inhibitors, calcium channel blockers, and anxiolytics).

51. **(1)** Lispro (Humalog) is the first analog of human insulin that has several advantages over regular insulin, including a more rapid onset and shorter duration of action. It reaches peak activity in 1−2 hours and has a 4-hour duration, as compared to 6−8 hours for regular insulin. It is convenient for many clients, as it can be injected immediately before eating (10−15 minutes). Because it has been on the market only since June 1996, there is no long-term safety profile established, and the teratogenicity is unknown. In addition, it is more expensive than insulin, and some third-party payers may not reimburse clients.

Musculoskeletal

Physical Examination & Diagnostic Tests

1. The primary examination techniques to use for assessing the musculoskeletal system are:

   1. Inspection and percussion.

   2. Auscultation and palpation.

   3. Inspection and palpation.

   4. Palpation and percussion.

2. What can the nurse practitioner use to confirm a diagnosis of polymyalgia rheumatica?

   1. Chest radiograph.

   2. Serum protein electrophoresis.

   3. Corticosteroid challenge.

   4. Erythrocyte sedimentation (ESR).

3. When performing an assessment, the nurse practitioner understands that the metacarpophalangeal (MCP) joints are frequently involved with:

   1. Gout.

   2. Rheumatic fever.

   3. Rheumatoid arthritis.

   4. Osteoarthritis.

4. In the evaluation of polyneuropathy, which study would not be recommended?

   1. Sedimentation rate.

   2. Complete blood count (CBC).

   3. Glycosylated hemoglobin A_{1c} (HgbA$_{1c}$).

   4. Electromyography (EMG).

5. In accurately assessing a client who reports back injury, it is critical to question:

   1. Family history of back problems.

   2. Previous injury.

   3. Personal history of chronic illness.

   4. Mechanism of injury.

6. Tinel's sign and Phalen's test are used in identifying a common workplace illness, which the nurse practitioner recognizes as:

   1. Lateral epicondylitis.

   2. Carpel tunnel syndrome.

   3. Dupuytren's disease.

   4. Thoracic outlet syndrome.

7. An elderly client complains of fatigue, weakness, lightheadedness, and anorexia. She also complains of hot, swollen proximal interphalangeal (PIP) and metacarpophalangeal (MCP) joints. These symptoms occurred 5 months ago and have reoccurred a few days ago. Which lab findings would be most conclusive of these assessments?

   1. Mean corpuscular volume (MCV) 104, low serum ferritin.

   2. MCV 92, high serum ferritin.

   3. Elevation in the uric acid level.

   4. Elevation in the white blood cell (WBC) count.

8. The nurse practitioner is assessing a preadolescent girl for scoliosis. She would:

   1. Have the girl bend at the waist and look for asymmetry in the back and hip area.

   2. Examine the child fully clothed, paying particular attention to the hips and back.

   3. Have the child walk heel-to-toe and observe the gait and pelvis.

   4. Place the child on her back and flex the knees and observe for misalignment.

Disorders

9. A middle-age client presents with a complaint of waking up yesterday morning with her big toe swollen and painful. The client reports she has never had anything like this before and has not had any previous health problems. Physical exam finds her big toe to be red, hot, and tender in the joint with inflammation extending into the surrounding tissue. Her temperature is 99.8°F and her WBC count

is mildly elevated. Needle aspiration of joint fluid reveals urate crystals. The best treatment choice the nurse practitioner could recommend for this client is:

   1. Bed rest, very-low-calorie diet, and increase fluid intake.

   2. Initiate pharmacologic therapy with allopurinal (Zyloprim) 200 mg PO qd and educate client on the need to remain on this medication for maintenance therapy once symptoms resolve.

   3. Start on naproxen (Naprosyn) 500 mg PO tid and instruct client to continue full dose until symptoms resolve and then taper and discontinue over 72 hours.

   4. Administer an injection of intra-articular corticosteroid therapy to the affected joint.

10. The nurse practitioner realizes that the most common cause of shoulder pain is:

    1. Frozen shoulder.

    2. Thoracic outlet syndrome.

    3. Impingement syndrome.

    4. Osteoarthritis.

11. A 45-year-old female complains of knee pain when kneeling and a "clicking" noise when walking up steps. On exam, there is a slight knee effusion and tenderness when palpating the patella against the condyles. The diagnosis for this client is:

    1. Anterior cruciate tear.

    2. Dislocated patella.

    3. Chondromalacia patella.

    4. Tendinitis.

12. A client has been diagnosed with a complete rotator cuff tear of the left shoulder. The nurse would expect the client to have difficulty in:

    1. Abducting the left arm.

    2. Supinating the left forearm.

    3. Shrugging the shoulders.

    4. Touching the left hand to the right shoulder.

13. A client has been diagnosed with polymyalgia rheumatica. The nurse practitioner understands that this disorder is:

    1. An autoimmune, multisystem problem where the body makes antibodies to its own proteins.

    2. A degenerative disorder with no inflammatory changes, and where joint cartilage wears away with age and eventually causes bone spurs.

    3. An inflammatory disorder involving the axial skeleton and large peripheral joints.

    4. An inflammatory connective tissue disorder that primarily affects older women and is associated with giant cell (temporal) arteritis.

14. In teaching a client about fibromyalgia, the nurse practitioner includes what information?

    1. Diagnostic studies such as ESR and CBC are important tools to confirm the progress of the syndrome.

    2. Avoid stretching exercises and daily low-impact aerobics.

    3. Take ibuprofen (Motrin) 200 mg q4–6h prn for pain and amitriptyline (Elavil) 10 mg 1–2 hours before bedtime.

    4. Apply heat or massage "trigger points" to reduce pain.

15. The nurse practitioner understands that chronic synovitis with pannus formation is the basic pathophysiologic finding in clients with:

    1. Systemic lupus erythematous (SLE).

    2. Ankylosing spondylitis.

    3. Rheumatoid arthritis.

    4. Osteoarthritis.

16. The nurse practitioner is examining a client who is complaining of pain in her hips and knees. She has a history of osteoarthritis. On examination, the joints are painful to movement and are warm to touch. The best immediate therapy for this client is:

    1. Physical therapy for range of motion of affected areas.

    2. Decreased physical activity and immobilizing splints for affected joints.

    3. Moist heat and/or cold therapy on painful joints.

    4. ESR to determine level of activity.

17. The history of a client who may have contracted Lyme disease includes:

    1. Erythematous rash on bridge of nose and cheeks with discoid patches on the trunk.

    2. Immediate development of arthritis symptoms, especially in the knees.

    3. Expanding rash with central clearing occurring within a month of being bitten.

    4. Early symptoms of meningitis and myocarditis.

18. The nurse practitioner understands that finding Heberden's nodes on a physical exam of a client is a cardinal sign of:

    1. Septic arthritis.

    2. Rheumatoid arthritis.

    3. Gouty arthritis.

    4. Osteoarthritis.

19. Diseases that often present as polyarthritic diseases include:

    1. Lyme arthritis, rheumatic heart disease, ankylosing spondylitis, and psoriatic arthritis.

    2. Rheumatoid arthritis, gout, Reiter's syndrome, and osteoarthritis.

    3. Gonococcal arthritis, SLE, and septic arthritis.

    4. Polymyalgi rheumatica, Lyme arthritis, pseudogout, and psoriatic arthritis.

20. Pain in lumbosacral strain typically begins:

    1. Immediately with the injury.

    2. 1–2 hours after injury.

    3. 6–8 hours after injury.

    4. 12–36 hours after injury.

21. Acute onset of pain that shoots down to the lower leg and foot of a 25-year-old obese adult is likely to be a symptom of:

    1. Lumbosacral strain.

    2. Herniated intervertebral disc injury.

    3. Osteomyelitis.

    4. Osteoporosis.

22. Which risk factor is associated with gout?

    1. Female gender.

    2. Over age 20.

    3. Ingestion of salicylate medications.

    4. Overuse of the extremity.

23. In a third-degree ankle strain there is:

    1. Moderate ecchymosis, moderate edema, and a stable joint.

    2. Moderate ecchymosis, moderate edema, and an unstable joint.

    3. Marked ecchymosis, marked edema, and a stable joint.

    4. Marked ecchymosis, marked edema, and an unstable joint.

24. A client with rheumatoid arthritis presents for follow-up. One of the best evaluative questions the nurse practitioner can ask that will help determine the severity of disease is:

    1. "Were you able to drive the car to your appointment today?"

    2. "Were you able to fix your dinner last night?"

    3. "How long does it take for your joints to loosen up after you get up in the morning?"

    4. "How many pounds can you carry?"

25. A 35-year-old female is seen with a complaint of diffuse musculoskeletal pain, stiffness, and fatigue for the past 3 months. The pain is worse in the morning and also with changes in weather. She states she wakes up in the morning feeling tired and unrefreshed. Physical exam is normal except for pain on digital palpation in 12

tender points. Laboratory results are unremarkable. The most likely diagnosis is:

    1. Fibromyalgia.

    2. Myofascial syndrome.

    3. Rheumatoid arthritis.

    4. Depression.

26. When counseling a postmenopausal female client on prevention of osteoporosis, all of the following are therapeutic recommendations **except**:

    1. Cessation of smoking.

    2. Daily intake of 200 mg of calcium and 40 IU of vitamin D.

    3. Continue hormone therapy indefinitely.

    4. Monitor bone loss by dual-energy x-ray absorptiometry (DEXA) every 1–2 years for women who are not on hormone replacement therapy but are at increased risk.

27. A client presents with a complaint of sudden pain and swelling in the knee. She also is complaining of chills and fever. Upon exam, the knee is warm, tender, and swollen with evidence of effusion. The family nurse practitioner would:

    1. Splint the affected joint.

    2. Obtain aspiration of synovial fluid from the affected joint.

    3. Initiate treatment with nonsteroidal anti-inflammatory drugs (NSAIDs).

    4. Recommend rest, ice, compression, and elevation of affected joint.

28. When determining the specific etiology of polyarticular complaints, the clinical clues most helpful for diagnosis are:

    1. Lab identification of antinuclear antibodies (ANA) and ESR.

    2. X-ray of affected joints.

    3. Affected joint pattern and presence of or lack of inflammation.

    4. Sexual history of client.

29. Which of the diet selections indicate the older client understands the health

education regarding the prevention of osteoporosis?

1. Chicken and baked potato.

2. A glass of skim milk and a toasted cheese sandwich.

3. Hamburger and salad.

4. Ice cream sundae with whipped cream.

30. During the history, which of the following questions would best assist the nurse practitioner in diagnosing osteoarthritis versus rheumatoid arthritis?

1. "Is your joint pain symmetrical and localized?"

2. "Does your morning stiffness usually last several hours?"

3. "Have you experienced fatigue, weakness, and weight loss?"

4. "Is your joint pain asymmetrical and worse with movement and relieved by rest?"

31. The number one cause of disability in adults under age 45 is:

1. Cancer.

2. Fracture.

3. Low back pain.

4. Migraines.

32. Which client is at highest risk for osteoporosis?

1. 55-year-old female, smoker, and retired athlete.

2. 60-year-old white, postmenopausal female switchboard operator weighing 105 lb.

3. 42-year-old African-American, female, intensive care nurse who is lactose intolerant.

4. 50-year-old white, obese female, wife of a dairy farmer, and mother of three.

33. A 53-year-old woman presents with complaints of morning stiffness in the neck and back, pelvic and shoulder pain, and fatigue. Her laboratory studies reveal an elevated ESR, a normal rheumatoid factor, a

normal creatine phosphokinase, and normochromic, normocytic anemia. Physical examination reveals an elevated temperature, bilateral pain, and stiffness of the pectoral and pelvic muscles. Based on this information, the best diagnosis is:

1. Polyarteritis nodosa.

2. Wegener's granulomatosis.

3. Polymyalgia rheumatica.

4. Rheumatoid arthritis.

34. A 55-year-old woman with a prior diagnosis of polymyalgia rheumatica presents with headache, low-grade fever, aching, stiffness, fatigue, malaise, and anorexia. Based on this information, the nurse practitioner would make a preliminary diagnosis of:

1. Influenza.

2. Pneumonia.

3. Temporal arteritis.

4. Rheumatoid arthritis.

35. Young adolescents with juvenile rheumatoid arthritis (JRA) must be screened regularly for:

1. Ulcerative colitis.

2. Iridocyclitis.

3. Diabetes mellitus.

4. Adrenal insufficiency.

Pharmacology

36. The primary drug of choice for a client with rheumatoid arthritis is:

1. Nonsteroidal anti-inflammatory drugs.

2. Aspirin.

3. Methotrexate.

4. Hydrocortisone.

37. A client with rheumatoid arthritis is placed on prednisone 5 mg PO qd. In teaching the client about her medication, it would be important for the nurse practitioner to include:

    1. When the symptoms of arthritis subside, she will be able to quit taking her medication.

    2. It is important to take the medication as prescribed, even after the redness and swelling decrease.

    3. Increased fluid intake is important to prevent renal damage by the steroids.

    4. The medication should be taken about 30 minutes before eating.

38. A correct medication and dose for the treatment of an adult with an acute episode of gout is:

    1. Indomethacin (Indocin) 25 mg PO prn.

    2. Naproxen (Naprosyn) 100 mg PO bid.

    3. Colchicine 0.6 mg qd.

    4. Indomethacin (Indocin) 50 mg q8h for six to eight doses then decrease to 25 mg PM q8h until gout episode has resolved.

39. Disease-modifying drugs for rheumatoid arthritis in adults include:

    1. Ibuprofen (Motrin, Advil), sulindac (Clinoril), salicylates (aspirin, Disalcid).

    2. Corticosteroids (prednisone, methylprednisolone).

    3. Misoprostol (Cytotec).

    4. Hydroxychloroquine (Plaquenil), sulfasalazine (Asulfidine), methotrexate, gold sodium thiomalate (Myochrysine).

40. Gold compounds are contraindicated in clients with all of the following **except**:

    1. Renal disease.

    2. Hepatic disease.

    3. Rheumatoid arthritis disease.

    4. Blood dyscrasia.

41. The most appropriate medication used to control pain for a client with osteoarthritis would include:

    1. Acetaminophen.

    2. Systemic corticosteroids.

    3. Gold salts.

    4. Misoprostol.

42. What is a serious side effect of ibuprofen in the elderly client?

    1. Rebound headaches.

    2. Impairment of renal function.

    3. Neuropathy.

    4. Liver failure.

43. A client has been on methotrexate (Rheumatrex) for 6 weeks. This was the medication of choice for her severe refractory rheumatoid arthritis. What parameters should the nurse practitioner monitor?

    1. Monthly platelet count, CBC, and differential.

    2. Urinalysis, blood sugar, and electrocardiogram every 2 weeks.

    3. Monthly CBC, urinalysis, and electrolytes.

    4. Coagulation studies, electrolytes, and CBC every week.

10 Answers & Rationales

Physical Examination & Diagnostic Tests

1. **(3)** The musculoskeletal system is examined by a visual inspection and palpation of bones, joints, and surrounding muscular tissue. Percussion is generally not done, and auscultation is not appropriate to the system being examined.

2. **(3)** Clients with polymyalgia rheumatica have a rapid, dramatic clinical response to corticosteroid therapy. The serum protein electrophoresis is used to rule out myeloma. The ESR is elevated in a number of diseases and is not specific to polymyalgia rheumatica. The chest radiograph is used to diagnose diseases affecting the lungs and thorax.

3. **(3)** The wrist, MCP, and PIP joints along with other small joints of the hands and feet are involved with rheumatoid arthritis. The great toe is most involved with gout. The large joints of the hip, knee, and shoulder along with the distal interphalangeal (DIP) joint and the base of the thumb are involved with degenerative joint disease (i.e., osteoarthritis).

4. **(2)** It would not be necessary to obtain a CBC. The HgbA$_{1c}$ would be ordered to evaluate the relative control of diabetes. The EMG is most often performed to evaluate both nerve conduction and needle electrode examination. Many toxins and inflammatory processes are involved with polyneuropathy, hence the sedimentation rate would be a helpful diagnostic tool.

5. **(4)** A thorough history is very important in assessing any client with injury, but in the event of a back injury, the mechanism of injury will provide the greatest clue as to the extent of injury and the proper path to take in diagnosis and treatment.

6. **(2)** Carpel tunnel syndrome, a compression of the median nerve at the wrist is commonly caused by repetitive finger motion and results in a positive Tinel's sign and Phalen's test. Tinel's sign is considered positive when tapping over the nerve with a reflex hammer causes tingling in the distribution of the nerve. Phalen's test is performed by fully flexing the wrist passively and noting tingling in the thumb or fingers.

7. **(2)** The clinical assessments point to a chronic inflammatory process such as rheumatoid arthritis. The dizziness, fatigue, lightheadedness, and weakness may be a problem with anemia. The anemia of chronic disease is either a microcytic or normocytic anemia. The value that differentiates the anemia of chronic disease from other anemias is the serum ferritin (iron stores). The value will be either normal or high. The MCV of 104 indicates a macrocytic anemia, which would not include the anemia of chronic disease. The low serum ferritin would not be considered a possibility with this disorder. The uric acid level would be elevated in gout, and the WBC count does not address the signs of anemia.

8. **(1)** The preadolescent should remove her shirt (leave on bra or swimsuit top) and bend at the waist. The nurse should examine for eneven hips and shoulders.

Disorders

9. **(3)** NSAIDs are recommended treatment for an acute gout attack in clients able to take NSAID therapy. Allopurinal (Zyloprim) is contraindicated in an acute attack and can even precipitate an attack in the early stages of treatment. Low-calorie diets increase the risk of gouty attacks. Joint injection would not be first-line choice of treatment; however, in refractory cases in clients unable to take oral medication, it may be an option.

10. **(3)** Impingement syndrome is usually caused by rotator cuff tendinitis, which is when internal/external rotation is impaired. Frozen shoulder can occur after a rotator cuff injury, especially if a sling is used for a prolonged period of time. Thoracic outlet syndrome would cause a decrease or loss of radial pulse when the client abducts arm and holds a deep breath while simultaneously hyperextending the neck and turning the chin toward the raised arm.

11. **(3)** The client's complaints are common symptoms of chondromalacia patella. With anterior cruciate tears, the client generally cannot bear weight on the extremity without it buckling or giving way. With a dislocated patella, there would be considerable effusion (loss of normal knee hollow on sides of patella) and possible patellofemoral compartment.

12. **(1)** With a complete rotator cuff tear (rupture of the supraspinatus tendon), the client would have difficulty abducting the arm and impaired internal/external rotation. Touching the hand to the opposite shoulder is adduction.

13. **(4)** Also, anemia is common in polymyalgia rheumatica, along with an elevated ESR, common complaint of morning stiffness, and rheumatoid factor is negative. Option #1 is characteristic of SLE, Option #2 is characteristic of osteoarthritis, and Option #3 is characteristic of ankylosing spondylitis.

14. **(3)** Diagnostic studies are of little value and benefit, except to rule out other causes, such as polymyalgia rheumatica, hypothyroidism, and the like. Treatment is symptomatic; usual drugs are amitriptyline (Elavil), NSAIDs, cyclobenzaprine (Flexeril), temazepam (Restoril), and triazolam (Halcion). Daily, slow, low-impact aerobic exercise, preferably in the late afternoon or early evening, is encouraged. Heat and massage are helpful, but not on the "trigger points."

15. **(3)** The chronic inflammatory disorder of rheumatoid arthritis has synovial hypertrophy from chronic synovitis and pannus formation, which results in progressive destruction of the cartilage, ligament, tendons, and bone. Ankylosing spondylitis usually involves the large peripheral joints (i.e., sacroiliac) and is characterized by extreme kyphosis. There is no inflammation with osteoarthritis. SLE has a distribution of symptoms similar to that of rheumatoid arthritis but no pannus formation.

16. **(3)** Moist heat or cold is appropriate to use on acutely affected joints, whichever relieves the pain more effectively. Physical therapy is recommended after the acute involvement of the joint, and care must be taken to decrease repetitive movements. Immobilization is avoided, as it tends to increase the stiffness of the joint. The ESR is not an appropriate indicator of activity of osteoarthritis.

17. **(3)** Option #1 describes the malar or "butterfly" rash of SLE. The arthritis symptoms and other complications (meningitis and myocarditis) occur later in the disease process, especially if the client is not treated with antibiotics (usually tetracycline, doxycycline, or amoxicillin).

18. **(4)** Deformities (bony protuberances) of the DIP are called Heberden's nodes and are cardinal signs of osteoarthritis. The DIP joints are seldom involved with rheumatoid arthritis. Gouty arthritis most often affects

the great toe. Joints are warm, red, tender, and swollen with septic arthritis.

19. **(1)** Lyme arthritis, rheumatic heart disease, ankylosing spondylitis, psoriatic arthritis, rheumatoid arthritis, Reiter's syndrome, osteoarthritis, gonococcal arthritis, SLE, and polymyalgia rheumatica commonly occur as polyarthritic diseases. Most often gout, septic arthritis, and pseudogout occur as monoarthritis.

20. **(4)** As the soft tissue swells, pain onset is usually about 12–36 hours after injury.

21. **(2)** Herniated intervertebral disc pain typically shoots to the lower leg and foot. Lumbosacral strain causes pain in the back, buttock, and sometimes thigh. Osteomyelitis must be preceded by an event that permits an infectious agent to enter the bone. Osteoporosis occurs most commonly in postmenopausal women.

22. **(3)** Gout generally affects men over 30 and is associated with obesity, lead intoxication, starvation, and use of some medications, including salicylates, diuretics, pyrazinamide, and alcohol.

23. **(4)** A third-degree strain is a complete tear of the ligament, resulting in marked edema, ecchymosis, pain, and an unstable joint.

24. **(3)** Morning stiffness on activity and the length of time it takes for maximal improvement is one of the American Rheumatism Association Classification criteria for rheumatoid arthritis and is a useful, measurable tool for effects of treatment. The other questions are good indicators of quality of activities of daily living but do not give a full, overall, measurable picture of the client's joint discomfort.

25. **(1)** The client meets classification criteria for fibromyalgia based on history of widespread pain, and pain in 11 of 18 tender points. Myofascial syndrome symptoms are more focal and there is no associated fatigue or sleep disorder. Rheumatoid disease would have abnormal serologic studies. Depression may cause musculoskeletal pain and fatigue but would not have reproducible tender points.

26. **(2)** This is a subtherapeutic amount of calcium and vitamin D. The other choices are recommendations for prevention of osteoporosis.

27. **(2)** Symptoms are indicative of septic arthritis, which is a medical emergency; if not treated promptly, the joint may be destroyed. Examination of the joint fluid is the single most important diagnostic test. Other choices may provide some symptomatic relief, but the first goal of treatment is to determine if the joint is septic.

28. **(3)** When developing the differential diagnosis, the history and physical exam will help narrow the differentiation. Other procedures are important in completing the evaluation, but the most important information is the pattern of joints affected and whether it is inflammatory or noninflammatory disease.

29. **(2)** The calcium intake is important in minimizing the development of osteoporosis. Both of these contain calcium. The other distractors are not focused on the calcium intake.

30. **(4)** Signs and symptoms of osteoarthritis include asymmetrical joint pain worse with movement and relieved by rest. Stiffness of short duration (<15 minutes) after inactivity, or in the morning. Pain may be described as aching and poorly localized. Options #1, #2, and #3 are indicative of rheumatoid arthritis.

31. **(3)** Low back pain is the number one cause of disability and accounts for 25% of disabling work-related injuries.

32. **(2)** This example demonstrates five of the risk factors for osteoporosis, which include female gender, Caucasian or Asian race, over age 45, low body weight, postmenopausal, sedentary lifestyle, low calcium intake, and smoker.

33. **(3)** Polymyalgia rheumatica is an inflammatory disorder of the proximal muscles presenting as described. Polyarteritis nodosa is an inflammatory disorder affecting the small arteries. It presents with muscle weakness, myalgias, headache, and subcutaneous nodules along the arteries in the extremities. Wegener's disease presents with mild anemia, dyspnea, cough, chest pain, hemoptysis, and abnormal urinalysis.

34. **(3)** Up to 40% of clients with temporal arteritis have a previous history of PMR. Presenting complaints include headache, low-grade fever, aching and stiffness of PMR, fatigue, malaise, and anorexia.

35. **(2)** Development of iridocyclitis may be insidious and asymptomatic, and if left untreated may cause blindness. Although young adolescents may develop any of these other diseases, there is no correlation with JRA.

Pharmacology

36. **(2)** Aspirin is the first choice. NSAIDs can be used, but the anti-inflammatory and antipyrectic effects of aspirin, plus low cost, make it the drug of choice. Methotrexate is used for severe cases that do not respond to either aspirin or NSAIDs. A steroid may be given, but it is not the drug of choice.

37. **(2)** The client needs to understand the importance of maintaining her dose of the steroids. When symptoms decrease, the medication is effective. It is not influenced by fluids and it should be taken with food.

38. **(3)** This is the only effective dose listed for the treatment of an acute episode of gout. The other doses are incorrect or insufficient as dosed.

39. **(4)** These drugs modify the disease when NSAIDs (ibuprofen, sulindac, salicylates) have not worked. Corticosteroids can be used until the disease-modifying agents begin to work. Misoprostol (Cytotec) is used to prevent ulcer development related to long-term medication use.

40. **(3)** Gold is indicated for treatment of rheumatoid arthritis and is contraindicated in the presence of these other diseases.

41. **(1)** Acetaminophen or NSAIDs are generally used for pain relief for clients with osteoarthritis. Systematic corticosteroids are not indicated in osteoarthritis. Gold salts may be one of several pharmacologic approaches to the treatment of rheumatoid arthritis. Misoprostol is used to minimize the development of NSAID-induced gastric ulcers.

42. **(2)** Renal function may be already reduced in the elderly, and ibuprofen can further impair renal function, which in turn can result in nephrosis, cirrhosis, and congestive heart failure.

43. **(1)** The client should be monitored for blood dyscrasias on a monthly basis. Women of child-bearing age should avoid pregnancy.

11 Neurology

Physical Examination & Diagnostic Tests

1. To evaluate the neurologic system for appropriate sensory system functioning in the geriatric client, stereognosis is determined. This is done by having the client:

   1. Rapidly touch the index finger and then the nose.

   2. Distinguish between a coin and key by touch.

   3. Stand with heels together and the eyes closed.

   4. Close the eyes and identify familiar odors.

2. To determine cerebellar functioning in the geriatric client, the practitioner evaluates:

   1. Ability of the client to balance on one foot and then the other.

   2. Discriminatory sensation between two familiar objects.

   3. Ability to recall names of three U.S. presidents.

   4. Range of motion and ability to move extremities.

3. What is considered a "soft" neurologic (or equivocal) sign?

   1. Positive Babinski's reflex in an adult.

   2. Mirroring hand movements of the extremities.

   3. Brudzinski's sign.

   4. Kernig's sign.

4. Which cranial nerve is being tested when the nurse practitioner asks the client to raise her eyebrows, smile, frown, or puff out her cheeks?

   1. Hypoglossal nerve.

   2. Acoustic nerve.

   3. Glossopharyngeal nerve.

   4. Facial nerve.

5. The nurse practitioner notes in a healthy individual an absent knee jerk reflex. What might the nurse practitioner ask the client to do?

   1. Lift both arms above the head and count to 5 slowly as the reflex is tested.

   2. Raise both legs slowly and then lower and immediately test for the reflex.

   3. Clench both hands together and pull while the reflex is tested.

   4. Close eyes and hold breath while the examiner tests for the reflex.

6. The nurse practitioner gently flexes a client's neck in the direction of the chin touching the chest. If there is pain and resistance to the flexion and the hips and knees flex at the same time, the nurse practitioner accurately describes this finding as:

   1. Phalen's sign.

   2. Romberg's sign.

   3. Kernig's sign.

   4. Brudzinski's reflex.

Disorders

7. The nurse practitioner understands that the most common form of facial paralysis in the adult client is:

   1. Facial nerve fasciitis.

   2. Trigeminal neuralgia.

   3. Bell's palsy.

   4. Herpes zoster.

8. A client has Parkinson's disease. The nurse practitioner is discussing safety measures for the home environment. It would be important for the nurse practitioner to include what information?

   1. Sleep on a firm mattress that is high off the floor to facilitate getting into and out of bed.

   2. Pour hot liquids with the cup of container placed on the table to avoid spilling.

3. Place a sheepskin pad on the bed to decrease the development of decubiti.

4. Perform passive and active range of motion twice daily to prevent contracture.

9. Many clients who suffer from recurrent headaches have similar symptoms with each episode. Which is a sign that a headache may be from a more serious cause?

   1. It occurs on the right side.

   2. Rhinorrhea occurs with the headache.

   3. The headache continuously becomes more and more painful.

   4. The client is able to sleep through the pain of the headache.

10. All of the following are included in the differential diagnosis of a client with facial paralysis **except**:

    1. Herpes zoster.

    2. Bell's palsy.

    3. Trigeminal neuralgia.

    4. Otitis media.

11. What would be appropriate to include in the treatment plan for health promotion in a client with a diagnosis of multiple sclerosis?

    1. Avoid aerobic exercise, due to muscle weakness.

    2. Keep warm (especially extremities) to improve neurologic function.

    3. Avoid antioxidants (vitamins C and E and β-carotene), as they contribute to loss of myelin sheath.

    4. Consume a low-fat, high-fiber diet, with daily cranberry juice, and calcium supplement.

12. A cerebrovascular accident client is incontinent of urine. The family should be taught to:

    1. Restrict fluid intake.

    2. Insert a Foley catheter.

3. Establish a scheduled voiding pattern.

4. Reposition the client often to reduce the discomfort of urgency.

13. Inflammation and swelling of the seventh cranial nerve with resultant unilateral facial muscle paralysis is called:

1. Bell's palsy.

2. Transient ischemic attack.

3. Facial droop.

4. Trigeminal neuralgia.

14. Many visits to emergency departments by adults are prompted by headaches. One symptom that may help the nurse practitioner differentiate a headache that is life threatening is:

1. It is preceded by an "aura."

2. It occurs mainly behind one eye and tends to be grouped.

3. The onset is sudden and accompanied by nuchal rigidity.

4. The headache occurs mainly on awakening.

15. An adult client presents with a complaint of facial paralysis that started suddenly. In making a diagnosis, the nurse practitioner considers the following symptoms of Bell's palsy:

1. Concurrent paralysis of the opposite arm and leg.

2. Pain in the ear that accompanies or precedes the paralysis.

3. Loss of bowel control.

4. Loss of hearing on the opposite side.

16. A student nurse practitioner studying for the nurse practitioner certification examination begins to have numbness and tingling in her hands and face. Convinced she is having a stroke from brain overload, she calls a fellow student to come to her aid. What should this friend offer her?

1. A ride to the emergency department.

2. A phone call to the local magnetic resonance imaging (MRI) facility.

3. A paper bag.

4. A different study source.

17. A recently diagnosed client with multiple sclerosis asks the nurse practitioner about the disease process. The nurse practitioner knows that:

1. 90% of all clients have a quickly progressive form of the disease.

2. 90% of all clients after the first onset of symptoms have relapses and remissions.

3. 10% of all clients will respond to corticosteroids.

4. 10% of all clients have problems with optic neuritis and sensory loss.

18. A 30-year-old female client has had several episodes of incontinence, weakness, visual loss, and some ataxia. Physical exam reveals slight swelling of the optic disc on funduscopic exam, difficulty in walking heel-to-toe, lower extremity weakness, and 2 ǀ deep tendon reflexes. The nurse practitioner suspects:

1. Multiple sclerosis.

2. Parkinson's disease.

3. Amyotrophic lateral sclerosis.

4. Postpolio syndrome.

19. A client has a history of recurrent headache for the past 3 years, occurring 1–2 times per month and lasting 12–18 hours for which she takes acetaminophen. The client has been using acetaminophen 6 gm in the past 12-hour period and has had no relief and presents to the clinic. The nurse practitioner would:

1. Refer the client to a neurologist for headache work-up.

2. Consider analgesic rebound relative to the dose of acetaminophen taken.

3. Order naproxen (Anaprox) for prophylactic treatment of the headaches.

4. Order an electroencephalogram (EEG) and MRI to rule out pathology.

20. A client returns to the clinic for a follow-up visit. She has a history of simple, partial seizures. When questioning the client regarding the recurrence of seizures, the nurse practitioner would identify the recurrence of this seizure activity if the client reported:

    1. Short episodes where she loses consciousness, but does not fall.

    2. No loss of consciousness, but jerking and tingling of her right leg then right hand.

    3. Auditory hallucinations, unconsciousness, and urinary incontinence.

    4. A short period of unconsciousness, followed by a period of confusion.

21. A client with a history of myasthenia gravis presents with ptosis, facial weakness, dysphagia, and generalized weakness. What is important for the nurse practitioner to establish initially?

    1. When did the symptoms first begin, and have they increased in severity?

    2. What medications is the client on and when did she last take them?

    3. What activity was the client participating in when the symptoms began?

    4. Has the client experienced any seizure activity with the increase in symptoms?

Pharmacology

22. An elderly client is diagnosed with herpes zoster. To reduce the occurrence of postherpetic neuralgia, the nurse practitioner orders which medication?

    1. Prednisone (Deltasone).

    2. Acyclovir (Zovirax).

    3. Ketorolac (Toradol).

    4. Carbamazepine (Tegretol).

23. A client is on antiepileptic medication. The nurse practitioner understands that antiepileptic medication:

    1. Must be taken indefinitely.

    2. Is usually discontinued after 4 years of no seizure activity, following an EEG test to confirm lack of seizure activity.

    3. Is usually given in combination with other antiepileptics or sedatives to reduce the seizure threshold.

    4. Must be given to all clients who experience a seizure.

24. A medication and dose that can be used for abortive therapy for an adult client with symptoms of a migraine headache are:

    1. Sumatriptan (Imitrex) 6 mg IM.

    2. Ergotamine (Ergostat) 2 mg SL.

    3. Ketorolac (Toradol) 100 mg IM.

    4. Amitriptyline (Elavil) 100 mg PO.

11   Answers & Rationales

Physical Examination & Diagnostic Tests

1. **(2)** Stereognosis is the ability to determine familiar objects by shape rather than visual identification. Option #1 determines fine motor movements and coordination. Option #3 determines proprioception (balance, posture) and Option #4 determines the functioning of the first cranial nerve (i.e., olfactory).

2. **(1)** The cerebellar area controls gross motor movements and balance, as well as fine motor movements of upper and lower extremities. Discriminatory sensations are controlled by the sensory system, and remote memory is tested by mental status examination, and involves the cerebral cortex.

3. **(2)** Soft neurologic signs involve slight deviations of the central nervous system (CNS), which are present occasionally or inconsistently. Examples are short attention span, clumsiness, frequent falling (disturbances of gait), hyperkinesis, left-handed but right-footed, language disturbances, anisocoria, and mirroring movements of the extremities (when one hand performs, the other is in motion). The other three options indicate a CNS problem that occurs consistently (i.e., Brudzinski's reflex and Kernig's sign indicate meningeal irritation; a positive Babinski's reflex in an adult may indicate an upper motor lesion, such as in the corticospinal tract).

4. **(4)** The facial nerve is tested by facial movement, taste, sensation, and corneal reflex. The hypoglossal nerve is tested by the client sticking out her tongue. The acoustic nerve is tested by a hearing test. The glossopharyngeal nerve is tested by taste, gag reflex, and giving the client a drink and asking her to swallow.

5. **(3)** Augmentation of the knee jerk reflex can be obtained by having the client isometrically tense muscles not directly involved with the reflex arc being tested. This is called Jendrassik's maneuver.

6. **(4)** This describes Brudzinski's reflex. Phalen's sign is elicited in carpal tunnel syndrome. Romberg's test is done to assess gross swaying by asking the client to stand with feet together and eyes closed for 5 seconds. Kernig's sign (inability to extend the lower leg when the leg is flexed at the hip or when there is resistance or pain during the process) along with Brudzinski's reflex indicates meningeal irritation and should be further evaluated.

Disorders

7. **(3)** The most common form of facial paralysis is Bell's palsy, which is a disorder affecting the facial nerve and characterized by muscle flaccidity of the affected side of the face. Trigeminal neuralgia is a disorder of cranial nerve V characterized by an abrupt onset of pain in the lower and upper jaw, cheek, and lips. Herpes zoster affects the dermatomes and does not cause a paralysis, but does cause pain and possible postherpetic neuralgia.

8. **(2)** Pouring liquids is frequently a complicated task for this client due to her tremors. If the cup or container in which the client is pouring the liquid is placed on the table, there is less chance of spilling the contents.

9. **(3)** If a headache becomes more and more severe, if there is new onset of severe headache in a client over 35 years old, if the headache's character or progression is different from other headaches, or if there is vomiting but no nausea, there could be a new and serious cause for the headache. The side on which the headache occurs, accompanying rhinorrhea, and sleeping through a headache may or may not be significant, depending on other symptoms.

10. **(3)** The differential diagnosis for facial paralysis includes numerous problems: bacterial infection of the ears, Lyme disease, herpes zoster, mumps, temporal bone fracture, acoustic neuroma, other types of tumors, and demyelinating diseases. Trigeminal neuralgia is associated with intense facial pain, not paralysis.

11. **(4)** In addition to the factors listed, keeping cool, not warm, is associated with improvement of neurologic function. A regular exercise program is encouraged along with daily intake of a multiple vitamin, antioxidants, and low-dose aspirin (81 mg). Maintaining ideal body weight, having rest periods or naps daily, and becoming informed about the disease process are also important aspects of promoting health.

12. **(3)** Re-establishing regularity will assist in maintaining bladder control A catheter exposes the client to infection. Fluids should not be restricted.

13. **(1)** The symptoms describe Bell's palsy, which is believed to be caused by a virus. This sudden onset of unilateral facial paralysis usually resolves within a couple of weeks but can endure for months. A few clients can have residual problems. Transient ischemic attacks last less than 24 hours. Facial droop occurs with Bell's palsy due to paralysis of the muscles innervated by the facial nerve (seventh cranial nerve). Trigeminal neuralgia is sudden pain along the fifth cranial nerve.

14. **(3)** Classic migraine headaches are accompanied by auras. Cluster headaches occur behind one eye and are grouped. Headaches associated with hypertension occur mainly on awakening. A sudden onset and nuchal rigidity may indicate a subarachnoid hemorrhage.

15. **(2)** Bell's palsy is typically preceded or accompanied by pain in the ear on the paralyzed side. The paralysis is confined to the face and there is no bowel involvement.

16. **(3)** Clients who are under stress have periods of hyperventilation in which they "blow off" more carbon dioxide than necessary. They experience numbness and tingling in their hands and faces and can experience syncope. Breathing into a paper bag increases the carbon dioxide level and relieves the symptoms of respiratory alkalosis.

17. **(2)** Multiple sclerosis is characterized by exacerbations and remissions of the symptoms. Only 10% have a progressive form of the disease from onset. Many clients (35–40%) have problems of optic neuritis, sensory loss, and weakness and do respond to corticosteroids.

18. **(1)** Involvement of more than one area of the CNS, age 15–60 years, two or more separate episodes of symptoms involving different sites, or a gradual progression over at least 6 months meets the criteria for multiple sclerosis.

19. **(2)** The recommended dose for acetaminophen is no more than 4 gm/day. This client may be experiencing analgesic rebound headache. Appropriate prophylactic medications for migraine include β-blockers (propanolol), tricyclic antidepressants (amitriptyline), selective serotonin reuptake inhibitors (fluoxetine), monoamine oxidase (MAO) inhibitors (phenelzine), and calcium channel blockers (verapamil). It is not necessary to order expensive tests for clients with migraine or tension headache. Usually, a careful, thorough history is sufficient.

20. **(2)** A simple partial seizure is characterized by unilateral paresthesia, numbness and tingling, and spastic movement of extremities (old term is Jacksonian seizure).

There is no loss of consciousness or incontinence of bowel or bladder.

21. **(2)** It is important to determine if the client has stayed on her medication schedule. The symptoms may be the result of missed medication, or may also occur due to too much medication. This is especially true with pyridostigmine bromide (Mestinon). This should be addressed first. The symptoms may also be exacerbated by exercise and heat.

Pharmacology

22. **(1)** Elderly clients are particularly susceptible to postherpetic neuralgia, which is pain at the site that may last for months or years. Management of discomfort is alleviated by pain medication. Systemic corticosteroids may reduce the occurrence of postherpetic neuralgia. Usually, 60 mg prednisone qd for 2 weeks with a rapid taper is prescribed. Acyclovir is used for immunocompromised clients.

23. **(2)** Although most medication is discontinued after 4 years of no seizure activity, this should be confirmed by an EEG. Not all seizure clients require medication; referral and monitoring by a neurologist are appropriate.

24. **(2)** The correct dose is ergotamine (Ergostat) 2 mg SL. Sumatriptan (Imitrex) is given SC or 100 mg PO. Ketorolac (Toradol) is dosed 30–60 mg IM. Amitriptyline (Elavil) is not used for abortive therapy.

12

Gastrointestinal & Liver

Physical Examination & Diagnostic Tests

1. The nurse practitioner is preparing to examine the abdomen of a client. What is the correct sequence in which to conduct the examination?

   1. Inspection, palpation, percussion, auscultation.

   2. Palpation, percussion, auscultation, inspection.

   3. Percussion, palpation, auscultation, inspection.

   4. Inspection, auscultation, percussion, palpation.

2. When obtaining a history from a client with abdominal pain, the following areas are to be examined:

   1. The quality, quantity, and location of the pain.

   2. The location, the way in which the pain developed (gradually over hours or suddenly), if the pain has changed since onset, and associated symptoms.

3. If the pain is referred to other sites, what aggravates or alleviates the pain and the client's past medical history and medication history.

   4. All of the above.

3. To test for a positive obturator sign in a client with abdominal pain, the nurse practitioner:

   1. Passively rotates the right hip from the 90-degree hip/knee flexion position.

   2. Asks the client to take a deep breath while applying pressure in the area of the gallbladder.

   3. Percusses over the costovertebral angles.

   4. Positions the supine client with hips flexed and auscultates for bowel sounds then palpates the abdomen, beginning with superficial palpation of nontender areas.

4. Serologic features* of acute hepatitis B are:

1. HBsAg, HBeAg, and a high titer of immunoglobulin M (IgM) anti-HBc.

2. HBeAg- and HBsAg-positive.

3. HBeAg- and HBsAg-negative.

4. IgM anti-HBc- (high titer) HBsAg-negative.

5. The nurse practitioner is performing a physical examination on a middle-aged woman. The history reveals the client's father died of colon cancer. What diagnostics are used to screen this client?

1. Barium enema and upper gastrointestinal (GI) series.

2. Carcinoembryonic antigen titer (CEA).

3. Proctoscopy and biopsy.

4. Colonoscopy and hemoccult.

6. The anti-HCV test indicates the client has:

1. Acute hepatitis C.

2. Chronic hepatitis C.

3. Resolved hepatitis C.

4. Acute, chronic, or resolved hepatitis C.

7. The diagnosis of early acute pancreatitis will be considered by the nurse practitioner based on physical findings and the following laboratory result:

1. A white blood cell (WBC) count of 10,300/mm^3.

2. A serum amylase of 75 U/L.

3. A serum amylase of 300 U/L.

4. A serum lipase of 75 U/L.

8. A middle-aged woman who is overweight has right upper quadrant pain that radiates to her right subscapular area, and that is severe and persistent. She is also experiencing anorexia, nausea, and has a fever. For her last meal, she ate a double quarter-pound hamburger with cheese, French fries, and a vanilla shake. Based on this information, the nurse practitioner

examines the abdomen and percusses for costovertebral angle tenderness. The abdomen is tender in the right upper quadrant; if there is a positive:

1. Obturator sign, the client has appendicitis.

2. Costovertebral angle tenderness, the client has a urinary tract infection.

3. Murphy's sign, the client has cholecystitis.

4. McBurney's sign, the client has a strangulated hernia.

9. A client complains of extreme pain in her abdomen and points to the right lower quadrant. In examining the acute abdomen, the nurse practitioner would:

1. Immediately order a WBC and abdominal x-ray.

2. Percuss the abdomen in all quadrants followed by auscultation and gentle palpation.

3. Palpate the right side of the abdomen first, paying close attention for guarding in the area of pain.

4. Palpate the left side of the abdomen then gently palpate the right side, noting guarding and tenderness.

Disorders

10. Diarrhea is often associated with:

1. Infectious gastroenteritis, inflammatory bowel disease, diverticulitis, and early intestinal obstruction.

2. Diseases of the colon or rectum.

3. Fever and abdominal pain in sexually transmitted diseases.

4. Dysuria and flank pain in urinary tract infections.

11. Esophageal pain may radiate to the:

1. Infrascapular area.

2. Right shoulder.

3. Neck and left arm.

4. Periumbilical area.

---

* HBeAg, hepatitis B e antigen; anti-HBc, antibody to hepatitis B core antigen; HBsAg, hepatitis B surface antigen.

12. The most important goal of assessing a client with abdominal pain is to:

    1. Palpate the area of pain right away.

    2. Rule out emergent conditions.

    3. Determine the exact etiology of the pain on the first visit for every client.

    4. Determine what tests to order.

13. When the nurse practitioner suspects peritonitis in a client, the best action is to:

    1. Percuss over the costovertebral angle and watch for signs of pain.

    2. Perform a rectal exam and test the stool for blood.

    3. Auscultate the abdomen for decreased bowel sounds.

    4. Palpate for a tense, hard abdomen and check for a positive obturator sign.

14. Which of the following suggests an emergent condition?

    1. Pain in an adolescent that is rated as 5 on a scale of 1–10 and relieved by having a bowel movement.

    2. Pain that is progressive, localized, and steady for more than 6 hours and accompanied by rebound tenderness and guarding.

    3. Pain in an adolescent girl that is sudden in onset and localized in the lower right or left quadrant and lasts 14–36 hours.

    4. Pain that follows the onset of vomiting and diarrhea.

15. Under what circumstances should peptic ulcer disease **not** be treated empirically before diagnostic studies are done? When the client's ulcer pain:

    1. Awakens him/her from sleep early in the morning.

    2. Can be relieved by food, antacids, or vomiting.

    3. Is worsened by food ingestion.

    4. Is atypical or occurring with anemia, blood in the stool, or weight loss.

16. A careful history of a client with a chief complaint of diarrhea reveals that this adult has recurrent abdominal pain and diarrhea that alternates with constipation. The most likely diagnosis is:

    1. Drug-induced diarrhea.

    2. Inflammatory bowel disease.

    3. Giardiasis.

    4. Irritable bowel syndrome (IBS).

17. Clients with dysphagia due to motility disorders:

    1. Usually have more difficulty swallowing solids than liquids.

    2. Can have a stricture due to esophagitis following a long history of reflux disorder.

    3. Usually complain cold liquids cause pain.

    4. Can have marked weight loss.

18. The pathogenesis of gastroesophageal reflux disease (GERD) is:

    1. Frequent and excessive retrograde movement of stomach contents into the esophagus due to an abnormal lower esophageal sphincter (LES) function.

    2. Due to a hiatal hernia that leads to the esophageal irritation and inflammation.

    3. Due to reflux of the gastric contents after meals when a client is in the upright position often after a period of vigorous exercise.

    4. Initiated by erosion of the gastrointestinal mucosa into the LES causing weakening of LES pressure and a burning sensation in the stomach.

19. The nurse practitioner's understanding of which principle will be helpful in educating clients with GERD?

    1. A hiatal hernia is always a coexisting and major contributing factor.

    2. The LES has become a poor antireflux barrier.

    3. The amount of acid reflux is dependent on a familial tendency for GERD.

    4. Overeating and use of caffeine and alcohol cause GERD.

20. Inflammatory toxigenic gastrointestinal illness is characterized by:

    1. Fecal leukocytes, dysentery, site: proximal small bowel.

    2. No fecal leukocytes, watery diarrhea, site: distal small bowel.

    3. Fecal leukocytes, secretory diarrhea, site: colon.

    4. Fecal leukocytes, watery diarrhea, site: colon.

21. Clinical features of IBS include which of the following?

    1. IBS affects men more than women.

    2. IBS affects children more than those in early adulthood.

    3. IBS affects women more than men.

    4. IBS predominantly affects elderly clients more than those in early adulthood.

22. The nurse practitioner understands that hepatitis B can be transmitted in blood and blood products. Another common mode of transmission of hepatitis B is:

    1. Respiratory contact.

    2. Contaminated fluid.

    3. Fecal–oral route.

    4. Perinatal exposure.

23. A young adult client presents to the nurse practitioner's office with a chief complaint of intermittent heartburn, which became worse 2 months ago from job stress. The discomfort is worse after eating and at night and is relieved temporarily by antacids. The client also states that several times in the last 14 days she has regurgitated very bitter tasting material into the mouth. The physical exam by the nurse practitioner is unremarkable. The nurse practitioner's most likely diagnosis is:

    1. Viral esophagitis.

    2. Irritable bowel syndrome.

    3. Gastroesophageal reflux disease.

    4. Carcinoma of the esophagus.

24. All of the following should be referred to an internist for management due to the high rate of chronic hepatitis **except**:

    1. Hepatitis A.

    2. Hepatitis B.

    3. Hepatitis C.

    4. Hepatitis D.

25. Which is true about enterobiasis?

    1. The parasite is in the soil and enters the body through the feet. It can cause anemia.

    2. The parasite causes pruritus around the anus because the gravid females exit through the anus at night and lay eggs on the skin. The human is the only host of this parasite.

    3. The eggs of this parasite enter the body by ingestion of dirt (pica) or dirt on unwashed vegetables that contain the eggs or through water containing eggs.

    4. This parasite is a protozoan. The source is usually contaminated water, but it is spread from person to person by oral–fecal contamination.

26. Nonpharmacologic management of GERD includes the following:

    1. Weight reduction, sleep with head of bed elevated 4–6 inches with blocks.

    2. Lying down and resting after meals, weight reduction.

    3. Drinking large amounts of fluids with meals, avoiding alcohol.

    4. Avoiding mint and orange juice, and consuming a high-energy diet.

27. An organism associated with the etiology of peptic ulcer disease is:

    1. *Streptococcus pneumoniae*.

    2. *Helicobacter pylori*.

    3. *Moraxella catarrhalis*.

    4. *Staphylococcus aureus*.

28. The most common cause of cirrhosis is:

    1. Hepatitis A.

2. Hepatitis B.

3. Hepatitis D.

4. Alcoholic hepatitis.

29. Prolapse of a vascular anal cushion through the anal canal with resultant entrapment by the internal anal sphincter describes a:

    1. Prolapse of the rectal mucosa.

    2. Hemorrhoid.

    3. Tumor.

    4. Hernia.

30. An acute febrile illness with jaundice, anorexia, and malaise; an incubation period of 45–160 days; having a chronic and an acute form; and transmitted by parenteral, sexual, and perinatal routes describes:

    1. Hepatitis A.

    2. Hepatitis B.

    3. Hepatitis C.

    4. Hepatitis D.

31. A client presents to the nurse practitioner's office with a history of cholelithiasis. Which client complaining of increased pain would require immediate admission to the hospital for possible prompt intervention?

    1. A client who is human immunodeficiency virus (HIV)-positive.

    2. A 75-year-old diabetic.

    3. A client who is 5 weeks pregnant.

    4. A client who is vomiting and has a slight fever.

32. An older adult female presents to the nurse practitioner complaining of weakness and vomiting. The client gives a history of "several" drinks per day for the past 12 years. The nurse practitioner observes that the client's lips appear to have dark blood on them. What emergent condition does the nurse practitioner suspect.

    1. Seizure disorder.

    2. Cerebral hemorrhage.

    3. Pancreatitis.

    4. Esophageal varices.

33. A usually benign diagnosis that can result in small bowel obstruction and infarction and which requires immediate referral to a surgeon is:

    1. Gastric ulcer.

    2. Endometriosis.

    3. Hernia.

    4. Ectopic pregnancy.

34. A young adult female presents to the nurse practitioner for evaluation of 2 days of increasing crampy, abdominal pain. She states that she also has some mild nausea, anorexia, and a low-grade fever. The client states that the pain is periumbilical. Her STAT complete blood count (CBC) reveals a slightly elevated white count but is otherwise normal. The nurse practitioner's next step for the care of this client is:

    1. Referral to a gynecologist for evaluation of a possible ectopic pregnancy.

    2. Referral to a surgeon for evaluation of possible appendicitis.

    3. Observe the client overnight and reassess the next day.

    4. Place the client on a clear liquid diet and have her watch for increasing symptoms.

35. A previously benign condition that can cause a client severe rectal pain and be the cause of an emergency visit to the nurse practitioner is:

    1. Hookworms.

    2. Pinworms.

    3. Thrombosed hemorrhoid.

    4. Cystitis.

36. An elderly client presents with fever, leukocytosis, left lower quadrant pain, and diarrhea alternating with constipation. The nurse practitioner would make the diagnosis of:

    1. Appendicitis.

    2. Diverticulitis.

    3. Irritable bowel syndrome.

    4. Pancreatitis.

37. Which clients would be the lowest risk for developing diverticular disease?

    1. Vegetarians.

    2. Type A personality.

    3. The elderly.

    4. Fad dieters.

38. The nurse practitioner knows that the following symptom is characteristic of left-sided colon cancer:

    1. Anemia.

    2. Tenesmus.

    3. Bright red rectal bleeding.

    4. Change in bowel habits.

39. The nurse practitioner knows that a history of pancolonic ulcerative colitis requires careful surveillance because of an increased risk of:

    1. Colon cancer.

    2. Anemia.

    3. Depression.

    4. Perforation.

40. The nurse practitioner identifies which of these conditions as most conducive to the development of metabolic alkalosis in a child?

    1. Severe anxiety resulting in hyperventilation.

    2. Excessive vomiting related to gastroenteritis.

    3. Depressed respirations from excessive narcotics ingestion.

    4. Decreased renal function with glomeruli damage.

41. The symptoms of abdominal discomfort associated with meals, diarrhea or constipation, anorexia, weight loss, failure to grow, and failure to develop sexually are most associated with:

    1. Ulcerative colitis.

    2. Irritable bowel syndrome.

    3. Carcinoma of the colon.

    4. Crohn's disease.

42. What is the most consistent finding in clients with acute appendicitis?

    1. An elevated WBC count.

    2. High fever.

    3. Periumbilical dull pain.

    4. Nausea and vomiting.

Pharmacology

43. Which of the following would be prescribed as initial treatment for uncomplicated peptic ulcer disease (PUD)?

    1. Cimetidine (Tagamet) 400 mg bid.

    2. Doxepin (Sinequan) 25 mg qhs.

    3. Omeprazole (Prilosec) 20 mg qd.

    4. Pirenzepine 50 mg tid.

44. Which drug would be most useful for the nurse practitioner to prescribe for a client to prevent ulcers due to nonsteroidal anti-inflammatory drugs (NSAIDs)?

    1. Misoprostol (Cytotec).

    2. Cimetidine (Tagamet).

    3. Doxepin (Sinequan).

    4. Pirenzepine.

45. After percutaneous or permucosal exposure to an HBsAg-positive source:

    1. In an unvaccinated person, begin the hepatitis B series.

    2. In a known hepatitis B responder with an adequate response, no treatment is necessary.

    3. In a known hepatitis B responder with inadequate anti-HBsAG, give hepatitis B immunoglobulin and initiate a new hepatitis B vaccine series.

    4. In an unknown hepatitis B responder who completed the entire hepatitis B vaccine series, give a hepatitis B booster.

46. *Helicobacter pylori* has been found to be a causative factor in many cases of PUD. Successful treatment requires therapy with which regimen?

    1. Combination of histamine$_2$ (H$_2$) blockers, antacids, and omeprezole (Prilosec).

    2. Combination of Pepto-Bismol, amoxicillin (Amoxil), and metronidazole (Flagyl).

    3. Combination of lifestyle changes, Pepto-Bismol, and cimetidine (Tagamet).

    4. Combination of H$_2$ blocker, amoxicillin (Amoxil), and antacid.

47. A primary therapy for clients with mild ulcerative colitis is:

    1. Metronidazole (Flagyl).

    2. Sulfasalazine (Azulfidine).

    3. Amoxicillin (Amoxil).

    4. Cephalexin (Keflex).

48. The stepwise approach to management of GERD is:

    1. Lifestyle changes and antacids as needed and cimetidine (Tagamet) 800 mg qd at bedtime.

    2. Lifestyle changes and antacids as needed followed by lifestyle changes plus ranitidine (Zantac) 150 mg bid.

    3. Lifestyle changes and antacids as needed followed by lifestyle changes plus omeprazole (Prilosec) 20 mg qd.

    4. Cisapride (Propulsid) 10 mg taken 15 minutes before meals and at bedtime. Lifestyle changes can be added if this therapy is not effective.

49. After exposure to household or sexual contacts with hepatitis A, the nurse practitioner would:

    1. Give immunoglobulin 0.02 ml/kg as soon as possible but no later than 2 weeks after exposure.

    2. Give hepatitis B immunoglobulin (HBIG) × 1 and immunoglobulin 0.02 ml/kg as soon as possible.

    3. Give immunoglobulin 0.02 ml/kg and HBIG × 2.

    4. Understand that no injections are needed.

50. Shigellosis is treated by:

    1. No medication intervention, careful toileting and bathroom sanitation, and keeping the perineal area clean.

    2. Symptomatic treatment and antidiarrheal agents.

    3. Symptomatic treatment and trimethoprim-sulfamethoxazole (Septra) dosed for age and weight bid × 5 days.

    4. Boiling water and quinacrine HCl (Atabrine) 100 mg PO tid × 5 days.

51. Pharmacologic management of nausea and vomiting includes:

    1. Emetrol 15–30 ml PO in adults.

    2. Promethazine (Phenergan) 25 mg for children over 6 years old and adults.

    3. Hydroxyzine hydrochloride (Vistaril) 1 mg IM for adults and children 12 years old and older.

    4. Trimethobenzamide (Tigan) 10 mg PO prn for adults.

52. A young woman presents with a history of recent unprotected sexual activity with a partner now diagnosed with hepatitis B. She is currently asymptomatic and she does not recall having a vaccine in the past. The best action for the nurse practitioner is:

    1. Draw blood for a hepatitis B e antibody test (anti-HBe).

    2. Administer one dose of HBIG.

    3. Administer two doses of HBIG and initiate vaccination.

    4. Administer one dose of HBIG and initiate vaccination.

53. What condition is a contraindication for the administration of the hepatitis B vaccine?

    1. Pregnancy.

    2. Lactating mothers.

    3. Severe hypersensitivity.

    4. Age >60 years.

54. A 78-year-old client is diagnosed with enterocolitis and the physician prescribes vancomycin (Vancocin) 125 mg PO qid. The nurse practitioner will follow the progress of the client. What areas will be monitored with regard to the medication tolerance?

    1. CBC, platelet count, clotting studies.

    2. Serum creatinine, blood urea nitrogen, hearing changes.

    3. Serum electrolytes, urinalysis, ataxia.

    4. Changes in bowel habits, diarrhea, electrocardiographic changes.

12 ▷ Answers & Rationales

Physical Examination & Diagnostic Tests

1. **(4)** Inspection and auscultation should be conducted first in order to prevent undue guarding. If the examination is painful initially, the client is going to be very uncomfortable with allowing the examiner to continue.

2. **(4)** All of the information is important in sorting out the cause of abdominal pain. The location and character may help identify the origin of the pain. Abrupt onset of pain usually has a different etiology than pain that develops over hours. Whether or not the pain has changed since onset can help in determining if a larger area of the abdomen is becoming involved or if the pain is subsiding. Both visceral and parietal pain can be referred to remote sites along shared nerve pathways. Aggravating and alleviating factors can provide clues as to the origin of the pain. Fever, chills, vomiting, diarrhea, constipation, and urogenital-associated symptoms are important in determining the cause of the abdominal pain. Past medical history and medication history can give clues to known conditions and to medications that may be causing the symptoms or are being used for conditions that can cause abdominal pain. For example, a client taking ranitidine (Zantac) may fail to mention a history of GERD.

3. **(1)** If abdominal pain results from passive internal rotation of the right hip from the 90-degree hip/knee flexion position, the client has a positive obturator sign, which is suggestive of appendicitis. In a positive Murphy's sign (Option #2), pain and a brief inspiratory arrest result when a client takes a deep breath while the examiner applies pressure over the gallbladder. This is suggestive of cholecystitis. Percussion over the costovertebral angles that elicits pain is suggestive of pyelonephritis. Positioning the client in the supine position with hips flexed and then auscultating and palpating the abdomen, beginning with light palpation in nontender areas, is the sequence for examining the abdomen.

4. **(1)** HBsAg is found in active or chronic hepatitis B disease. HBeAg indicates active replication of the virus. IgM anti-HBsAg indicates chronic disease. Positive HBsAg indicates chronic disease, and negative HBsAg indicates prior exposure.

5. **(4)** These are standard diagnostics used for screening a client with a high risk for colon cancer. CEA is used more to determine recurrence of cancer; barium enema, upper GI, and proctoscopy do not provide as reliable information for detecting the malignancy.

6. **(4)** This is the surface marker for hepatitis C; at present there is no way to differentiate the diffuse forms of hepatitis C, as the viremia level is well below the threshold of most assays.

7. **(3)** Options #2 and #3 are almost identical. (*Note: use the testing strategy; both are wrong or one is the correct answer*). In acute pancreatitis the serum amylase increases within 3–6 hours of onset. The serum lipase elevates after the increase in amylase. (Normal levels of serum amylase in adults are 50–180 U/L; those of serum lipase, 55–417 U/L.)

8. **(3)** The history, right upper quadrant pain that radiates to the right subscapular area, and a positive Murphy's sign are all commonly associated with cholecystitis. A positive obturator sign at McBurney's point is a sign associated with appendicitis. Clients with strangulated hernias have colicky abdominal pain, nausea, vomiting, abdominal distention, and hyperperistalsis. Those with reducible hernias are asymptomatic or have only mild pain.

9. **(4)** Always palpate the nontender areas first, before going to the area of pain and tenderness. Option #2 is not described in the correct order of assessing an abdomen, which is inspection, auscultation, percussion, and palpation. Although Option #1 may be done, it does not answer what the question is asking.

Disorders

10. **(1)** Diarrhea is a common symptom in infectious gastroenteritis, inflammatory bowel disease, diverticulitis, and early intestinal obstruction. Diseases of the colon or rectum are often associated with constipation that clearly precedes the onset of abdominal pain. With sexually transmitted diseases, abdominal pain can often occur with vaginal discharge or bleeding and sometimes irregular menses. Dysuria, flank pain, hematuria, and urinary frequency are common signs and symptoms of upper or lower urinary tract infections or ureteral calculi.

11. **(3)** Esophageal pain may radiate to the neck and left arm. Gallbladder pain can radiate to the infrascapular area, diaphragm pain to the right shoulder, and the pain of appendicitis to the periumbilical area.

12. **(2)** The most important goal in evaluating a client who presents with abdominal pain is to rule out emergent conditions. Palpation is done after auscultation. Begin in an area away from the site of the pain. It is important to rule out emergent causes and ideal to make an exact diagnosis every time. However, due to the sometimes complicated nature of abdominal pain, it is not always possible to do this. Ordering appropriate laboratory tests is important but is not the most important goal.

13. **(4)** A tense, hard abdomen, verbal refusal or severe pain when asked to jump, or a positive obturator sign are positive peritoneal signs. Costovertebral angle tenderness is a sign of a renal disorder. Stool for occult blood is not a test for peritonitis. Decreased bowel sounds could be present in appendicitis or bowel obstruction but is not a peritoneal sign.

14. **(2)** Localized pain that steadily increases for 6 or more hours with rebound tenderness and guarding could be caused by an emergent condition, such as appendicitis or ruptured ectopic pregnancy. Pain in an adolescent girl that is relieved by having a bowel movement could be constipation; pain that is sudden in onset and in the right lower quadrant and lasting 14–36 hours could be mittelschmerz, if the girl is midway through her menstrual cycle. Pain that follows the onset of vomiting and diarrhea usually occurs in gastroenteritis.

15. **(4)** Atypical pain or pain that occurs with hematochezia, anemia, or weight loss could be caused by a disorder other than peptic ulcer, such as gastric cancer, or the client's ulcer could be bleeding. Pain that awakens a client early in the morning from sleep or is relieved or worsened by food ingestion is typical of peptic ulcer pain.

16. **(4)** Irritable bowel syndrome presents with abdominal pain and/or altered bowel habits. These symptoms can be aggravated by psychological stresses. Symptoms disappear while sleeping. Bacterial or viral gastroenteritis presents as abdominal pain with diarrhea and vomiting of abrupt onset. Drug-induced diarrhea follows initiation of drug therapy, and in this situation, there is no mention of previous drug therapy. In

inflammatory bowel disease, nocturnal diarrhea and abdominal pain are often accompanied by rectal fistula, fever, and/or skin lesions. Diarrhea occurring with giardiasis is malodorous. Weight loss occurs over a period of weeks.

17. **(3)** Cold liquids causing pain, dysphagia for both liquids and solids, and repeated swallowing or performance of a rapid Valsalva maneuver that helps food or liquid pass into the stomach are experiences reported by clients with dysphagia caused by a motility disorder. Those with dysphagia due to obstruction have more difficulty swallowing solids than liquids, can have a stricture due to esophagitis resulting from longstanding esophageal reflux, and may report marked weight loss if a tumor is present.

18. **(1)** Esophageal inflammation caused by excessive reflux that overpowers the normal mucosal defense mechanism leads to symptoms of reflux. People with and without a hiatal hernia can experience gastroesophageal reflux. Physiologic or normal reflux occurs in most people after eating when they are in an upright position, especially during vigorous exercise; however, its low frequency and small volume do not lead to symptoms. Symptoms of peptic ulcer disease are initiated by erosion of the gastrointestinal mucosa.

19. **(2)** The factor contributing most to reflux is an abnormal antireflux barrier, the LES. Hiatal hernia is not believed to play an important factor in the etiology of reflux. Reflux occurs postprandially in the upright position and may be exacerbated by meals, but overeating is not a direct cause. Alcohol and excessive use of caffeine may affect the LES pressure.

20. **(3)** The etiologic agents that produce inflammation and cause diarrhea are characterized by positive fecal leukocytes. Viral diarrhea is free of pus, thus no fecal leukocytes would be found on the smear. Noninflammatory diarrhea is usually caused by a rotavirus. Toxigenic bacteria cause diarrhea by elaborating toxins that have been released after bacterial growth in the intestines. These poisonous substances result in secretory diarrhea.

21. **(3)** The female-to-male ratio for IBS is 4:1. It is a disease of young or middle-aged adults, frequently appearing at age 20–25.

22. **(4)** A common means of hepatitis B transmission is from mother to baby, perinatally. Other mechanisms of transmission are by infected body fluids, sexual contact, and parenterally. Hepatitis E virus is spread in contaminated water. Hepatitis A's mode of transmission is fecal–oral and person-to-person.

23. **(3)** The client is presenting with the most reliable symptoms of GERD. GERD is most often related to inappropriate relaxation of the LES, which allows reflux of gastric acid and pepsin into the distal esophagus. Common presentations of IBS are differentiated by cramping, abdominal pain, or altered bowel habits predominating. Clients with esophagitis complain of the acute onset of chest pain, dysphagia, and odynophagia. Bleeding is associated with carcinoma.

24. **(1)** Hepatitis A and E do not have a chronic stage and generally resolve without any long-term effects.

25. **(2)** These parasites reside in the intestine. Females lay eggs on the skin outside the anus, resulting in extreme pruritus. The only host is humans. Hookworm larvae reside in the soil, enter the body through the feet, and can cause anemia. When dirt containing roundworm eggs is ingested due to pica or on unwashed vegetables, or when contaminated water is consumed, an intestinal infestation occurs. Giardiasis results from ingestion of the protozoan *Giardia lamblia* through contaminated water or via oral–fecal transmission.

26. **(1)** A high-energy diet is used for clients with anorexia. Management of GERD includes weight reduction, avoidance of lying down after meals, avoidance of large meals, avoidance of exercise after meals, and elevating the head of the bed. Certain foods and drinks, such as alcohol, mint, and orange juice, should be avoided, as they may cause symptoms of heartburn.

27. **(2)** *Helicobacter pylori* has been implicated in the etiology of peptic ulcer disease. The other organisms listed are implicated in other types of infections, such as acute otitis media and skin infections.

28. **(4)** Alcohol is the most important cause of cirrhosis in the United States. Especially in men, one six-pack of beer or four to six glasses of wine significantly increases the risk for long-term hepatic injury leading to cirrhosis. This amount is about half for women. Hepatitis A is a self-limited infection without a known chronic state. Hepatitis B and D acute infections do not directly result in a high incidence of cirrhosis.

29. **(2)** A hemorrhoid results when a vascular anal cushion prolapses through the anal canal and is entrapped by the internal anal sphincter. In a rectal mucosa prolapse, the wall of the rectum prolapses. A tumor is not a vascular anal cushion.

30. **(2)** These characteristics describe hepatitis B. Hepatitis A has similar symptoms but can be transmitted by the oral–fecal or oral–genital route and has an incubation period of 15–50 days and no chronic form. Hepatitis C infection rarely causes jaundice. It is transmitted parenterally and has an incubation period of 14–140 days and a chronic form. Hepatitis D coexists with hepatitis B, is transmitted parenterally, and can also become chronic. Hepatitis E is characterized by oral–fecal transmission associated with contaminated food and water, an incubation period of 14–60 days, and no chronic disease state.

31. **(2)** While most clients need eventual intervention, those who are elderly and diabetic are at increased risk and should be hospitalized for prompt diagnosis, intravenous fluids, pain control, and surgical consultation.

32. **(4)** Clients with a history of heavy alcohol intake are at increased risk for cirrhosis and portal hypertension, which may result in variceal bleeding. These clients often present clinically with bleeding, hypotension, and eventual shock.

33. **(3)** A strangulated hernia is irreducible and the blood supply to the trapped bowel is compromised, resulting in bowel infarction. Ulcers, endometriosis, and ectopic pregnancy can cause abdominal pain and can be surgical emergencies, but they do not cause bowel obstruction.

34. **(2)** Increasing crampy abdominal pain that starts as periumbilical pain, anorexia, and fever are classic symptoms of appendicitis. The client should be evaluated by a surgeon to decrease the risk of rupture of the appendix. While ectopic pregnancy should always be a consideration in young females with abdominal pain, the characteristics of the pain and other symptoms are not typical of an ectopic pregnancy.

35. **(3)** Thrombosed hemorrhoids can cause severe pain for clients and should be quickly decompressed. Although they are irritating and cause itching, pinworms do not cause rectal pain. Hookworms penetrate the soles of the feet, and cystitis usually causes lower abdominal pain, not rectal pain.

36. **(2)** Diverticular disease presents with change in bowel habits (diarrhea alternating with constipation or both) and blood in stool. If diverticulitis develops, flatus, low-grade fever, and leukocytosis may be present. The majority of clients with diverticulosis may have no symptoms; some may have abdominal pain in the left lower quadrant. Appendicitis may present with pain in the right lower quadrant and may not be severe until perforation occurs. Other signs may include nausea and vomiting, leukocytosis, and fever may or may not be present. Irritable bowel syndrome may present with aching or cramping periumbilical or lower abdominal pain often precipitated by meals and relieved by defecation. Pain may radiate to the left chest or arm, and there are alternating episodes of diarrhea and constipation. Pancreatitis may present with epigastric pain or tenderness that lasts for hours and may radiate to the back; there may also be fever, nausea and vomiting, mental confusion, and jaundice.

37. **(1)** A high-fiber diet is the treatment for this disease and vegetarians eat increased amounts of fruits, vegetables, grains, and cereals. Options #2, #3, and #4 are at higher risk because they do not address the concept of fiber.

38. **(4)** Colorectal cancer occurs most commonly in individuals over age 50. A change in bowel habit with reduced caliber of stool and blood mixed with the stool are characteristic of left-sided colon cancer, which is the most common site. Anemia is found with right-sided lesions. Bright red rectal bleeding and tenesmus are characteristic of rectal cancer.

39. **(1)** Colon cancer risk in pancolonic ulcerative colitis increases by 2% per year after the tenth year of diagnosis.

40. **(2)** Excessive vomiting with loss of acid is a common problem with metabolic alkalosis. Respiratory problems do not precipitate primary metabolic acid-base imbalance, and renal disease most often causes metabolic acidosis.

41. **(4)** In irritable bowel syndrome abdominal pain predominates. Altered bowel habits with either diarrhea or constipation are also seen. Clinical findings associated with carcinoma of the colon include mild, occult blood loss with intermittent episodes of acute bleeding. Clinical features of Crohn's disease include severe weight loss, abdominal pain, growth failure, and weight loss. Clinical features of ulcerative colitis include diarrhea, rectal bleeding, and moderate weight loss.

42. **(3)** Appendicitis usually begins as dull periumbilical pain accompanied by anorexia and nausea, but not necessarily vomiting. Within a few hours there may be low-grade fever. Most laboratory tests are normal. A WBC count of >15,000/mm^3 is often noted but neither confirms nor excludes the diagnosis of appendicitis.

Pharmacology

43. **(1)** Goals of PUD treatment include relief of pain, healing of ulcer, and cost effectiveness.

The H$_2$ receptor antagonists heal 90% of duodenal ulcers and 70% of gastric ulcers. The proton pump inhibitors such as omeprazole are recommended for ulcers unresponsive to the receptor antagonists after 8–12 weeks with full dosing and GERD. The anticholinergic drugs doxepin (Sinequan) and pirenzepine are useful when used with the H$_2$ receptors but are limited by side effects, and are used only in Canada and Europe at this time.

44. **(1)** The prostaglandins, such as misoprostol (Cytotec), are used to decrease recurrent ulcerations in clients who require NSAIDs. They have not, however, been shown to increase ulcer healing. Cimetidine (Tagamet) has been shown to increase healing. Doxepin (Sinequan) and pirenzepine are not prescribed in the United States as of this date.

45. **(2)** If a person exposed to a client known to be positive for hepatitis B has sufficient immunity to hepatitis B, no treatment is necessary. If this same person had not been vaccinated, in addition to initiation of the hepatitis B vaccine series, HBIG 0.06 ml/kg IM is also administered. If an exposed person has had an inadequate immune response to the hepatitis B vaccine series, a hepatitis B booster is given. There is no need to repeat the series. If the response to the hepatitis B vaccine series is unknown, test the exposed person's hepatitis B surface antigen level and decide what intervention, if any, is needed.

46. **(2)** Clients with refractory ulcers due to *H. pylori* are most successfully treated with the triple-drug therapy of Pepto-Bismol, amoxicillin or tetracycline, and metronidazole (Flagyl). Less effective but well-tolerated regimens consist of omeprazole (Prilosec) and amoxicillin.

47. **(2)** Sulfasalazine (Azulfidine) therapy for clients with mild ulcerative colitis results in symptomatic improvement in 50–75% of cases. If no response is seen after 2–4 weeks, the addition of prednisone is recommended. This drug prevents relapse of ulcerative colitis once remission is induced. The other drugs listed are not recommended as first-line treatment.

48. **(2)** Since 25% of clients are effectively treated with lifestyle changes, therapy should begin with use of these measures. If these are not completely effective, an H_2 receptor antagonist can be added. Twice-daily dosing is recommended. Omeprazole (Prilosec) is recommended only for refractory cases. Cisapride (Propulsid) can be effective, but lifestyle changes and antacid tablets as needed is the recommended starting point for therapy.

49. **(1)** To minimize the risk of a contact developing hepatitis A, immunoglobulin 0.02 ml/kg should be given as soon as possible after exposure. It has not been shown to be effective if administered more than 2 weeks after exposure.

50. **(3)** Treatment with trimethoprim-sulfamethoxazole shortens the course and prevents further spread of the organism. Prevention of dehydration that can result from the diarrhea is accomplished through symptomatic treatment (clear liquids for 24–48 hours, no dairy products, electrolyte-rich sports drinks, advance diet as tolerated). Antidiarrheal medications are not recommended because intestinal motility is important in recovery. Option #4 would be appropriate treatment for nonpregnant adults who have giardiasis.

51. **(1)** The Emetrol dose for adults is 15–30 ml. Phenergan 25 mg can be given to children over 12 years old (not 6 years old) and adults. The older child and adult dose for hydroxyzine hydrochloride (Vistaril) is 25–100 mg. Trimethobenzamide (Tigan) is dosed at 200 mg, not 10 mg.

52. **(4)** For clients with exposure to hepatitis B and who are unvaccinated, administer one dose of HBIG and initiate the vaccine. If the client thinks they may have been vaccinated but does not know if they responded, the nurse practitioner may have a prevaccination antibody testing done. The HBe antibody is tested for to determine the potential for transmission; it generally appears about 3 months after the onset of the infection.

53. **(3)** The only contraindication to the hepatitis B vaccine is prior anaphylaxis or severe hypersensitivity to the vaccine or components of the vaccine.

54. **(2)** This medication causes problems with nephrotoxicity and ototoxicity (eighth cranial nerve). Laboratory tests to monitor renal function should be determined on a regular basis. The client should be frequently evaluated for any hearing loss. The geriatric client is particularly susceptible to the complications and toxicity.

13

Hematology

Physical Examination & Diagnostic Tests

1. On physical examination, a palpable, firm, nontender, supraclavicular lymph node is noted on the left side of the body. This information is consistent with a diagnosis of:

    1. Bacterial infection draining from the internal jugular chain.

    2. Thoracic or abdominal malignancy.

    3. Inflammation of the tonsils and adenoids.

    4. Non-Hodkin's lymphoma.

2. The nurse practitioner describes a "shotty" lymph node as:

    1. Tender, mobile, and >5 mm.

    2. Small and pellet-like.

    3. Discrete and cystic.

    4. Irregular, soft, and fixed to surrounding tissue.

3. A macrocytic, normochromic anemia is diagnosed in an elderly woman. The next test(s) that should be ordered is(are):

    1. Serum iron and total iron-binding capacity TIBC levels.

    2. Bone marrow biopsy.

    3. Colonoscopy.

    4. Vitamin B_{12} and red blood cell (RBC)-folate levels.

4. After confirming the diagnosis of iron deficiency anemia in an adult client based on standard laboratory values (complete blood count [CBC], peripheral smear, serum iron, TIBC, serum ferritin), what would be the next essential test for the nurse practitioner to order?

    1. Stool guaiac $\times$ 3.

    2. Prothrombin time and partial thromboplastin time.

    3. Liver function tests.

    4. Endoscopy.

5. Evaluation of an elderly female client reveals a macrocytic, normochromic anemia. Subsequent testing shows a folate level that is normal and a decreased vitamin B_{12} level. Further evaluation should include:

   1. Referral to a hematologist for a bone marrow biopsy.

   2. Schilling's test.

   3. Upper gastrointestinal (GI) series.

   4. No tests are indicated at this time.

6. The most sensitive test for the diagnosis of sickle cell anemia is:

   1. CBC with a peripheral smear.

   2. Bone marrow biopsy and aspiration.

   3. Hemoglobin electrophoresis.

   4. Hemoglobin and hematocrit.

7. In evaluating the laboratory findings on a young adolescent with iron deficiency anemia, the nurse practitioner expects:

   1. MCV 80 and reticulocyte count low.

   2. MCV 120 and hemoglobin 12 gm.

   3. MCV 99 and hematocrit 34%.

   4. MCV 96 and normal reticulocyte count.

8. An elderly female presents to the nurse practitioner's office with complaints of fatigue, dizziness, decreased activity tolerance, and occasional bounding heart rate. Physical examination reveals pallor (including mucous membranes), tachycardia, and general appearance of lethargy. The following tests are ordered: CBC with differential, peripheral smear, serum iron, TIBC, and serum ferritin. These tests are ordered because there is a high index of suspicion of:

   1. Sideroblastic anemia.

   2. Pernicious anemia.

   3. Folic acid deficiency anemia.

   4. Iron deficiency anemia.

9. Anemia of chronic disease would reveal which of the lab findings?

   1. Decreased iron, decreased TIBC, and decreased serum ferritin.

   2. Decreased iron, decreased TIBC, and increased serum ferritin.

   3. Decreased iron, increased TIBC, and decreased serum ferritin.

   4. Decreased iron, increased TIBC, and increased serum ferritin.

Disorders

10. Sickle cell anemia is caused by:

    1. Exposure to ionizing radiation.

    2. A genetically induced production of abnormal hemoglobin S.

    3. A deficiency of dietary folic acid.

    4. Long-term use of thiazide diuretics.

11. An adult client presents to the nurse practitioner with a history of erythrocytosis. One common complaint that could cause a serious complication for this client is:

    1. A laceration.

    2. Vomiting and diarrhea.

    3. Coughing.

    4. Dizziness.

12. A young adult female has a folic acid deficiency anemia. The nurse practitioner teaches the client to eat foods rich in folic acid such as:

    1. Green leafy vegetables, nuts, and liver.

    2. Carrots, salmon, and avocados.

    3. Cottage cheese, yogurt, and skim milk.

    4. Lima beans, brussel sprouts, and potatoes.

13. Which of the changes occur in the RBC indices for pernicious anemia?

    1. Microcytic, normochromic.

    2. Microcytic, hypochromic.

3. Normocytic, normochromic.

4. Macrocytic, normochromic.

14. Iron deficiency anemia is an example of:

    1. Macrocytic, normochromic anemia.

    2. Macrocytic, hypochromic anemia.

    3. Microcytic, hypochromic anemia.

    4. Normocytic, normochromic anemia.

15. A client with pernicious anemia may present with which signs/symptoms?

    1. Paresthesias, unsteady gait, lethargy and fatigue.

    2. Hepatomegaly, jaundice, and right upper quadrant pain.

    3. Hypertension, angina, and peripheral edema.

    4. Blurred vision, diplopia, and decreased visual acuity.

16. A young female client presents to the clinic for a routine checkup. History is unremarkable, and on physical exam, an enlarged (2-cm) mobile, nontender and rubbery lymph node is palpated on the left posterior cervical chain. The nurse practitioner's next step is:

    1. Order a throat culture and monospot.

    2. Referral to a surgeon for a lymph node biopsy.

    3. Order a STAT chest x-ray.

    4. No intervention is necessary at this time.

17. In teaching a client with anemia to include foods rich in iron in her diet, the nurse practitioner encourages the client to eat:

    1. Cheese, milk, and yogurt.

    2. Red beans, whole-grain bread, and bran cereal.

    3. Tomatoes, cabbage, and citrus fruits.

    4. Beef, spinach, and peanut butter.

18. Anemia of chronic disease is associated with:

    1. Malnutrition and vitamin B_{12} deficiency.

2. Infections, inflammation, and neoplasms.

3. Traumatic injuries and folate deficiency.

4. Excessive menstrual flow, trauma, and heredity.

19. The nurse practitioner is counseling a client who has a child with sickle cell disease. The client asks, "If my child has sickle cell disease, does that mean that I am at an increased risk for developing the same problems?" The nurse practitioner's response would be based on what principle of sickle cell disease?

    1. The mother is at an increased risk, because the condition is inherited; she probably has the condition and has not had an active episode.

    2. There is no risk for the mother developing the condition, as males are the carriers of the trait.

    3. There is a 25% chance that the mother will be affected by the disease, especially at times of stress.

    4. The parents are both carriers of the trait, but they do not have the active disease; each child has a 25% chance of having the condition.

20. Anemia of chronic disease is a:

    1. Normochromic, normocytic anemia.

    2. Normochromic, microcytic anemia.

    3. Hypochromic, microcytic anemia.

    4. Hypochromic, macrocytic anemia.

21. The nurse practitioner understands that most adult clients with Hodgkin's disease present with:

    1. Nausea, vomiting, and diarrhea.

    2. Night sweats, weight loss and fever.

    3. Painless, movable mass in the neck, axilla, or groin.

    4. Hepatosplenomegaly with a painful mass in the mediastinum.

22. What is the most common leukemia found in the older adult and is typically asymptomatic and characterized by a median survival rate of approximately 10 years?

    1. Acute myelogenous.

    2. Chronic myelogenous.

    3. Acute lymphocytic.

    4. Chronic lymphocytic.

Pharmacology

23. The nurse practitioner determines that an adult female client has an iron deficiency anemia, and has ruled out GI bleeding as the cause. The nurse practitioner:

    1. Refers the client to a hematologist.

    2. Refers the client to a GI specialist.

    3. Prescribes ferrous sulfate 300 mg PO tid, and has the client return in 1 month for a repeat CBC, serum iron, and TIBC.

    4. Has the client return in 6 months for additional stool guaiac testing.

24. Teaching clients regarding the treatment of vitamin B_{12} deficiency includes:

    1. The client will receive vitamin B_{12} tablets given twice daily for 1 year.

    2. Oral folic acid supplements will be given daily for the client's lifetime.

    3. Monthly cyanocobalamin (vitamin B_{12}) injections will be given for the client's lifetime (after being given weekly for the first month).

    4. Iron supplementation and monthly blood transfusions will be required until the deficiency is corrected.

25. Treatment of anemia of chronic disease should include:

    1. A folic acid supplement, 1 mg PO qd.

    2. Iron sulfate ($FeSO_4$) supplement, 300 mg PO tid.

    3. Treatment of the underlying condition.

    4. Weekly epoetin alfa (Epogen) injections.

13 Answers & Rationales

Physical Examination & Diagnostic Tests

1. **(2)** A Virchow's node in the left supraclavicular region is of concern due to the high correlation with abdominal or thoracic malignancy. Infections and inflammatory conditions produce tender, inflamed lymph nodes.

2. **(2)** Shotty, or small and pellet-like, lymph nodes that are movable, cool, nontender, discrete, and up to 3 mm in diameter are usually considered normal.

3. **(4)** It is important to determine which type of macrocytic anemia a client has, so that the appropriate therapy can be ordered. Therefore, the vitamin B_{12} and RBC-folate levels would be ordered. These tests would determine if the client has a pernicious anemia (the most common type) or a folate deficiency (also common in the elderly). Serum iron and TIBC would be ordered if an iron deficiency anemia was suspected (it is not in this case because it is a microcytic anemia). There is no indication for a colonoscopy. It would be premature to order a bone marrow biopsy at this point, without performing initial testing and potentially overlooking an easily treated condition (i.e., pernicious anemia, folate deficiency anemia).

4. **(1)** Stool guaiac would identify blood loss from the GI tract, the most common cause of iron deficiency anemia. The other tests should be done if the stool guaiacs are positive. Finding the cause of the iron deficiency is paramount, and the stool guaiac is an easy, noninvasive method of ruling out bleeding as the cause.

5. **(2)** A Schilling's test will determine the cause of the vitamin B_{12} deficiency. It will distinguish between inadequate intake, an intrinsic factor deficiency, or a malabsorption problem. This will allow the practitioner to prescribe the most appropriate therapy for the client. A bone marrow biopsy and an upper GI series is not indicated at this time.

6. **(3)** Normal and abnormal hemoglobins can be detected by electrophoresis, which matches hemolyzed red cell material against standard bands for the various known hemoglobins, including hemoglobin S (the abnormal hemoglobin that is associated with sickle cell anemia). CBC with peripheral smear, and hemoglobin/ hematocrit would not yield enough information to diagnose sickle cell anemia. Bone marrow biopsy would not be necessary and would not indicate the presence of hemoglobin S.

7. **(1)** The findings associated with iron deficiency anemia include a low mean corpuscular volume (MCV) (<90), decreased hemoglobin and hematocrit, and a low reticulocyte count. An elevated MCV is associated with macrocytic anemias (i.e., pernicious anemia).

8. **(4)** This client's clinical picture is a classic presentation for anemia. Further testing would be needed to determine the type of anemia involved. The most common cause in elderly males is GI bleeding, which would cause an iron deficiency anemia. The tests that were ordered would confirm or rule out this diagnosis; the peripheral smear is especially important in diagnosing the specific type of anemia. If the smear ruled out the diagnosis of iron deficiency anemia, it would lead the practitioner to other diagnoses (including the remaining choices) and appropriate laboratory tests required for confirmation.

9. **(2)** Normal to increased iron stores (serum ferritin) with concurrent low serum iron is the hallmark finding of anemia of chronic disease. The serum iron is decreased along with the TIBC. Options #1 and #4 contain incorrect information for the anemias. Option #3 contains the findings for iron deficiency anemia.

Disorders

10. **(2)** Sickle cell anemia is a genetic disorder characterized by the production of hemoglobin S, an anemia secondary to shortened erythrocyte survival, microvascular occlusion by sickle-shaped erythrocytes, and an increased susceptibility to certain infections. Exposure to ionizing radiation has been associated with the development of certain malignancies, especially leukemia. A deficiency of dietary folic acid does not cause sickle cell anemia, although folic acid is used in the treatment of these clients to help increase hematopoiesis and aid in recovery from aplastic events. Long-term use of thiazide diuretics has been implicated in the development of hemolytic or aplastic anemias. in very rare cases.

11. **(2)** Erythrocytosis (or polycythemia) can be worsened by dehydration from any cause. Coughing and dizziness will have no effect on the condition and a laceration may actually improve the symptoms due to the blood loss.

12. **(1)** Green leafy vegetables, nuts, and liver are excellent sources of folic acid. Also,

cereals and breads are now fortified with folic acid. The other foods are not significant sources of folic acid.

13. **(4)** A macrocytic (MCV >100), normochromic anemia resulting from atrophic gastric mucosa not secreting intrinsic factor is the definition for pernicious anemia. These indices could also include folic acid deficiency anemia. Options #1 and #2 could include iron deficiency anemia or anemia of chronic disease. Option #3 could also include anemia of chronic disease.

14. **(3)** Iron deficiency anemia is a microcytic, hypochromic anemia. The red blood cells are smaller (microcytic) due to the decrease in hemoglobin production caused by inadequate amounts of iron. This also makes the cell appear pale (hypochromic). The other selections describe other types of anemia, and would be determined by the peripheral smear.

15. **(1)** A deficiency in vitamin B_{12} can cause neurologic signs and symptoms including paresthesias, an unsteady gait, lethargy, and fatigue. These findings are specific to pernicious anemia, and so must always be assessed for in any client who presents with an anemia. The other signs and symptoms are not characteristic of pernicious anemia.

16. **(2)** Lymphadenopathy as described, without evidence of infection, should always be referred to a surgeon for biopsy, because biopsy is the only definitive test to rule out a malignancy (a frequent cause of lymphadenopathy, not caused by infectious processes). There are no signs or symptoms to suggest the need for a throat culture, monospot, or chest x-ray. Not intervening is not appropriate because the cause of lymphadenopathy needs to be determined.

17. **(4)** Beef, spinach, and peanut butter are iron-rich foods. The remaining selections are examples of foods rich in calcium, fiber, and vitamin C, respectively.

18. **(2)** Anemia of chronic disease is associated with infections (i.e., tuberculosis), chronic inflammatory conditions (i.e., systemic lupus erythematosus, rheumatoid arthritis), and malignancies. Excessive blood loss from menstrual flow or traumatic injuries would more likely cause an iron deficiency anemia.

Malnutrition can contribute to iron, vitamin B_{12}, and folate deficiencies.

19. **(4)** Sickle cell disease is transmitted by two parents who have the sickle cell trait but do not show symptoms of the disease. Each pregnancy carries a 25% chance of sickle cell disease and 25% chance of the child carrying the trait.

20. **(1)** Anemia of chronic disease is a chronic normochromic, normocytic anemia. There is normal production of hemoglobin, along with normal maturation of red blood cells.

21. **(3)** Most clients present a painless, movable mass in the neck, axilla, or groin. Older clients may present with fatigue, weight loss, or persistent fever, and night sweats. Often, there is pain in diseased areas after consuming alcohol (an unexplained finding). Hepatosplenomegaly presents with advanced disease.

22. **(4)** Chronic lympocytic leukemia (CLL) is found primarily in the middle and older adult; fewer than 10% of all clients are under the age of 50. Acute myelogenous leukemia (AML) incidence increases with age and approximately 50% are younger than 50 years of age. Chronic myelogenous leukemia (CML) occurs most often at a median age of 45. Acute lymphocytic leukemia (ALL) is most common in children and gradually increases in frequency in later life.

Pharmacology

23. **(3)** Treatment with iron orally for at least 6 months is necessary to correct both the anemia and the depleted body stores. The client should have the hemoglobin, hematocrit, iron, and TIBC rechecked after 1 month on iron supplementation. If there is not improvement in all parameters, most notably a rise in the hemoglobin by 1 gm/dl, the client should be referred to a hematologist. There is no need to refer to a GI specialist or repeat the guaiac, because there is no indication that this client's condition is caused by bleeding.

24. **(3)** If the deficiency is not due to inadequate intake, the client will require lifetime supplementation of vitamin B_{12}. It must be given in the form of an intramuscular or subcutaneous injection to ensure absorption. Oral folic acid, iron, and blood transfusions would not treat the cause of the deficiency, and therefore the resulting anemia would not be corrected.

25. **(3)** Treatment of the underlying condition leads to resolution of the anemia of chronic disease. Folic acid and iron supplements are indicated for folate and iron deficiency anemias, respectively. Epoetin alfa (Epogen) injections are indicated for those conditions that affect erythropoiesis, namely, chronic renal failure, chemotherapy-induced anemia, and acquired immunodeficiency syndrome.

14

Urinary

Physical Examination & Diagnostic Tests

1. When taking a history on voiding patterns in adults, the nurse practitioner knows:

   1. Adults normally void q2–3h in a 24-hour period (8–12 times a day).

   2. The first sensation to void occurs when the bladder fills to 200–30 ml.

   3. Normally, 15–20 minutes passes between the first urge to void and when the functional capacity is reached.

   4. Adults typically reach functional (comfortable) capacity at 200–300 ml and may experience some leakage if voiding is delayed.

2. A urinalysis that suggests a urinary tract infection shows:

   1. Protein only.

   2. Alkaline pH and positive nitrite and leukocyte esterase.

   3. Hematuria and pyuria only.

   4. Red color without the presence of red blood cells.

3. An intravenous urography and voiding cystourethrography assists in diagnosing:

   1. Congenital anomalies, stone formation, or foreign bodies.

   2. Renal size and the presence of stone.

   3. A problem in the urethra, prostate, or bladder.

   4. Visualization of the ureter and renal pelvis.

4. According to the Agency for Health Care Policy and Research (AHCPR) Guideline Panel, the basic continence evaluation for the primary care provider includes:

   1. History, physical examination, measurement of postvoid residual volume, and urinalysis.

   2. Measurement of postvoid residual volume, blood urea nitrogen (BUN), serum creatinine, and urinalysis.

   3. History, physical examination, serum glucose, BUN, serum creatinine, and urinalysis.

   4. Urodynamic, endoscopic, and imaging tests; urinalysis and serum creatinine.

5. The nurse practitioner expects which findings on examination of an older client with dehydration?

   1. Tongue furrows and skin tenting on the forehead.

   2. Specific gravity of urine 1.004.

   3. Pulse rate, 58, strong and regular; blood pressure (BP) 100/62.

   4. Geographic tongue and reduced saliva pool.

6. A young adult comes to the student health clinic complaining of severe abdominal discomfort and bloody urine. Priority in the diagnostic work-up should include:

   1. Intravenous pyelogram (IVP) to rule out a kidney stone.

   2. Straining all urine.

   3. Microscopic urine exam.

   4. A 24-hour urine culture.

Disorders

7. An older adult female client explains to the nurse practitioner that she has been having frequent and painful urination. The nurse practitioner orders a clean-catch urine for routine urinalysis and culture and sensitivity. The laboratory culture and sensitivity report is as follows: 10^5 *Escherichia coli* and 10^4 *Staphylococcus epidermidis* per milliliter. The nurse practitioner would:

   1. Treat the *E. coli*.

   2. Order penicillin.

   3. Treat the *S. epidermidis*.

   4. Encourage citric fruit juices.

8. An elderly female client is incontinent of urine. What should the nurse practitioner advise the family caretaker to avoid using on the skin in the perineal area?

   1. Petrolatum.

   2. Moisture-barrier films.

   3. Mild soap and water.

   4. zinc oxide ointment.

9. Which plan would be most appropriate for an older client with functional incontinence?

   1. Evaluate need for pads.

   2. Limit fluid intake in the evenings.

   3. Perform Credé's maneuver.

   4. Provide a bedside commode.

10. The usual clinical presentation of an adult client with cystitis is:

    1. No symptoms noted.

    2. Acute onset of chills, fever, flank pain, headache, malaise, and costovertebral angle tenderness.

    3. Complaints of dysuria, urgency, frequency, nocturia, and suprapubic heaviness.

    4. Signs and symptoms of fever, irritability, decreased appetite, vomiting, diarrhea, constipation, dehydration, and jaundice.

11. A possible cause of transient urinary incontinence, which can be reversed, is:

    1. Poor pelvic support causing hypermobility of the base of the bladder in females.

    2. Lower urinary tract problems, such as carcinoma.

    3. Cystocele or uterine prolapse in women.

    4. Ingestion of certain medications, such as sedatives, diuretics, anticholinergic agents, and α-adrenergic agents.

12. Functional incontinence is:

    1. Leakage of urine during activities that increase abdominal pressure, such as coughing, sneezing, laughing, or other physical activities.

    2. Mainly caused by factors outside the urinary tract, such as dementia or immobility that prohibit proper toileting habits.

3. Characterized by the inability to delay urination with an abrupt and strong desire to void.

4. The occurrence of incontinence with overdistention of the bladder.

13. The two most common pathogens in community-acquired urinary tract infections are:

1. *Klebsiella penumoniae* and *Proteus mirabilis*.

2. Staphylococcus saprophyticus and *Escherichia coli*.

3. *Proteus mirabilis* and *Staphylococcus saprophyticus*.

4. *Escherichia coli* and *Proteus mirabilis*.

14. Recurrent urinary tract infections in older adult females are due to relapse or reinfection. The nurse practitioner understands that relapse:

1. Is less common than reinfection and occurs within 2 weeks of the completion of drug therapy for the infection.

2. Is responsible for most recurrent urinary tract infections in females.

3. May occur due to residual urine after voiding due to a prolapsed uterus or bladder or to lack of estrogen.

4. Can be treated with the same medication regimen as the original infection.

15. A client has a renal stone that consists of uric acid. What is the best diet to order for this client to decrease the incidence of the stone formation?

1. Alkaline ash diet and low purine.

2. High purine and an acid ash diet.

3. Increased fluid intake and high doses of vitamin C.

4. High complex carbohydrate and decreased protein.

16. The nurse practitioner understands that the treatment of pyelonephritis:

1. In females is suggestive of a structural problem.

2. Requires hospitalization, parenteral antibiotic therapy, and an IVP in males.

3. In females requires hospitalization, parenteral antibiotic therapy, and an IVP.

4. Requires no follow-up.

17. A client is diagnosed with renal failure and the origin of the problem is thought to be postrenal. What would the nurse practitioner identify as a possible precipitating cause of this client's renal failure?

1. History of myocardial infarction with severe hypotensive episode.

2. Advanced prostate hypertrophy with hematuria.

3. Renal vascular changes secondary to a long history of diabetes.

4. Exposure to carbon tetrachloride on his job site.

18. Urinary incontinence associated with conditions such as Parkinson's disease, Alzheimer's disease, and stroke is termed:

1. Stress incontinence.

2. Urge incontinence.

3. Frequency incontinence.

4. Overflow incontinence.

19. A female client presents with complaints of blood in her urine; it is painless and she has no difficulty with voiding. The nurse practitioner obtains a urinalysis to confirm the presence of blood and there is no bacteria present. What is the priority diagnosis that must be ruled out on this client?

1. Postrenal failure.

2. Prerenal failure.

3. Renal calculi.

4. Cancer of the bladder.

20. The nurse practitioner is taking a history on a client who has been diagnosed with renal calculi. What information in the history would the practitioner identify as a precipitating factor in the development of renal calculi?

    1. Increased incidence of urinary tract infections over the past 3 years.

    2. Drinking 6–8 oz of milk daily.

    3. History of fractured femur and prolonged bed rest.

    4. High intake of citrus fruit and high-fiber carbohydrates.

21. A nurse practitioner recognizes what factors as contributing to the development of prerenal failure?

    1. History of an anaphylactic reaction that rendered the client unconscious.

    2. Extended treatment of an infection with gentamicin (Garamycin).

    3. Acute pyelonephritis and consequently glomerulonephritis.

    4. Renal vascular changes that occur secondary to atherosclerotic disease.

22. The nurse practitioner is teaching a female client some guidelines regarding bladder health which include all **except**:

    1. Drink at least six to eight glasses of water per day.

    2. Avoid doing Kegel's exercises.

    3. Avoid constipation.

    4. Consider estrogen replacement after menopause.

Pharmacology

23. The nurse practitioner has selected nitrofurantoin (Macrodantin) for treatment of a chronic urinary tract infection in a female geriatric client. What parameter should be evaluated prior to the administration of this medication?

    1. Determine creatinine clearance to be >50 ml/min.

    2. Evaluate levels of serum alanine aminotransferase (ALT).

    3. Any current medications that include anticoagulant agents.

    4. History of allergic reactions to sulfa-based medications.

24. Which of the following agents can be useful for stress incontinence?

    1. Propantheline (Pro-Banthine) 7.5–30 mg, three to five times a day.

    2. Oxybutynin (Ditropan) 2.5–5 mg tid to qid.

    3. Doxepin (Sinequan) 10–25 mg qd/bid/tid initially to a maximum total daily dose of 25–100 mg.

    4. Conjugated estrogen (Premarin) 0.3–1.25 mg/day orally or vaginally, medroxyprogesterone (Progestin) 2.5–10 mg/day either continuously or intermittently.

25. In order to decrease the production of uric acid stones, the nurse practitioner orders what medication?

    1. Allopurinol (Zyloprim).

    2. Potassium citrate (Urocit-K).

    3. Bethanechol (Urecholine).

    4. Phenazopyridine (Pyridium).

26. A 70-year-old woman is treated with oxybutynin (Ditropan) for her urinary frequency and urgency. The nurse practitioner would explain to the client she will probably experience:

    1. Increased sensitivity to sunlight.

    2. Dizziness when she stands up.

    3. A dry mouth and increased thirst.

    4. Increased bruising.

27. All of the following medications can cause urinary incontinence in the older adult **except**:

    1. Hypnotics.

    2. Antibiotics.

3. Sedatives.

4. Antidepressants.

28. A 46-year-old female with a history of renal calculi presents with complaints of severe flank pain radiating to her groin area. She is also experiencing nausea and vomiting. Her temperature is 99°F. What is the best initial order for the nurse practitioner to give at this time?

   1. Morphine sulfate 10 mg SC now.

   2. Ibuprofen (Advil) 600 mg PO now and q6h.

   3. Increase fluid intake and strain all urine.

   4. Trimethobenzamide (Tigan) 250 mg PO now.

29. The nurse practitioner is prescribing nitrofurantoin (Macrodantin) for a woman who is experiencing problems with urinary tract infections. What specific directions are given to this client regarding the administration of this medication?

   1. Medication should be taken with food and anticipate the urine to have brown discoloration.

2. Do not take medication with milk products and take on empty stomach for better absorption.

3. Take the medication four times a day until the symptoms have subsided for at least 24 hours.

4. Acetaminophen (Tylenol) and/or ibuprofen (Advil) should not be taken with this medication.

30. A young woman presents with complaints of burning on urination, frequency, and urgency. Phenazopyridine (Pyridium) is prescribed by the nurse practitioner. What specific directions are given to the client regarding this medication?

   1. May discolor contact lens; if sclera begin to turn yellow, return to the office.

   2. Always take the medication on an empty stomach to increase absorption.

   3. Do not take any medication containing aspirin or salicylate.

   4. May interfere with effectiveness of minipill for birth control.

14   Answers & Rationales

Physical Examination & Diagnostic Tests

1. **(2)** Adults normally void four to six times in a 24-hour period (q4–6h). Most usually do not get up in the middle of the night, unless they have a medical problem (e.g., urge incontinence). The feeling of the bladder filling occurs around 90–150 ml, with first urge occurring at 200–300 ml. Normally, 1–2 hours passes between the first urge to void and when the functional capacity is reached. Adults typically reach functional (comfortable) capacity at 300–600 ml and should *never* experience leakage if voiding is delayed.

2. **(2)** These are results indicating the presence of a urinary tract infection. Proteinuria alone suggests glomerulonephritis. Hematuria and pyuria without bacteria may indicate chlamydia, gonorrhea, viral infection or, less commonly, tuberculosis. If a dipstick test is negative for red blood cells but the urine color is red, a substance that can change the color of the urine is likely the cause.

3. **(1)** In an intravenous urography and voiding cystourethrography, congenital anomalies, stone formation, or foreign bodies can be identified. Renal size and the presence of stones can be seen in flat plate and upright films of the abdomen. In a cystoscopy, the urethra, prostate, and bladder can be visualized. A urethroscopy can visualize the ureter and renal pelvis.

4. **(1)** The 1996 AHCPR Guideline Panel encourages primary health care providers to initiate the basic evaluation of urinary incontinence by performing a history and physical examination, measurement of postvoid residual volume, and urinalysis. The other tests may be performed based on the findings from the initial evaluation.

5. **(1)** The classic sign of dehydration in the older adult is lack of skin turgor along with skin tenting on the forehead, concentrated urine (specific gravity >1.025), oliguria, sunken eyes, lack of axillary moisture, orthostatic blood pressure changes, tachycardia, dry mucous membranes of the mouth and nose, and absent or small saliva pool. It is important to examine the mouth, as it reveals reliable assessment data in the older adult suspected of having dehydration. A geographic tongue (patchy papillary loss giving rise to a map-like appearance) should not be confused with tongue furrows and tongue coating.

6. **(3)** The nurse practitioner suspects a urinary tract infection and needs to confirm with a microscopic urinalysis exam to identify presence of white blood cells (WBCs) and bacteria.

Disorders

7. **(1)** *E. coli* is the most common organism causing urinary tract infections in the young adult female and counts of 10^5 are diagnostic and should be treated with trimethoprim-sulfamethoxazole (Bactrim DS) or any suitable, sensitive anti-infective

agent. *S. epidermidis* is more often a contaminant due to inappropriate clean-catch specimen collection technique.

8. **(2)** Although moisture-barrier films may protect the skin from urine, they often contain alcohol and can further burn and irritate denuded skin. Cleansing with a mild soap and water helps prevent infections. Petrolatum and zinc oxide, which are types of moisture-barrier ointments, are used to prevent or treat irritant dermatitis.

9. **(4)** Functional incontinence is an inability to toilet appropriately due to impaired mobility. Providing physical assistance and guidance such as with wheelchairs, bedside commodes, that can be removed easily, and accessible facilities are effective with this type of incontinence. Evaluating the need for pads is effective with stress incontinence. Limiting fluid intake in the evenings to reduce nocturnal incontinence is appropriate for urge incontinence. Performing Credé's maneuver is appropriate for overflow incontinence.

10. **(3)** Cystitis in adults usually presents with dysuria, urgency, frequency, nocturia, and suprapubic heaviness. Acute onset of chills, fever, flank pain, headache, malaise, and costovertebral angle tenderness are common in pyelonephritis in adults.

11. **(4)** Sedative hypnotics, diuretics, anticholinergic agents, α-adrenergic agents, and calcium channel blockers can cause transient reversible urinary incontinence. Poor pelvic support is a possible cause of stress incontinence. Urge incontinence, or the inability to delay urination with a sudden and powerful urge to void, is a possible result of lower tract problems. A prolapsed uterus or bladder can cause overflow incontinence with overdistention of the bladder.

12. **(2)** Functional incontinence results from a client's inability to toilet appropriately. Stress incontinence is leakage from the bladder during activities that increase intra-abdominal pressure and, therefore, increase the pressure on the bladder, forcing some urine out. An inability to delay urination with a strong, abrupt urge to void is urge incontinence and is due to bladder hyperactivity or a hypersensitive bladder. The client often has little warning before urine passes out of the bladder. Incontinence with overdistention of the bladder is called overflow incontinence and is due to an underactive detrusor or one that will not contract or to bladder outlet or urethral obstruction. It is characterized by frequent urination in small amounts.

13. **(2)** *Escherichia coli* is the pathogen in 80–90% of community-acquired infections. Gram-positive *Staphylococcus saprophyticus* is the second most common pathogen. *Klebsiella pneumoniae* and *Proteus mirabilis* are also possible common pathogens. In hospital settings, *Escherichia coli* is less prevalent.

14. **(1)** Relapse is an uncommon cause of recurrent urinary tract infections in women and occurs within 2 weeks of completion of antibiotic therapy. It may need to be treated for 2–12 weeks. Reinfection is the cause of most urinary tract infections in women and may be due to residual urine due to a prolapsed uterus or bladder or to lack of estrogen in perimenopausal women. If the client has two or fewer urinary tract infections in a year, the single-dose or 3-day regimen of antibiotic therapy may be used.

15. **(1)** With an acid stone, the rule of thumb is to promote a diet that will render the urine more alkaline, which is an alkaline ash diet. A high-purine diet contributes to the development of the renal stones, so the client needs decreased purine. Foods that are high in purines include liver, spinach, chicken, and dried peas. Milk is allowed on an alkaline ash diet. An increased fluid intake is recommended in all stones, but does not particularly correlate with vitamin C intake. High carbohydrates do not contribute to the stone formation.

16. **(2)** Pyelonephritis in men is suggestive of a structural abnormality and is usually an indication for hospitalization, parenteral antibiotics, and an IVP. Pyelonephritis in women is usually a result of invasion of the urinary tract by bacteria that have ascended the urethra from the introitus of the urethra. If bacteremia is suspected, women need to be hospitalized, also. Suggested follow-up is by telephone contact within 12–24 hours of initiation of antibiotic therapy and at 2 weeks and 3 months for posttreatment urine cultures.

17. **(2)** Postrenal failure is the development of a complication that presents an obstructive problem distal to the kidney. The hypotensive episode is prerenal, and the vascular changes due to diabetes and the exposure to nephrotoxic chemicals are both intra-renal.

18. **(2)** Urge incontinence is associated with conditions that involve the central nervous system causing detrusor motor and/or sensory instability.

19. **(4)** Painless hematuria is the most common symptom in the client with bladder cancer. This often occurs early, and it may be the only symptom the client will exhibit. There is no evidence of renal failure; renal calculi are characterized by flank pain.

20. **(3)** Sedentary lifestyle or episodes of immobilization can predispose a client to the development of stones. Urinary infections usually do not precipitate problems with stones; however, presence of stones will predispose the client to urinary tract infections. Six to 8 oz of milk daily is not excessive, and the increased intake of citrus and high-fiber carbohydrates is good.

21. **(1)** The precipitating factor in prerenal failure is most often an incident that precipitated renal ischemia, most often a shock situation. Nephrotoxic medications, pyelonephritis, and renal vascular changes are all causes of intrarenal failure.

22. **(2)** Kegel's (pelvic floor) exercises keep the bladder support strong. Weak pelvic floor muscles contribute to urinary incontinence, especially with activity. In addition, the teaching should include avoiding bladder irritants, such as caffeine, alcohol, and spicy foods.

Pharmacology

23. **(1)** If there is any impairment of renal function, the antibacterial concentration in the urine is inadequate and there is increased risk of toxicity. With normal doses, there should be no serum or tissue accumulation of the medication. Liver function studies may be indicated if the client experiences adverse reactions to the medication. Anticoagulants and sulfa-based medications have not been reported as producing any significant drug interactions.

24. **(4)** Combination hormone replacement therapy can be useful for management of stress incontinence. Propantheline and oxybutynin may be useful in urge incontinence; research is limited on the use of these drugs for urge incontinence.

25. **(1)** To decrease the formation of uric acid stones, a urinary alkylating agent such as allopurinol (Zyloprim) is frequently used.

26. **(3)** Oxybutynin produces anticholinergic side effects. Dry mouth is very common. Other reactions are not consistent with oxybutynin.

27. **(2)** Sedatives and hypnotics lead to sedation and muscle relaxation. Antidepressants have anticholinergic effects and lead to sedation. Antibiotics have not been implicated in the development of incontinence in the older adult.

28. **(1)** The severe pain of renal calculi should be addressed prior to other treatments or diagnostics. The ibuprofen may be used for beginning pain, but severe pain needs to be treated with morphine or meperidine (Demerol). Tigan can be used, but only after the pain relief has been initiated.

29. **(1)** The most common side effect is gastrointestinal upset. This can be decreased if the medication is taken with food or milk. The discoloration of the urine is a very common occurrence. The medication should be taken for at least 3 days after sterile urine is obtained.

30. **(1)** Yellow discoloration of the sclera may indicate poor renal excretion. Pyridium should be administered with food, and there is no drug interaction with aspirin or with birth control pills.

Women's Health

Physical Examination & Diagnostic Tests

1. When obtaining a cervical specimen for a Pap smear, the nurse practitioner:

   1. Lubricates the speculum with a water-soluble lubricant to assist in the insertion of the instrument.

   2. Utilizes the cervical brush when obtaining the cervical cells on a prenatal client due to the presence of the cervical mucous plug.

   3. Uses warm water to lubricate the speculum to assist in the insertion of the instrument.

   4. Completes the bimanual portion of the examination first in order to determine the relative position of the cervix to assist in a comfortable insertion of the speculum.

2. To promote client comfort prior to performing a pelvic exam, the nurse practitioner:

   1. Asks the client to bear down slightly as the speculum is inserted.

   2. Has the client empty her bladder.

   3. Explains each step of the procedure in a calm manner.

   4. Carefully reassures the client that the exam will only take a few minutes.

3. What finding is considered a normal surface characteristic of the cervix?

   1. Small, yellow, raised round area on cervix.

   2. Red patchy areas with occasional white spots.

   3. Friable, bleeding tissue at opening of cervical os.

   4. Irregular, granular surface with red patches.

4. The primary role of a breast ultrasound is:

   1. As a screening test for breast cancer.

   2. For definitive diagnosis of breast cancer.

   3. To determine if a breast lesion is cystic or solid.

   4. To locate small lesions prior to surgery.

5. The optimal time to perform a hysterosalpingogram (HSG) is:

   1. During menses.

   2. Immediately after ovulation.

   3. After menses, but before ovulation.

   4. 3–4 days prior to menses.

6. Which statement about mammography is **false**?

   1. Mammography detects all breast cancers.

   2. Mammography should be accompanied by breast exam.

   3. Negative mammography should not delay biopsy of a clinically suspicious mass.

   4. Mammography is a cost-effective method to screen for breast cancer.

7. The use of potassium hydroxide (KOH) when doing a wet mount assists in the diagnosis of:

   1. Bacterial vaginosis and candida vaginitis.

   2. Trichomonas and chlamydia.

   3. Syphilis and gonorrhea.

   4. Herpes and condyloma.

8. The nurse practitioner is reviewing the lab results of an 18-year-old client seen recently for a Pap smear. The results are as follows: Classification—high-grade squamous intraepithelial lesion; endocervical cells seen; adequate smear. The nurse practitioner phones the client and tells her which of the following?

   1. "Your Pap smear was normal. Follow up in 1 year, sooner if problems arise."

   2. "Your Pap smear shows invasive cancer. I would like you to see a gynecologic oncologist for treatment."

   3. "Your Pap smear shows abnormal tissue that needs to be evaluated. Please schedule an appointment for a colposcopy."

4. "Your Pap smear shows a minor abnormality. Sometimes this can signify a disease process just beginning. Please schedule another Pap smear in 4 months for follow-up."

9. A 27-year-old client reports the desire to become pregnant. She and her husband have had regular, unprotected intercourse for more than 1 year. The nurse practitioner completes a thorough history and gynecologic exam, which appear normal. What diagnostic test might you order early in your work-up?

   1. Hysterosalpingogram.

   2. Tests for antisperm antibodies.

   3. Semen analysis.

   4. Endometrial biopsy.

10. When describing the findings from a normal breast examination, the nurse practitioner documents on the client record:

   1. Left nipple everted, several coarse black hairs arising from the areola, enlarged axillary lymph nodes palpated bilaterally, and tender nodes in supraclavicular area.

   2. No dimpling or retraction; 1-cm hard, fixed, stellate mass noted next to nipple with scant nipple discharge; no pain or tenderness of palpation.

   3. Right breast slightly larger and denser than left with no nipple discharge, right areola dark pink in color and inverted, left areola dark brown in color and everted, breasts tender to palpation with no axillary nodes noted.

   4. Pendulous breasts with no dimpling, retraction, nipple discharge, or areas of discoloration; numerous small nevi near areola with Montgomery's tubercles noted, no supraclavicular or axillary lymph nodes palpated.

11. In an infertility work-up, what is the best way to evaluate ovulation?

   1. Hysterosalpingogram.

   2. Postcoital test.

3. Endometrial biopsy.

4. Basal body temperature (BBT) chart.

12. The nurse practitioner is reviewing the lab work of a 61-year-old adult client seen recently for a Pap smear. She has been treated for breast cancer with mastectomy and tamoxifen (Nolvadex). She is not and never has been on hormone replacement therapy. The results of her Pap smear are as follows: Atrophic changes—scant endocervical cells; adequate smear. What is appropriate for the nurse practitioner to tell the client when she phones her with her result?

    1. "Your Pap smear is slightly abnormal. I would recommend the use of some estrogen vaginal cream nightly for 3 weeks, then return to the office to have the Pap smear repeated."

    2. "Your Pap smear is normal but shows a mild thinning of the tissue. This is to be expected in someone who is not on hormones and it does not pose a threat to your health. Please return to the office in 1 year for your annual exam, sooner if needed."

    3. "Your Pap smear shows that you don't have enough endocervical cells. Please make an appointment for endocervical curettage."

    4. "Your Pap smear is abnormal. This could signify a disease state of the cervix. Please schedule a colposcopy at your earliest convenience."

13. Which test is the "gold standard" for the diagnosis of chlamydia?

    1. Use of potassium hydroxide (KOH) wet mount "whiff" test.

    2. Presence of inflammatory cells in Pap smear.

    3. Direct fluorescent antibody (DFA).

    4. Culture with special media and collection technique.

14. The nurse practitioner is discussing mammography with a group of women. It is important for the nurse practitioner to advise the women:

    1. A mammogram should be done annually for all women of child-bearing age.

    2. All women over 40 years old should have a mammogram on an annual basis.

    3. A mammogram should be done annually after pregnancy, if the woman does not breast-feed.

    4. A mammogram should be done if there is any breast pain or nipple retraction.

15. Which is the most accurate statement regarding a reactive serologic test for syphilis?

    1. All reactive serologic tests require confirmation with a treponemal test.

    2. Reactive serologic tests are highly suspicious for active syphilis.

    3. A false-positive serologic test, though rare, can be unnecessarily traumatizing to a client.

    4. A reactive serologic test most likely implies the need for retreatment.

16. While working-up a client with secondary amenorrhea, the prolactin serum assay results show a level of 24 ng/ml. Appropriate management includes:

    1. Administering medroxyprogesterone acetate 10 mg bid × 5 days.

    2. Referring to an endocrinologist.

    3. Recording the results as within normal limits (WNL).

    4. Assessing for nipple discharge.

17. When evaluating a young adult with amenorrhea and normal secondary sex characteristics, the purpose of the progesterone challenge is determining the presence of:

    1. Endogenous estrogen.

    2. Thyroxine.

    3. Prolactin.

    4. Adequate body fat.

18. A client comes in with complaints of fatigue, breast tenderness, abdominal bloating, fluid retention, irritability and difficulty sleeping the week before onset of menses. This has been occuring for the past 4 months. What is most important in establishing a diagnosis of PMS in the client?

    1. Occurrence of symptoms in the menstrual cycle.

    2. Severity of the symptoms.

    3. Number and frequency of symptoms over past 4 months.

    4. Presence or absence of anxiety or depression.

Normal Gynecology

19. The endometrial cycle is often described in three phases. Select the correct phases:

    1. Follicular, menstrual, and luteal.

    2. Proliferative, luteal, and menstrual.

    3. Follicular, secretory, and menstrual.

    4. Proliferative, secretory, and menstrual.

20. The nurse practitioner understands that premenstrual syndrome occurs with the greatest frequency and severity in the:

    1. Late luteal phase.

    2. Follicular phase.

    3. Proliferative phase.

    4. Ovulatory phase.

21. Which hormone is **not** released from the anterior pituitary gland?

    1. Follicle-stimulating hormone (FSH).

    2. Luteinizing hormone (LH).

    3. Oxytocin.

    4. Prolactin.

22. The primary function of FSH is:

    1. Stimulate maturation of ovarian follicles.

    2. Milk secretion.

    3. Trigger ovulation.

    4. Inhibits release of LH from the pituitary gland.

23. In the ovarian cycle, what phase begins with ovulation and ends with the onset of menses?

    1. Follicular phase.

    2. Ovulation.

    3. Proliferative phase.

    4. Luteal phase.

24. Which is **not** a risk factor for heart disease in the postmenopausal female?

    1. Hyperlipidemia.

    2. Cigarette smoking.

    3. Hormone replacement therapy.

    4. Diabetes mellitus.

25. An adult client's last menstrual period (LMP) was 2 months ago. She has a Paragard T 380 intrauterine device (IUD) in place for the last 4 months. She is complaining of nausea, fatigue, breast tenderness, and abdominal bloating. Her physical exam reveals the following:

    - Abdomen: WNL
    - Pelvic: cervix—positive Chadwick's sign, IUD strings seen protruding from the
    - cerivcal os
    - Uterus: enlarged, approximately 7 weeks size, nontender
    - Adnexae: nontender, without mass, no cervical motion tenderness (CMT).

    The most likely diagnosis is:

    1. Uterine fibroid.

    2. Ovarian cancer.

    3. Dislodged IUD.

    4. Pregnancy.

26. What function do the Bartholin's glands have in reproduction?

    1. Prevent vaginitis by maintaining adequate pH.

2. Prepare the mucous plug, which occurs during early pregnancy.

3. Produce an alkaline secretion, which enhances sperm viability.

4. Produce small amounts of hormones necessary for ovulation.

27. Which is **not** a risk factor for osteoporosis?

    1. Cigarette smoker.

    2. Caucasian race.

    3. Alcohol consumption.

    4. Obesity.

28. A young woman complains to the nurse practitioner that she is experiencing headaches, irritability, decreased appetite, and fatigue about 1 week prior to her menses. Appropriate management includes:

    1. Treating the premenstrual syndrome (PMS) with increased protein and salt in the diet.

    2. Incorporating daily regular aerobic exercise into her lifestyle.

    3. Ordering a complete blood count (CBC), SMAC-12, and urinalysis.

    4. Supplementing the diet with an additional 1–2 gm of vitamin C.

29. A middle-aged female presents with dysfunctional uterine bleeding. A hormonal profile reveals increased FSH and LH levels. The most likely cause for these findings is:

    1. Hypothalmic disorder.

    2. Onset of climacteric.

    3. Premature ovarian failure.

    4. Anterior pituitary disorder.

30. While assessing a 16-year-old girl, the nurse practitioner was asked about douching. What information would be used in the nurse practitioner's teaching plan?

    1. Douching during menstruation is safe.

    2. Due to vaginal discharge, daily douching is important.

3. Hypoallergenic douches include flavored or perfumed types.

4. Douching removes natural mucus and upsets normal vaginal flora.

31. A 29-year-old female client presents to the family planning clinic for her annual exam. She had a tubal ligation postpartum 6 months ago. She has been feeling tired and nauseated, and is slowly gaining weight. She had one menses postpartum, 4 months ago. The nurse practitioner notes the following on physical exam:

    - Abdomen: bowel sounds × 4, soft, no HSM, palpable mass in lower abdomen, measures 14 cm, no tenderness
    - Pelvic: BUS normal
    - Cervix: os closed, smooth, pink mucosa
    - Bimanual: uterus enlarged, nontender, smooth contours, no CMT
    - Adnexae: not palpable

    What is the likely diagnosis?

    1. Pregnancy.

    2. Uterine fibroid.

    3. Premature menopause.

    4. Colon cancer.

Gynecologic Disorders

32. During a yearly physical examination, a nurse practitioner asks a woman if she has any problems or questions about sexual function or activity. Initially, the client hesitates, but with further questioning and discussion, she states that she is unsure if she has ever experienced an orgasm before. The nurse practitioner suspects:

    1. Vaginismus.

    2. Primary orgasmic dysfunction.

    3. Secondary orgasmic dysfunction.

    4. Dyspareunia.

33. The nurse practitioner is talking with a young woman who has been diagnosed with herpes simplex type 2 (genital). In discussing her care, it would be important for the nurse practitioner to include what information?

    1. The initial lesions are usually worse than lesions that occur with outbreaks at a later time.

    2. Her sexual partner will not contract it, if she does not have sex when the lesions are present.

    3. This condition can be treated and cured, if she takes all of the antibiotics for 2 weeks.

    4. If in the future she becomes pregnant, she will have to have a cesarean delivery.

34. The definition of bacterial vaginosis is:

    1. A syndrome resulting from homeostatic disruption in the vagina.

    2. Vaginitis caused by flagellated protozoan.

    3. A bacterial sexually transmitted disease that can be symptomatic or asymptomatic.

    4. A virus characterized by recurrent outbreaks and remissions.

35. A 22-year-old married client complains of severe dysmenorrhea. Her gynecologic exam is normal. Which management protocol is preferred?

    1. Assess for contraceptive interest and, if interested, suggest use of oral contraceptives (OCs).

    2. Suggest use of prostaglandin synthetase inhibitor (PGSI).

    3. Suggest over-the-counter use of ibuprofen.

    4. Assess exercise patterns and use of relaxation techniques.

36. Which is **not** a criteria for the diagnosis of bacterial vaginosis?

    1. Positive amine test (whiff test).

    2. Presence of clue cells.

    3. Vaginal pH >4.5.

    4. The presence of pseudohyphae.

37. A client with a history of dilatation and curettage (D&C) after a first-trimester spontaneous abortion and subsequent amenorrhea would lead the nurse practitioner to suspect which problem?

    1. Polycystic ovarian syndrome.

    2. Asherman's syndrome.

    3. Hypogonadism.

    4. Premature ovarian failure.

38. The LH/FSH ratio in polycystic ovarian syndrome (Stein-Leventhal syndrome) is:

    1. 1.5:1.

    2. 3:1.

    3. 6:1.

    4. 1:3.

39. What is a criterion for diagnosing polycystic ovarian syndrome?

    1. Weight loss.

    2. Hyperprolactinemia.

    3. Laboratory evidence of increased estradiol.

    4. Chronic anovulation.

40. The most common cause of dysfunctional uterine bleeding is:

    1. Thyroid disorder.

    2. Blood dyscrasia.

    3. Anovulation.

    4. Uterine tumor.

41. A 30-year-old female presents with scant pubic hair, minimal breast development, absent cervix, and uterus with a 46, XY karyotype. Your diagnosis is:

    1. Turner's syndrome.

    2. Müllerian agenesis.

    3. Testicular feminization.

    4. Gonadal dysgenesis.

42. The most common cause of a breast mass in clients aged 15–25 is:
    1. Fibroadenoma.
    2. Intraductal papilloma.
    3. Infiltrating lobular carcinoma.
    4. Fibrocystic breast syndrome.

43. An effective treatment for primary dysmenorrhea is:
    1. Nonsteroidal anti-inflammatory analgesics.
    2. Tranquilizers.
    3. Progestins.
    4. Steroids.

44. What is a cause of secondary amenorrhea?
    1. Testicular feminization.
    2. Hypogonadotropic hypogonadism.
    3. Congenital absence of uterus.
    4. Extreme exercise.

45. A young woman comes into the clinic for a well-woman checkup. She states that about 3 weeks ago she had a sore on her labia that went away. It was not particularly painful, did not itch, and there did not seem to be any residual problems from it. The nurse practitioner treats this woman by:
    1. Ordering the treponemal specific test (FTA-ABS).
    2. Swabbing the area of the lesion for a viral culture.
    3. Advising her to notify her sexual contacts to determine if they have had any symptoms.
    4. Ordering nystatin (Mycostatin) cream to be applied to the area three or four times a day.

46. A high school athlete presents to the clinic with concerns regarding her menstrual periods. She states she has not had a period in the past 2 months. She has been in training and running about 3 miles a day for the past 3 months. She has lost approximately 15 lb. She is about 63 inches tall and currently weighs 100 lb. The best response by the nurse practitioner is to:
    1. Determine the client's percentage of body fat and body mass.
    2. Obtain FSH serum levels.
    3. Determine serum levels of human chorionic gonadotropin (hCG.)
    4. Order thyroid function tests.

47. Which is **not** a risk factor for the development of cervical cancer?
    1. Human papillomavirus (HPV).
    2. Virginal status.
    3. Multiple sexual partners.
    4. Previous high-grade squamous intraepithelial lesions (HSIL).

48. A young woman is complaining of tenderness and burning of her vulva. On examination the vulva is edematous and excoriated. The nurse practitioner performs a wet mount prep of the vaginal secretions. It reveals pseudohyphae and spores. The diagnosis for this client is:
    1. Vulvovaginal candidiasis.
    2. *Chlamydia trachomatis.*
    3. Bacterial vaginitis.
    4. Gonorrhea.

49. The leading cause of death in female genital cancers, excluding breast, is:
    1. Ovarian cancer.
    2. Endometrial cancer.
    3. Cervical cancer.
    4. Vulvar and/or vaginal cancer.

50. A young woman presents with complaints of an irritation in the vaginal area. This is the first time it has occurred. On vaginal examination, the cervix is inflamed and friable. Flagellated protozoa are seen on the wet prep. The most likely diagnosis is:

    1. Trichomoniasis.

    2. Mucopurulent cervicitis.

    3. Chlamydia.

    4. Bacterial vaginosis.

51. A 26-year-old female client presents to the emergency room and is seen by the nurse practitioner. The client had a gradual onset of abdominal pain, starting in the periumbilical region, now in the right lower quadrant. It is accompanied by nausea, anorexia, constipation, and low-grade fever. The physical exam confirms the diagnosis of acute appendicitis. What diagnostic studies are **least** useful in confirming this diagnosis?

    1. CBC, with differential.

    2. Flat plate of abdomen, kidney-ureter-bladder (KUB).

    3. Pelvic ultrasound.

    4. Pregnancy test.

52. Which is **not** a risk factor for endometrial cancer?

    1. Obesity.

    2. Birth control pill use.

    3. Unopposed estrogen use.

    4. Advancing age, >50 years.

53. Which statement is true regarding the diaphragm?

    1. May be inserted up to 24 hours prior to intercourse.

    2. May be inserted any time up to 6 hours prior to intercourse.

    3. Should be removed within 1 hour after intercourse.

    4. May be left in place only up to 12 hours.

54. A contraceptive method that is associated with an increase in urinary tract infection is the:

    1. Intrauterine device.

    2. Diaphragm.

    3. Norplant.

    4. Oral contraceptive pills.

55. Which is **not** a risk factor for ovarian cancer?

    1. Family history of ovarian cancer.

    2. Advancing age, >50 years.

    3. Birth control pill use.

    4. Positive BRCA 2 gene.

56. What is the most common female genital malignancy, excluding the breast?

    1. Ovary.

    2. Endometrium.

    3. Cervix.

    4. Vulva/vagina.

57. A 20-year-old female college student presents to urgent care with new onset of painful sores in the vulva. These erupted yesterday and are associated with exquisite pain, fever, flu-like symptoms of headache, general body aches, and mild dysuria. The examination reveals vesicular lesions covering the labium; extreme tenderness to palpation of the external genitalia; normal Bartholin's, Skene's, and urethral glands; normal vaginal inspection with a mild leukorrhea; normal cervical mucosa; and slightly tender minimally enlarged inguinal lymph nodes bilaterally. What is the likely diagnosis?

    1. Gonorrhea.

    2. Chlamydia.

    3. Herpes simplex virus.

    4. Lymphogranuloma venereum.

58. A 21-year-old female client is seen for her annual gynecologic exam. She is sexually active, rarely uses condoms for sexually transmitted disease (STD) prevention, and

has multiple sexual partners. She smokes one pack per day, admits to sedentary lifestyle, eats two meals per day, most often at fast food restaurants. Her exam is negative for any abnormality. Her family history and personal medical history are negative for major disease. There are no menstrual abnormalities, her LMP was 1 week ago. The nurse practitioner has done her Pap smear. Which would **not** be appropriate for this client?

1. Cultures for gonorrhea and chlamydia.

2. Lab testing: glucose, cardiac risk profile, and TSH.

3. Human immunodeficiency virus (HIV) titer and rapid plasma reagin (RPR).

4. Counseling on safe sex practice and contraceptive information.

59. Which is **not** considered to be a risk factor in the development of breast cancer?

1. Early menopause.

2. High-fat diet.

3. Advancing age.

4. Early menarche.

60. A 32-year-old female client, G2 T1 P1 A0 L2, is seen in the clinic by the nurse practitioner for her annual exam and is requesting information on preconception counseling. She has been on oral contraceptives for 3 years without complications. During the past year, she has started an exercise program at a health club 5 days a week and is eating three nutritionally sound meals daily. She has lost 33 lb and is now at her ideal body weight. She quit her job as a postal worker and now stays home with her children. As part of her preconception care, what should the nurse practitioner recommend?

1. Start prenatal vitamins with folic acid.

2. Discontinue exercise.

3. Update measles-mumps-rubella (MMR) vaccine.

4. Genetic counseling due to advanced maternal age.

61. The initial work-up for dysfunctional uterine bleeding (DUB) should include:

1. Referral for diagnostic D & C.

2. Referral for endometrial biopsy to rule out cancer.

3. CBC, pregnancy test, endocrine studies.

4. Coagulation studies, STD cultures.

62. Which is **not** a risk factor for breast cancer?

1. History of maternal breast cancer— premenopausal onset.

2. First pregnancy after age 35.

3. Late menopause after age 54.

4. Fibrocystic breast disease.

63. A 20-year-old female client presents for her first well-woman exam; she is not sexually active and never has been. Her family history and past medical history are negative for any gynecologic diseases. Her menses occur every 28 days, lasting 5 days with a relatively moderate flow, and no significant abdominal cramps. Her physical exam/visit today should include which tests?

1. Pap smear.

2. Cultures for gonorrhea and chlamydia.

3. Stool hemoccult.

4. Baseline mammogram.

64. What is the leading cause of death for females in the United States?

1. Breast cancer.

2. Colon cancer.

3. Heart disease.

4. Stroke.

65. During a gynecologic exam at the family planning clinic, an underweight 17-year-old presents with bruising around her upper torso and genitalia. She is minimally interactive and avoids eye contact as much as possible. Priority intervention should focus on:

    1. Lab work to rule out bleeding disorder.

    2. Nutritional assessment to determine possible anemia.

    3. Determination of possible physical abuse.

    4. Finding out if she has a support system.

66. Reactive cellular changes noted on a Pap smear are most often associated with:

    1. Inflammation.

    2. Use of estrogen vaginal cream.

    3. Drying artifact.

    4. Use of oral contraceptives.

67. Risk factors for cervical disease include:

    1. Pregnancy after 35 years of age.

    2. Viral exposure.

    3. Low parity.

    4. Prolonged contraceptive use.

68. What is the most common cancer in females in the United States?

    1. Breast cancer.

    2. Colon cancer.

    3. Malignant melanoma.

    4. Lung cancer.

69. A 48-year-old female client presents to the clinic with the following list of complaints: hot flashes, no menses for 14 months, insomnia, crying spells, irritability, decreased libido, and fatigue. At the end of her history and physical exam, she begins to cry and tells the nurse practitioner that she thinks she is going crazy; she then begs the nurse practitioner to tell her what is wrong. What is **inappropriate** for the nurse practitioner to advise the client at this point?

    1. Obtain lab tests including FSH and LH.

    2. Discuss hormone replacement, including risks and benefits, and short- and long-term treatment strategies.

    3. Start antidepressant therapy and refer for counseling sessions for depression.

    4. Provide the client with written information regarding menopause and the options for treatment of symptoms.

70. Follow-up care for a client with chancroid should include:

    1. Screening for HIV as well as syphilis.

    2. Mandatory notification and treatment of all sexual partners.

    3. Screening for lymphogranuloma venereum.

    4. Culture for gonorrhea.

71. During her annual exam, a 39-year-old female complains of recent breast changes. She states that her breasts are painful and frequently feel "lumpy." Because of this, she has stopped doing monthly breast self-examination (BSE), feeling that it is a waste of time. What would be the most appropriate advice to offer her?

    1. Stress the importance of continuing monthly BSE to detect unusual lumps because she knows the feel of her breasts.

    2. Suggest she at least do BSE every 2 months.

    3. Suggest she start getting mammograms to establish some baseline data about her breasts.

    4. Determine when her breasts are nontender and least "lumpy" and change her schedule for BSE.

72. During a breast exam on a young adult female, a 2-cm painless lobular mass in the right breast that is firm and freely mobile is noted on palpation. Appropriate management includes:

    1. Continued observation and rechecking in 3 months.

2. Referral for a mammogram.

3. Referral for probable surgical excision.

4. Detailed family history to determine breast cancer risk.

73. A woman with bilateral breast implants asks if it is really necessary to do monthly BSE because she does not know what to feel for. The most appropriate response would be:

1. Suggest she involve her sexual partner in assessing her breasts on a regular basis.

2. Review the steps in BSE until she feels comfortable with the process.

3. Acknowledge the difficulty of doing BSE after implant surgery.

4. Explain the usefulness of regular mammograms for implant clients.

74. An adult client comes to the clinic complaining of abnormal vaginal discharge (dark watery brown) along with postcoital bleeding. The nurse practitioner suspects the possibility of cancer of the cervix. During the vaginal exam, suspicious physical results would be:

1. Soft, sill-shaped cervix.

2. Very firm cervix with an ulcer.

3. Vague lower abdominal discomfort.

4. Tender, enlarged lymph nodes.

75. A postmenopausal female is worried about pain in the upper outer quadrant of her left breast. The nurse practitioner should:

1. Do a breast exam and order a mammogram.

2. Explain that pain is related to hormone fluctuations and order laboratory studies.

3. Reassure the client that pain is not a presenting symptom of breast cancer and check for proper fit of the brassiere.

4. Teach the client BSE.

76. A 22-year-old female client comes to the nurse practitioner's office with a complaint of 1 day of fever of 102°F, a diffuse macular rash, vomiting, headache, and decreased urinary output. The history obtained by the nurse practitioner must include:

1. Whether the client's immunizations are up to date.

2. Whether the client is currently menstruating.

3. Whether the client has a history of tuberculosis.

4. What type of contraception the client uses.

77. A young female client presents to the nurse practitioner's office with a complaint of abdominal pain. In the United States, this diagnosis results in about 1 death per 1000 and therefore must be considered early in the decision process:

1. Irritable bowel syndrome.

2. Appendicitis.

3. Pyelonephritis.

4. Ectopic pregnancy.

78. A young adult female client presents with a history of vaginal itching and heavy white discharge. The client gives a history of no sexual activity. On exam, the nurse practitioner finds a red, edematous vulva and white patches on the vaginal walls. There is no odor to the discharge. The nurse practitioner expects what factors in the client's history?

1. A vegetarian diet.

2. Recent diarrhea.

3. Early menopause.

4. Recent antibiotic use.

79. A young female client comes to the office complaining of vaginal bleeding. The client states that she has used five tampons in the past 3 hours. She admits to sexual activity and takes oral contraceptives. On further questioning, the client states that she started her last pack of contraceptives "about 2 weeks late." The nurse practitioner should:

    1. Perform a stat urine pregnancy test.

    2. Perform a stat CBC.

    3. Discuss proper use of oral contraceptives.

    4. Send the client for a pelvic sonogram.

80. The nurse practitioner knows that the majority of breast cancers occur in which area of the breast?

    1. Upper inner quadrant.

    2. Upper outer quadrant.

    3. Beneath the nipple and areola.

    4. Lower outer quadrant.

81. The client presents with dysfunctional uterine bleeding and has been found to have endometrial cancer. She returned to the nurse practitioner because she does not understand how this is possible when the Pap smear 6 months ago was negative. The best response is:

    1. Uterine cancer develops quickly.

    2. Pap smears are difficult to read and mistakes can happen.

    3. Pap smears are not useful in detecting uterine cancers in most cases.

    4. The previous Pap smear did not have an adequate sample of tissue.

Pharmacology

82. A 42-year-old female client presents to the office with complaints of dysuria, urinary frequency and urgency. These symptoms began early this morning. She leaves a clean-catch midstream urine which shows the following: white blood cells (WBCs) too numerous to count (TNTC)/high-power field (HPF), 4–5 red blood cells (RBCs)/HPF, positive nitrites. A urine culture is set up and will be ready in 3 days. Which is **not** a correct treatment for an uncomplicated lower urinary tract infection?

    1. Phenazopyridine (Pyridium) 200 mg 1 tab PO tid × 2 days.

    2. Trimethoprim-sulfamethoxazole (Bactrim DS) 1 tab PO bid × 5 days.

    3. Ceftriaxone (Rocephin) 1 gm IM.

    4. Nitrofurantoin (Macrobid) 1 tab PO bid × 5 days.

83. A 46-year-old female client is being seen in the clinic by the nurse practitioner. She was last seen 2 weeks ago for an upper respiratory tract infection and was treated with amoxicillin (Amoxil) 250 mg PO tid × 10 days. She completed her medication last week but now is aware of vaginal itching and a cottage cheese–like vaginal discharge. She states that she has never experienced such intense itching before. She is in a mutually monogamous relationship. Her LMP was 2 weeks ago. Her partner had a vasectomy 2 years ago. Wet mount with KOH shows negative whiff test, rare clue cells, positive lactobacilli, positive hyphae and spores, few WBCs, and no trichomonads. She is leaving tomorrow for a week-long cruise. She is not on any medications, and has no known drug allergies. Your treatment for this problem is:

    1. Metronidazole (Flagyl) 500 mg PO bid × 7 days.

    2. Clindamycin (Cleocin) vaginal cream one applicator full vaginally qhs × 7 days.

    3. Fluconazole (Diflucan) tablet 150 mg 1 tab PO one time.

    4. Hydrocortisone (Cortaid) 1% cream apply sparingly bid × 7 days.

84. A 25-year-old female client presents with complaints of a malodorous vaginal discharge described as white and watery. She douches with vinegar and water every 2 weeks. She uses a diaphragm for

contraception. She and her boyfriend have been sexually active for 2 years, using condoms for STD prevention with every act of coitus. She denies any dyspareunia. Her LMP was 1 week ago, and there are no noted changes in her normal menstrual pattern. Her wet mount with KOH results show positive whiff test, TNTC clue cells/HPF, no lactobacilli, no hyphae or spores, no trichomonads, and few WBCs. Treatment for this client is:

1. Doxycycline (Vibratabs) 100 mg PO bid × 10 days.

2. Terconazole (Terazol 7 cream) one applicator full per vagina qhs × 7 days.

3. Acyclovir (Zovirax) 200 mg 1 PO q4h × 5 days.

4. Metronidazole (Metrogel) vaginal cream one applicator full per vagina qhs × 5 days.

85. A 55-year-old female client is being seen in the clinic for her annual exam. She went through a natural menopause 5 years ago and has never been interested in hormonal therapy. She smokes one pack per day, does no formal exercise. She is a G2 T2 P0 A0 L2. Her family history is positive for osteoporosis in her mother, myocardial infarction in her father, and negative for any cancers. She had a normal physical exam today and had a negative mammogram yesterday. She is interested now in hormonal therapy but wants to know what her alternatives are. Which choice has **not** been clinically proven for prevention of osteoporosis or cardiovascular disease?

1. Conjugated equine estrogen (Premarin) 0.625 mg 1 tablet PO qd and medroxyprogesterone acetate (Provera) 2.5 mg 1 tablet PO qd.

2. Weight-bearing exercise three times weekly, calcium 1500 mg PO qd.

3. Discontinue cigarette smoking.

4. Wild Mexican yam cream; apply to skin three times daily.

86. A young female is seen in the STD clinic. She noticed some itchy bumps in the vulvar area and is concerned that they

could be cancer. On careful inspection the nurse practitioner notes the following: five cauliflower-like, warty, pinkish colored lesions in the lower introitus; two smaller lesions nestled anterior to the hymeneal ring of the vagina and cervix fail to reveal any abnormalities. A wet mount with KOH is negative. A culture for gonorrhea and chlamydia was obtained, Pap smear done, and HIV titer and RPR drawn. Which is **not** an appropriate treatment for this client?

1. Podophyllin (Podoben) application, wash off in 6 hours with soap and water.

2. Trichloroacetic acid application, do not wash off.

3. Cryotherapy with liquid nitrogen to lesions.

4. Benzathine penicillin 2.4 million units IM weekly × 3 weeks.

87. A young adult female client is being seen in the urgent care unit by the nurse practitioner. She is complaining of vaginal itching, thick yellow mucous discharge, and urinary discomfort. She is sexually active and uses condoms with one of her partners, but not both. On physical exam, the abdomen is negative. The pelvic exam reveals the BUS WNL, the cervix has a mucopurulent discharge exuding from the os, and the mucosa is friable to palpation. The bimanual exam is negative. Cultures were taken but are not yet available. Wet mount with KOH reveals negative whiff test, few clue cells, TNTC WBCs, no yeast, no trichomonads. What is the likely diagnosis and appropriate treatment?

1. Chlamydia; give azithromycin (Zithromax) 1 gm PO single dose.

2. Chlamydia; give ceftriaxone (Rocephin) 125 mg IM.

3. Herpes simplex virus; give acyclovir (Zovirax) 200 mg 1 cap PO q4h × 5 days.

4. Trichomoniasis; give metronidazole (Flagyl) 2 gm PO single dose.

88. An adult female client is seen in the family planning clinic for a consultation on contraception. She is using birth control pills but forgets to take them because her work schedule changes every week. She is looking for an effective method that will be easy to remember. She has been married for 14 years, is G2 T2 P0 A0 L2, and is a nonsmoker. She has a negative past history for any major diseases and has a negative gynecologic history for abnormalities. She has never been treated for an STD and is in a mutually monogamous relationship. She is needle phobic and faints when she has to have blood drawn. What contraceptive method would be a good choice for the client?

    1. Depo-Provera injection every 3 months.

    2. Norplant implantation system for 5 years.

    3. Intrauterine device.

    4. Diaphragm.

89. A young adult female client is being seen at the family planning clinic by the nurse practitioner. The client wants birth control pills but has heard that they are dangerous to one's health. When asked for clarification, she lists the following: weight gain, ovarian cancer, heavy or irregular periods, and infertility. The nurse practitioner tells her: "I can see that you are concerned about your health...."

    1. "There are a lot of fallacies about birth control pills. They actually are felt to reduce the risk of ovarian cancers, help to regulate the bleeding, and are not associated with causing infertility. There can be a minor increase in body weight of 3–5 lb."

    2. "Perhaps you would be better off trying the Norplant system of Depo-Provera."

    3. "What you have heard is true. They can be dangerous to your health and many people experience these problems."

    4. "There are a lot of fallacies about birth control pills. While ovarian cancer and infertility are risks that are taken with the use of the birth control pill, they do not cause weight gain or bleeding changes on periods. Pap smears done every year will detect such things as ovarian cancer."

90. A 41-year-old female client is seen in the family planning clinic. She is seeking information about contraceptive methods because her Norplant system is due for removal next month. She is in a new sexual relationship and plans to use condoms for STD prevention. She is in excellent health, is a nonsmoker, and is nulliparous. Her menses are every 28 days, light flow. Which is **inappropriate** for the nurse practitioner to recommend?

    1. Oral contraceptives.

    2. Intrauterine device.

    3. Norplant system.

    4. Depo-Provera injections.

91. An adult female client is on oral contraceptive agents. She calls into the clinic with complaints of bleeding through the first $2\frac{1}{2}$ weeks of every package of pills. She has been on this pill for 4 months and takes them at the same time every day. Her present pill is a low-dosage monophasic pill. She is not on any other medications and denies any adverse effects to the birth control pills. She would like to remain on oral contraceptives if possible. The nurse practitioner's advice should include:

    1. Discontinue the pills and do not restart them. An alternative contraceptive method should be used.

    2. Change to a higher dosage, higher progestational agent.

    3. Try taking the pills first thing in the morning on an empty stomach to improve metabolism of the agents.

    4. There is no cause for concern; breakthrough bleeding is a normal side effect of oral contraceptives.

92. An adult female client is seen by the nurse practitioner at the family planning clinic. The client notes heavy, irregular menses. There has been an increase in facial acne and facial/abdominal hair growth over the past few years. She is G1 T1 P0 A0 L1, and not planning future pregnancies. After a normal pelvic exam, the client decides she wants oral contraceptives. A good pill choice would be:

1. Loestrin 1/20.

2. Triphasil.

3. Demulen 1/35.

4. Birth control pills are inappropriate for this client.

93. A 41-year-old female client is seen for her 6-weeks-postpartum exam by the nurse practitioner. She is breast-feeding without difficulty and plans to continue for a year. She wants to begin using a contraceptive and plans no further pregnancies. Which is an **inappropriate** choice for this client?

1. Depo-Provera 150 mg IM injection every 3 months.

2. Intrauterine device.

3. Progestin-only oral contraceptive.

4. Combined oral contraceptive.

94. A 38-year-old female client is seen for her 6-weeks-postpartum exam by the nurse practitioner. The client was breast-feeding for a short time but discontinued 4 weeks ago. Her menses have resumed. She is contemplating another pregnancy in a year or so; if she became pregnant before that she would not mind. She is seeking contraception. She smokes 1 pack per day. Her exam is normal, with the uterus being well involuted. Which is **contraindicated** in this client?

1. Progestacert IUD.

2. Oral contraceptive agents.

3. Depo-Provera injection.

4. Condoms and spermicide.

95. A 25-year-old female client is seen by the nurse practitioner for her annual exam. The client is interested in contraceptive choices. She just quit smoking and is well motivated to remain a nonsmoker. She is on phenobarbital and phenytoin (Dilantin) for seizure control. She is G3 T2 P0 A1 L1. She may be planning future pregnancies but is unsure at this time. She is in good health other than the seizure disorder, and has a normal exam. What contraceptive method is contraindicated in this client?

1. Diaphragm.

2. Depo-Provera injection.

3. Intrauterine device.

4. Norplant implantation system.

96. A 22-year-old female client presents to the urgent care department and is seen by the nurse practitioner. She is complaining of abdominal pain, low-grade fever, and mucopurulent vaginal discharge. Her symptoms began 3 days ago, and are getting worse. She has a new sexual partner, and has not used condoms with him yet. Her menses just ended; she is on oral contraceptive agents. She denies nausea, vomiting, or anorexia. Her exam reveals findings consistent with pelvic inflammatory disease (PID). Cultures were taken for gonorrhea and chlamydia. Which represents an **inappropriate** treatment plan for the nurse practitioner to follow?

1. Ceftriaxone (Rocephin) 250 mg IM.

2. Doxycycline (Vibratabs) 100 mg PO bid × 10 days.

3. CBC, erythrocyte sedimentation rate (ESR).

4. Hospitalization.

97. An older female client is seen by the nurse practitioner for her annual exam. She has been on hormone replacement therapy (HRT) for 6 months, having started herself on the pills left over by her deceased mother. She brings the pills with her, as she wants to remain on these and requests a prescription for Estrace 1 mg daily. She has an intact uterus, is in excellent health, and denies any complaints. She does not have any contraindications to the use of HRT. Her exam is normal. Which represents an **incorrect** and potentially dangerous plan for the nurse practitioner to follow?

1. Endometrial biopsy.

2. Prescription for Estrace 1 mg daily; plus medroxyprogesterone acetate (Provera) 2.5 mg daily.

3. Prescription for Estrace 1 mg daily.

4. Instruct the client on the risks and benefits of HRT.

98. An older adult female client is seen for follow-up to discuss her HRT with the nurse practitioner. She is seeking a refill on her HRT but is not sure it is working right. She continues to feel hot flashes, moodiness, and decreased libido, and has many sleep disturbances. She is on Premarin 0.625 mg daily, and Provera 2.5 mg daily. She denies any vaginal bleeding. Which is **not** an acceptable choice for the client?

    1. Premarin 0.9 mg 1 tab PO qd and Provera 5 mg 1 tab PO qd days 1–12.

    2. Premarin 0.9 mg 1 tab PO qd and Provera 5 mg 1 tab PO qd days 16–25.

    3. Premarin 0.3 mg 1 tab PO qd and Provera 2.5 mg 1 tab PO qd.

    4. Premarin 1.25 mg 1 tab PO qd and Provera 10 mg 1 tab PO qd days 1–12.

99. Which is **not** a contraindication to the use of HRT in the postmenopausal female?

    1. Recent deep vein thrombosis.

    2. Chronic active hepatitis.

    3. Controlled hypertension.

    4. Undiagnosed abnormal genital bleeding.

100. A young adult female client presents to the clinic with complaints of a malodorous, yellowish vaginal discharge and vulvovaginal itching. She has never had a gynecologic exam and is extremely apprehensive. She is sexually active and has had a new sexual partner for 2 months. She states that they use condoms most of the time and are not interested in alternate forms of contraception at this time. Her LMP was 1 week ago. Her wet mount with KOH reveals few clue cells, moderate lactobacilli, few WBCs, no yeast, and TNTC mobile trichomonads. Appropriate treatment for this client would include:

    1. Metronidazole (Flagyl) 2 gm PO single dose.

    2. Metronidazole (Metrogel) vaginal cream one applicator full per vagina qhs × 5 days.

    3. Fluconazole (Diflucan) 150 mg PO single dose.

    4. Terconazole (Terazol) vaginal cream one applicator full per vagina qhs × 7 days.

101. Which dose of conjugated equine estrogen (Premarin) is the minimal effective dose to prevent osteoporosis?

    1. 0.3 mg.

    2. 0.625 mg.

    3. 0.9 mg.

    4. 1.25 mg.

102. A single woman presents for contraceptive counseling expressing preference for a diaphragm. Which factor in her history would make a diaphragm a poor choice?

    1. Three urinary tract infections in the past year.

    2. Strong desire to avoid pregnancy.

    3. Last two Pap smears showed atypical cells.

    4. Nulliparous cervix.

103. Combination oral contraceptive pills prevent pregnancy primarily by:

    1. Decreasing fallopian tube motility.

    2. Thinning of cervical mucus.

    3. Suppressing ovulation.

    4. Causing inflammation of the endometrium.

104. A young adult client is hesitant to be fitted for an IUD because of strong antiabortion views and asks your opinion. Which explanation most accurately describes the probable action of an IUD?

    1. Slows transport of ovum through the fallopian tube, causing it to age and die in transit.

    2. Prevents effective implantation of a fertilized ovum.

    3. Action is no different than that of spermicide.

    4. Mechanically blocks sperm from entering uterus.

105. What is a unique advantage of a Progesterone T IUD?

    1. Lowest failure rate of IUDs.

    2. May be left in place for up to 10 years.

    3. Decreases menstrual blood loss and dysmenorrhea.

    4. Must be replaced annually.

106. An older female client is seen by the nurse practitioner for her annual exam and needs a refill on her hormone replacement therapy. She is feeling well and has not voiced concerns. The client had a total abdominal hysterectomy and bilateral salpingo-oophorectomy 2 years ago for benign fibroids. Her exam is normal. She takes conjugated estrogen (Premarin) 0.625 mg days 1–25 and medroxyprogesterone acetate (Provera) 10 mg from days 16–25. What changes would be appropriate for the nurse practitioner to make in the HRT regimen?

    1. No changes needed; the client is doing well on the present regimen.

    2. Premarin 0.625 mg daily; discontinue the Provera.

    3. Premarin 0.625 mg daily; Provera 2.5 mg daily.

    4. Premarin 0.625 mg days 1–25; Provera 5 mg days 16–25.

107. Which statement about progestin only pills is true?

    1. Women who are breast-feeding should not use progestin only pills.

    2. Ovulation suppression is as effective with progestin only pills as with combined oral contraception pills.

    3. There is an increased incidence of functional ovarian cysts.

    4. The risk of ectopic pregnancy is lowered for women using progestin only pills.

108. Before prescribing HRT, which clinical approach should have the highest priority?

    1. The decision about use should rest primarily with the client after providing appropriate education and counseling.

    2. For most women the benefits of HRT far outweigh any possible side effects, so HRT should be actively encouraged.

    3. Involving the sexual partner in the counseling session is likely to lead to a higher compliance rate for HRT.

    4. Education regarding HRT should include a thorough review of risk factors and possible side effects in order to avoid liability issues.

109. The most common side effect associated with depo-medroxyprogesterone (DMPA; Depo-Provera) is:

    1. Nausea.

    2. Acne.

    3. Menstrual cycle changes.

    4. Increased menstrual cramps.

110. The beneficial effects of estrogen on high-density (HDL) and low-density (LDL) lipoprotein fractions include:

    1. An increase in HDL and an increase in LDL.

    2. A decrease in HDL and a decrease in LDL.

    3. An increase in HDL and a decrease in LDL.

    4. A decrease in HDL and an increase in LDL.

111. The nurse practitioner is teaching a client about taking alendronate (Fosamax); her information includes:

    1. Take it midmorning.

    2. Take with food.

    3. Take with a full glass of orange juice.

    4. Remain upright after taking medication.

112. The addition of a progesterone to an estrogen regimen in a postmenopausal woman with a uterus reduces the risk of:

    1. Endometrial cancer.

    2. Cervical cancer.

    3. Gallbladder disease.

    4. Breast cancer.

113. The treatment of choice for trichomoniasis is:

    1. Azithromycin (Zithromax) 1 gm PO single dose.

    2. Ofloxacin (Floxin) 500 mg PO single dose.

    3. Metronidazole (Flagyl) 2 gm PO single dose.

    4. Clindamycin (Cleocin) 300 mg PO single dose.

114. A 25-year-old woman comes into the office with complaints of profuse malodorous discharge. The nurse practitioner's diagnosis is bacterial vaginosis. The nurse practitioner would:

    1. Advise the client to notify her sexual contacts regarding the diagnosis.

    2. Treat the problem with metronidazole (Flagyl) 2 gm for one dose.

    3. Initiate a treatment with doxycycline (Vibramycin) 100 mg PO bid × 7 days.

    4. Determine the presence of pregnancy prior to initiating a course of treatment.

115. A young woman who is taking a low-dose OC calls the clinic in a panic stating that she forgot her pill 2 days ago. She is taking phenytoin (Dilantin) for seizure activity and has been seizure free for over a year. She asks, "What should I do about my pills?" The most appropriate response should be:

    1. Advise her to take the forgotten dose today along with the regular dose.

    2. Refer her to her physician for advice about the Dilantin.

    3. Advise her to continue pills, but to use another contraceptive through the rest of this cycle.

    4. Advise her to come to the clinic for a "morning-after" pill.

116. A vaginal culture has confirmed the presence of chancroid in a Haitian homeless woman who presented with a painful genital ulcer. The treatment regimen of choice should be:

    1. Ceftriaxone (Rocephin) 250 mg IM in a single dose.

    2. Erythromycin (E-Mycin) 500 mg PO qid × 7 days.

    3. Metronidazole (Flagyl) 2 mg PO in a single dose.

    4. Clindamycin (Cleocin) cream 2% one full applicator (intravaginally × 5 days.

117. A young adult female presents to the office for evaluation of abdominal pain. The client admits to recent sexual activity and states that she does not have her partner use condoms. On exam the nurse practitioner finds vaginal discharge and CMT. Other than sending cultures to the lab, the nurse practitioner would treat this client with:

    1. Penicillin G 2.4 million units IM.

    2. Metronidazole (Flagyl) 500 mg PO bid × 7 days.

    3. Ceftriaxone (Rocephin) 125 mg IM and azithromycin (Zithromax) 1 gm PO.

    4. Acyclovir (Zovirax) 400 mg PO bid × 7 days.

118. When assisting the woman to decide whether to initiate HRT, which statement is true?

    1. Estrogen replacement delays the onset of menopause.

    2. Estrogen and progesterone cause vasomotor symptoms.

    3. Estrogen increases HDL cholesterol levels.

    4. Estrogen replacement with progesterone increases the risk of ovarian cancer.

Answers & Rationales

Physical Examination & Diagnostic Tests

1. **(3)** Lubricants, such as Vaseline or K-Y gel, should not be used if a cervical specimen is being obtained for analysis. The cervical brush should not be used on pregnant clients. The bimanual exam is performed after the internal vaginal exam.

2. **(2)** To aid in the examination, an empty bladder will provide for client comfort and will assist the nurse practitioner in making a more accurate assessment during the bimanual portion of the exam. Options #1 and #3 help reduce the client's anxiety, which ultimately may assist in the achievement of comfort.

3. **(1)** A nabothian cyst is a small, white or yellow, raised round area on the cervix. The surface of the cervix should be smooth and may have a symmetrical, reddened circle around the os (squamocolumnar epithelium). The other options are all unexpected, abnormal findings.

4. **(3)** A breast ultrasound is used to determine if a lesion is solid or cystic. Ultrasound misses 50% of lesions <2 cm. The test is not sensitive enough to be used for routine screening and cannot replace mammography. The definitive diagnosis of breast cancer is the breast biopsy.

5. **(3)** The HSG is used to document the presence of a normal uterine cavity and patency of the fallopian tubes. A contrast dye is injected into the uterus and x-rays are taken to assess anatomy. The best time to do this test is 2–5 days after menses but before ovulation.

6. **(1)** Approximately 10% of breast cancers are not seen mammographically.

7. **(1)** KOH lyses epithelial cells and WBCs, making it easier to visualize *Candida* (yeast). *Candida* cells are resistant and remain intact. KOH also assists with diagnosing bacterial vaginosis by alkalinizing vaginal discharge, causing a distinct fishy odor. This is a positive amine or whiff test.

8. **(3)** The Pap smear is a screening test for cervical cancer and precancerous states. The diagnostic test needed to confirm the diagnosis of a high-grade lesion is the colposcopy with guided biopsies. The results to this test are clearly abnormal and must be acted upon. Waiting a year could be deleterious to the client's health. This is not the Pap smear report that one would choose to redo in 4 months; the client needs a diagnostic test, not another screening test. This is not a diagnosis of cervical cancer on this Pap smear; therefore, a referral to a gynecologic oncologist is premature at this time.

9. **(3)** All of the above tests may be included in the work-up for infertility. Because male factors account for 35–40% of infertility, a semen analysis should be done early in the work-up. HSG and an endometrial biopsy are tests that require scheduling at specific times of the menstrual cycle. Tests for antisperm antibodies would be done if the postcoital test revealed abnormalities.

10. **(4)** The abnormal finding in Option #1 is the enlarged lymph nodes. The abnormal finding in Option #2 is the fixed, stellate mass with nipple discharge. In Option #3, asymmetrical size is normal but not the different colors of the areola and unilateral nipple inversion. Longstanding nevi and Montgomery's tubercles are normal in Option #4.

11. **(4)** The BBT chart is one of the most important ways to evaluate ovulation. Clients should be instructed on the first visit how to use the special BBT thermometer and record the findings on the BBT chart. The remaining answers, which are possibly part of an infertility work-up, are not methods to evaluate ovulation.

12. **(2)** Atrophic changes on the cervix of a postmenopausal female are to be expected, as is the paucity of endocervical cells. Due to her past medical history of breast cancer, she is not a candidate for the use of estrogen vaginal cream, nor is the Pap smear interpretation abnormal. Endocervical curettage is used as a biopsy technique for sampling tissue from the endocervical canal; however, it is not appropriate to recommend this invasive procedure for someone with scant endocervical cells, but rather for one with abnormal endocervical cells. Since this Pap smear report really is not classified as abnormal, there is no need to recommend a diagnostic procedure for the client.

13. **(4)** Culture and DFA are both used. The culture is the only certain or definitive method of diagnosis. It is a collected cervical specimen, and it takes about 2–6 days to obtain the results. The DFA is fast and has good sensitivity and specificity.

14. **(2)** Mammography should be done on a regular basis, baseline screening around age 35, then every 2 years. After age 40, it should be done on an annual basis. It should be done regardless of breast-feeding, and the client should not wait until a mass or other symptoms are present.

15. **(1)** Serologic tests are good screening tests, but positive results require following up with a treponemal test to detect specific antibodies.

16. **(2)** Serum prolactin assay levels >20 ng/ml indicate need for medical referral, usually to an endocrinologist. The most common cause of hyperprolactinemia and galactorrhea (milky breast discharge) is a pituitary tumor or lesion of the hypothalamus. Other causes may be hypothyroidism, medications (narcotics, tranquilizers, antihypertensives), and oral contraceptives.

17. **(1)** The initial work-up for this client includes determining the prolactin level by evaluating serum concentrations and determining the presence of endogenous estrogen. If the woman experiences withdrawal bleeding after the administration of PO or IM progesterone and the prolactin level is normal, this woman is producing estrogen and can be considered anovulatory. Absence of withdrawal bleeding with a normal prolactin level requires further work-up.

18. **(1)** The occurrence of the symptoms in the menstrual cycle will assist the nurse practitioner to make a diagnosis of PMS. The client should keep track on a calendar as to when each symptom occurs and disappears, and the onset and completion of menstrual flow.

Normal Gynecology

19. **(4)** Inside the uterus the lining first proliferates and begins preparation for implantation. During the secretory phase glandular epithelium develops, further enhancing the lining. If no fertilized egg arrives for implantation, the lining sloughs off; this is the menstrual phase.

20. **(1)** Premenstrual syndrome occurs approximately 5–11 days prior to the onset of menses (late luteal phase) and is gone within 1–2 days of the onset of menses. This phase is progesterone dominant. The follicular phase is estrogen dominant.

21. **(3)** Oxytocin is released from the posterior pituitary. FSH, LH, and prolactin are all released from the anterior pituitary gland. The other hormones released from the anterior pituitary are TSH, adrenocorticotropic hormone (ACTH), and growth hormone.

22. **(1)** FSH stimulates the maturation of ovarian follicles, resulting in a dominant follicle. Milk secretion is dependent on prolactin. The production and release of LH is regulated by estrogen. LH is responsible for ovulation.

23. **(4)** The ovarian cycle is divided into three phases. The follicular phase begins on the first day of menses and continues until day 14, when ovulation usually occurs. Immediately after ovulation, the empty follicle begins to enlarge and develops into a corpus luteum, which releases increasing amounts of progesterone. If implantation does not occur, the corpus luteum regresses, causing the onset of menses. This phase from ovulation to menses is the luteal phase.

24. **(3)** Hormone replacement therapy reduces the risk of heart disease in the postmenopausal female.

25. **(4)** Pregnancy is the most likely diagnosis in this client, given the list of symptoms and physical findings. She certainly could have a uterine fibroid; however, it is not contributing to the symptoms listed. Ovarian cancer could present with nausea, fatigue, and abdominal bloating; however, it would not cause the uterus to be enlarged, nor would it cause the positive Chadwick's sign. A dislodged IUD will usually change the position of the IUD, thereby causing the strings to be less visible or causing the IUD itself to be expelled into the vagina or endocervical canal.

26. **(3)** Maintaining an alkaline pH is important to promote viability of sperm that is deposited into the vaginal vault.

27. **(4)** Obesity is not a risk factor for osteoporosis. Cigarette use, Caucasian race, and alcohol consumption, in addition to others not listed here, are considered to be risk factors for osteoporosis.

28. **(2)** Conservative management for PMS includes daily exercise, support and reassurance that her problems are not uncommon, and education about symptoms that can help the client obtain some type of control to assist her to adapt to the situation. A low-salt diet is encouraged and a diuretic (HCTZ) may be ordered to deal with water retention along with vitamin B_6 (50–100 mg/day) and vitamins A and E for breast symptoms.

29. **(2)** As the function of the ovaries declines and the amount of circulating estrogen begins to fall, the middle-aged female may begin to experience the symptoms commonly associated with menopause. The body's feedback system will attempt to stimulate the ovaries and increase the estrogen level. FSH and LH levels rise in response to these efforts.

30. **(4)** The vagina naturally cleanses itself; therefore, douching is not necessary unless prescribed by a health care provider to treat a medical condition. Douching should be avoided during menses to prevent infection.

31. **(1)** Pregnancy is the most likely diagnosis, requiring a pregnancy test and pelvic ultrasound to confirm it. Even though she has had a tubal ligation, failure rates of 1 in 300 have been quoted. This client could have uterine fibroids; however, they do not generally present with this symptom complex and are not associated with amenorrhea, but they do cause uterine enlargement. Premature menopause could cause all these symptoms, including amenorrhea, but not the enlarged uterus. Colon cancer can present with these symptoms, and could certainly be responsible for an abdominal mass, but not uterine enlargement or amenorrhea.

Gynecologic Disorders

32. **(2)** Primary orgasmic disorder is when an individual has never achieved orgasm, usually a lifelong problem. Dyspareunia is painful intercourse and vaginismus is painful vaginal spasms upon penetration. Secondary orgasmic dysfunction refers to an acquired problem of loss of orgasmic function after an individual has experienced orgasm.

33. **(1)** The initial outbreak is usually the worst. It can be transmitted even when there is no lesion present and it cannot be cured. Vaginal delivery is allowed, if there are no genital lesions at the time of labor.

34. **(1)** Bacterial vaginosis results when the normal environment in the vagina is disrupted. The normal vaginal lactobacilli are decreased or absent, and there is an overgrowth of many different types of anaerobic bacteria. Trichomoniasis is caused by a flagellated protozoan and gonorrhea is caused by a bacteria and may be asymptomatic. The virus that causes recurrent outbreaks of genital lesions is herpes genitalis type 2 (HSV-2).

35. **(1)** OCs will reduce prostaglandin production, which is thought to be the primary cause of dysmenorrhea.

36. **(4)** The criteria for the diagnosis of bacterial vaginosis are characteristic milky homogeneous discharge, pH >4.5, amine odor (positive whiff) with addition of KOH, and the presence of epithelial cells studded with coccibacilli that obscure the borders (clue cells). Pseudohyphae are present in candidiasis.

37. **(2)** In Asherman's syndrome, a normally functioning uterus has been damaged and scarred secondary to instrumentation, usually a D&C. Ovulation may be occurring normally, but there is no healthy endometrial lining to shed, so clients do not menstruate. Asherman's syndrome is a problem with the uterus. The others, polycystic ovarian syndrome, hypogonadism, and premature ovarian failure are problems with the ovaries.

38. **(2)** The LH/FSH ratio in polycystic ovarian syndrome is 3:1. The normal LH/FSH ratio is 1.5:1.

39. **(4)** The criteria for the diagnosis of polycystic ovarian syndrome are onset of menstrual irregularity, increased body weight, physical and laboratory evidence of androgen excess, chronic anovulation, and normal prolactin levels. Estradiol is not increased but may be decreased.

40. **(3)** 90% of dysfunctional uterine bleeding is caused by anovulation. The lack of progesterone allows asynchronous, excessive proliferation of the endometrium. This tissue is fragile and the normal hemostatic mechanism is altered. Thyroid disease, blood dyscrasias, and uterine tumors can mimic dysfunctional uterine bleeding and must be excluded.

41. **(3)** A female-appearing person with a 46, XY karyotype is referred to as having androgen insensitivity syndrome, or testicular feminization. This maternal X-linked recessive disorder accounts for approximately 10% of all cases of amenorrhea, and these appear normal until puberty. These clients present with amenorrhea, scant or absent pubic hair, and abnormal or no breast development. Persons with Müllerian abnormalities have a normal XX karyotype with abnormalities of fallopian tubes, uterus, and upper vagina occurring in fetal development. In Turner's syndrome, there is congenital absence of ovaries due to loss of one X chromosome.

42. **(1)** The most common breast mass in young women less than 30 years old is the fibroadenoma. This benign breast mass is the third most common breast mass after fibrocystic changes and carcinoma. Fibrocystic breast changes are seen most commonly in women 30–50 years old. Intraductal papilloma is a wart-like growth located in the mammary duct and occurs in women 40–50 years old. Malignant breast neoplasms occur most frequently in women over 40 and are rarely seen in women 15–25 years old.

43. **(1)** Nonsteroidal anti-inflammatory analgesics inhibit prostaglandin synthesis and are effective agents in primary

dysmenorrhea. The other agents listed have not demonstrated effectiveness in primary dysmenorrhea. Other measures to decrease discomfort are exercise, relaxation techniques, heat application, and low-dose OCs.

44. **(4)** Secondary amenorrhea is defined as no menses for three cycle lengths or 6 months in a woman with previously established menses. Exercise can cause an increase in estrogen and endorphin levels, which influence the release of gonadotropin releasing hormone (GnRH). Without appropriate GnRH release, FSH and LH are not released appropriately, resulting in anovulation, which may lead to amenorrhea. The other conditions listed are causes of primary amenorrhea.

45. **(1)** This has the characteristics of a syphilitic lesion and needs to be evaluated. Only after determining the presence or type of STD can it be treated effectively. The herpes viral culture should be done while the lesion is present and the fluid from the vesicles can be obtained.

46. **(3)** Pregnancy is the most common cause of amenorrhea in young women. It is important to rule out pregnancy in female clients with a problem of amenorrhea, even if she is very athletic. Interviewing the client regarding her sexual practices is unreliable. The presence or absence of pregnancy should be determined prior to other diagnostic studies.

47. **(2)** A person who has never engaged in coital activity is not considered to be at risk for cervical cancer, due to the unlikelihood of exposure to HPV. In addition to others not listed here, the presence of HPV, multiple sexual partners, and/or previous HSIL are considered to be risk factors in the development of cervical cancer.

48. **(1)** The pseudohyphae and spores on the wet mount (KOH) are diagnostic for *Candida*. Chlamydia trachomatis is diagnosed by direct immunofluorescence assay (DFA, or by chlamydia culture). Gonorrhea is diagnosed by a cervical culture, and bacterial vaginitis shows clue cells on the wet mount prep.

49. **(1)** Cancer of the ovary is the leading cause of death due to female genital cancer, excluding the breast, in the United States.

50. **(1)** Flagellated protozoan confirms the diagnosis of trichomoniasis. The DFA test confirms chlamydia. Mucopurulent cervicitis is characterized by vaginal discharge and dysuria. Bacterial vaginosis is confirmed by gram stain and malodorous discharge with a fishy odor.

51. **(3)** The pelvic ultrasound is not a useful test for appendicitis, as it will not allow for adequate examination of the appendix. The CBC with differential is useful due to the expected rise in WBCs seen in this inflammatory state. The flat plate of the abdomen and KUB are very helpful to determine the extent of the problem and rule out other diagnoses. Since pregnancy can cause these symptoms if complicated by an ectopic, the practitioner should consider it as part of the differential diagnosis.

52. **(2)** Birth control pills have been shown to reduce the risk of endometrial cancer. Obesity, unopposed estrogen use, and advanced age, in addition to others not listed here, are considered to be risk factors for developing endometrial cancer.

53. **(2)** The diaphragm may be inserted any time up to 6 hours prior to intercourse and should be removed no sooner than 6 hours after intercourse. The diaphragm should be left in place for no longer than 24 hours.

54. **(2)** Urethral discomfort and recurrent urinary tract infections are associated with diaphragm use and are the most common reasons for discontinuing use and changing birth control methods.

55. **(3)** Birth control pill use has been shown to reduce the risk of ovarian cancer. Family history of ovarian cancer, advancing age, and positive BRCA 2 gene, in addition to others not listed here, are considered to be risk factors for developing ovarian cancer.

56. **(2)** Endometrial cancer is the most common female genital cancer.

57. **(3)** Herpes simplex virus type 2 commonly presents dramatically in the newly infected primary outbreak. Gonorrhea generally is associated with a mucopurulent vaginal discharge, and is not accompanied by vesicular lesions. Chlamydia can be associated with dysuria, and unless accompanied by PID, is not generally accompanied by fever or body aches, nor is it associated with vesicular lesions. Lymphogranuloma venereum is a rare disease classically accompanied by pustular enlargement of the lymph nodes, particularly the inguinal nodes. It is not associated with vesicles, but with bubos.

58. **(2)** Screening lab blood work for glucose, cardiac risk profile, and TSH in this age group without any stated risk factors is not cost effective, and is of little value. The client can be better served by a discussion regarding diet and exercise. Since this client is at risk for STDs, counseling and testing for these is a reasonable approach. Contraceptive information educates the client and allows her to make wiser choices in her family planning.

59. **(1)** Early menopause has not been associated with the development of breast cancer. High-fat diet, advancing age, early menarche, and others not listed here have been identified as risk factors in the development of breast cancer.

60. **(1)** The use of prenatal vitamins with folic acid preconceptually has been found to reduce the risk of neural tube defects in the fetus. It is important for the client to continue her exercise program, although some discussion about the type of exercise and any limitations are important once pregnancy is achieved. Since the client has had two previous pregnancies, it is likely that her rubella immune status has been determined; if she is found to not be immune to rubella, then a MMR vaccine should be recommended. This client is not of advanced maternal age and therefore does not require genetic counseling.

61. **(3)** Baseline lab work should be obtained to determine presence of anemia, possible pregnancy, and/or endocrine dysfunction.

62. **(4)** Fibrocystic breast disease is not a risk factor for breast cancer. In addition to others, those listed above are considered to be risk factors for breast cancer.

63. **(1)** The recommended age for a female to begin screening Pap smears is at the onset of sexual activity or at 18 years old. Since this client is 20 years old and has not had her first Pap smear yet, this would be the most appropriate test to perform. It is not necessary to perform STD screening on clients who have not been sexually active. Stool hemoccult testing and mammography are not recommended as screening procedures in the young adult.

64. **(3)** Heart disease remains the leading cause of death for females in the United States.

65. **(3)** Presence of bruising, particularly on genitalia, should raise suspicion of abuse. Combined with nonverbal behavior, the nurse practitioner should explore the possibility of abuse.

66. **(1)** Reactive cellular changes are most commonly associated with inflammation, including typical repair. Other causes include atrophy with inflammation (atrophic vaginitis), IUD use, radiation, and diethylstilbestrol exposure in utero. Oral contraceptives do not cause reactive changes, and estrogen vaginal cream may be used to improve atrophy.

67. **(2)** The exact cause of cervical disease is unknown. Evidence is increasing that sexually transmitted agents act as carcinogens. Viral exposure to herpes genitalis, HPV, and HIV are, therefore, considered risk factors. Other risk factors are related to sexual activity, such as sex prior to 18 years of age, first pregnancy prior to 18 years of age, multiple sexual partners, high parity, and partners with carcinoma in situ (CIS) of the penis.

68. **(4)** Lung cancer is the most common cancer in females in the United States.

69. **(3)** These symptoms are classic for menopausal syndrome, although it is true that there are some depressive symptoms listed. Antidepressant therapy and counseling for depression at this stage of

treatment is not appropriate. Testing, teaching, and treatment in this case should be aimed at the menopause. The depressive symptoms will undoubtedly improve with greater understanding and treatment of the menopausal symptoms.

70. **(1)** Chancroid is well established as a cofactor for HIV transmission.

71. **(4)** Monthly BSE is the most effective way to detect early breast changes. Educate her regarding increased tenderness during the last half of the menstrual cycle. BSE should be done 7 days after cycle ends.

72. **(2)** Symptoms are most likely indicative of benign fibroadenoma. Mammography is indicated. Surgical excision is unlikely for a young woman.

73. **(2)** The client needs to become more knowledgeable about the normal feel of implants as well as her own breast tissue. Mammography is not a substitute for BSE.

74. **(2)** A very firm cervix along with a cervical lesion/ulcer is suspicious for cancer of the cervix, which can be confirmed with a Pap smear.

75. **(1)** This complaint is an indication for breast exam and mammography. Although pain is not a common presenting symptom, it can be. Teaching BSE is important but not the most important action in this situation; hormone levels can explain breast pain but should not be the first place to look for an explanation.

76. **(2)** Toxic shock syndrome occurs primarily in menstruating women age 12–24 who use tampons. The diagnosis is made with the presence of fever over 102°F, macular rash, hypotension, and involvement of three or more organ systems.

77. **(4)** Over 16% of ectopic pregnancies present as surgical emergencies. In the United States, 1 in 1000 deaths from ectopic pregnancies occur as the result of blood loss.

78. **(4)** Almost half of all vaginal infections are due to candidiasis. The majority of women who develop the disease have recently taken antibiotics. It is not a sexually transmitted disease.

79. **(1)** It is important to evaluate the client for threatened abortion as soon as possible. It is most likely too soon for the CBC to reflect blood loss. A pelvic sonogram will take longer than a urine pregnancy test, and it is imperative that the client be immediately referred for a D&C, if her pregnancy test is positive.

80. **(2)** The most common site for breast cancer occurrence is the upper outer quadrant, followed by the area beneath the nipple.

81. **(3)** Pap smears are crucial for the detection of cervical cancer but do not diagnose uterine cancer. In the early stages, uterine cancer can be asymptomatic and would not be detectable even on bimanual examination.

Pharmacology

82. **(3)** Rocephin is a very effective drug for complicated urinary tract infection, but is unnecessary in the uncomplicated lower urinary tract infection. Bactrim DS and Macrobid are both very effective for urinary tract infection treatment. Pyridium will help to make the client more comfortable until the antibiotic reaches effective levels for treatment.

83. **(3)** Fluconazole is now approved for single-dose oral treatment of uncomplicated vulvovaginal candidiasis. It is most convenient for this client, who is unlikely to be extremely compliant with vaginal creams, given the upcoming travel. She does not have any contraindications to its use. Metronidazole and clindamycin are treatments for bacterial vaginosis and not for candida infections. Hydrocortisone is a topical steroid used for inflammatory dermatologic conditions and, while it may help the itching, it would not treat the candidiasis.

84. **(4)** Metronidazole vaginal cream is the treatment of choice for bacterial vaginosis. The newest recommendations allow for its use once daily for 5 days. The use of doxycycline listed here is for treatment of uncomplicated vaginal *Chlamydia trachomatis*. Terconazole vaginal cream is used for vaginal candidiasis; acyclovir is used for treatment of herpes simplex infections.

85. **(4)** While some authors may recommend herbal treatments for menopausal symptoms, there have not been any controlled studies regarding prevention of disease with this substance. Traditional medicine supports the use of HRT for prevention of osteoporosis and cardiovascular disease. The use of weight-bearing exercise and calcium intake has been shown to help maintain bone health. Cigarette smoking increases the risk for both osteoporosis and cardiovascular disease. This client can significantly reduce her risk of these two diseases by quitting her tobacco habit.

86. **(4)** Benzathine penicillin 2.4 million units IM is the treatment of choice for syphilis, but this client has condyloma acuminatum, not lata. The topical use of podophyllin, trichloroacetic acid, or cryotherapy are all accepted treatment modalities for condyloma acuminatum.

87. **(1)** Chlamydia will often present this way; take note of the dysuria, mucopurulent discharge, and cervical friability. The treatment of choice in ambulatory care settings is single-dose therapy with azithromycin 1 gm PO. The treatment listed in Option #2 is the treatment for gonorrhea, not chlamydia. Herpes simplex virus will present with painful vesicles in the vulvovaginal region and is treated with acyclovir 200 mg 1 cap PO q4h for 5 days for recurrences. Trichomoniasis can present this way; however, the absence of trichomonads on the wet mount is the key; the suggested treatment for trichomoniasis is metronidazole 2 gm PO in a single dose.

88. **(3)** The IUD would be a good choice for this client because it is extremely effective (>99%). There is not much she has to do to maintain it and there are no injections involved for the insertion or removal. The Depo-Provera injections, while being extremely effective (>99%), require an injection every 3 months, which could lead to decreased compliance for the client. The Norplant system of implants is also very effective (>99%), but it too requires injections for insertion and removal, and she is trying to avoid that. The diaphragm is a noninvasive contraceptive, and is effective (88%), but it requires her to be a more active participant in its use. None of these methods are contraindicated for this client, but an attempt should be made to help her choose one with which she is likely to be comfortable.

89. **(1)** Try to find out what the client has heard and dispel the fallacies if possible. Recent research supports the protective benefit provided by oral contraceptives from ovarian cancer as well as endometrial cancer. There is generally a reduction in the amount of menstrual bleeding and a regulation of the cycle. Minimal weight fluctuations are reported. Infertility is not associated with oral contraceptive use. To suggest either Norplant or Depo-Provera injections to someone who voices concerns about irregular menses or weight gain is sure to lead to an unhappy client, for these are quite common side effects of both methods. Option #3 and #4 are incorrect and misleading; Pap smears do not screen for ovarian cancer.

90. **(2)** The IUD is not recommended for use by individuals who are nulliparous or not in a stable, mutually monogamous relationship, due to the increased risk of complications. The use of oral contraceptives in a 41-year-old nonsmoker in good health is acceptable without concern. The client is already familiar with Norplant and may not be aware that she could have a new set of implants inserted when she has the others removed. Depo-Provera would be equally appropriate for this client.

91. **(2)** Very often, changing to a pill with a stronger progestational agent, or a different progestational agent, will resolve the problem of bleeding irregularities on oral contraceptives. There are so many choices one can make in the dosage or strength of a birth control pill that it is

likely that her problem can be resolved with a different pill. Taking them at a different time of day or on an empty stomach will do nothing to resolve the stated problem. The problem stated is not breakthrough bleeding, but rather prolonged bleeding likely secondary to poor endometrial support. If a change is not made in the pills, the client will continue to bleed in this fashion and may eventually develop anemia as a consequence.

92. **(3)** A pill such as Demulen 1/35 is a good choice for one with more androgenic characteristics due to the ability of this pill to exhibit a strong estrogenic effect with a moderate progestational effect. The Loestrin 1/20 is a poor choice for several reasons: the weaker dose of estrogen and progestin may not be adequate to support her endometrium, nor will it have a positive effect on the androgenic characteristics displayed by this client. Triphasil is a triphasic pill and does have a positive progestational effect that should support the endometrium well; however, the progestin in this pill tends to be slightly more androgenic, which is undesirable in this client.

93. **(4)** The use of combined oral contraceptives is not recommended for breast-feeding mothers due to the potential effect it can have on decreasing milk quantity and quality. Progestin only oral contraceptives are cleared for use in nursing mothers because there has not been any proven deleterious effect on either milk quantity or quality. Depo-Provera and the IUD are also accepted contraceptive methods for use in lactating females.

94. **(2)** Oral contraceptives are contraindicated for use in a cigarette smoker who is 35 years or over. There is no contraindication to the use of Depo-Provera injection in the cigarette smoker. The Progestacert IUD would probably be a good IUD choice for this client because it is only approved for 1 year's use and is safe in a cigarette smoker as well. The only contraindications to the use of condoms and spermicide is allergy to either substance.

95. **(4)** The Norplant implantation system is contraindicated in the person with a seizure disorder on phenobarbital or Dilantin because there is potential for either reduced anticonvulsant effect or reduced contraceptive effect. This does not occur with Depo-Provera, allowing the client to use this method freely, without concern. The IUD is not contraindicated for use with anticonvulsant medications, and the client is a good candidate for its use. The diaphragm is not contraindicated with the use of anticonvulsant therapy.

96. **(4)** It is not necessary to hospitalize the client with acute PID who is not vomiting or pregnant. If she does not respond well to outpatient treatment, then hospitalization can be recommended. The medications listed are the accepted treatment of choice for outpatient management of PID and should be started before the results of the lab tests are available, based on the clinical presentation of the client. The CBC and ESR are helpful to track the WBC and inflammatory response of the body.

97. **(3)** The use of unopposed estrogen in the client with an intact uterus could put her at risk for endometrial hyperplasia or cancer. The addition of a progestin protects the endometrium adequately. The client is an excellent candidate for endometrial biopsy, to document the status of the endometrium. This client also needs to be educated on the risks and benefits of HRT.

98. **(3)** The regimen of Premarin 0.3 mg has not been proven to be effective for prevention of osteoporosis or heart disease. In addition, lowering the dosage of the estrogen would not help the client's symptoms. The other dosage regimens listed are all acceptable choices for this client, proving that there are many effective ways for one to utilize HRT, allowing for individualization of the regimen to the client.

99. **(3)** Well-controlled hypertension is not a contraindication to the use of HRT.

100. **(1)** Metronidazole 2 gm PO in a single dose is the treatment of choice for trichomoniasis. Metronidazole vaginal cream does not effectively treat vaginal trichomoniasis. Fluconazole and terconazole are treatments for vaginal candidiasis.

101. **(2)** 0.625 mg of conjugated equine estrogen (Premarin) is the minimal effective dose to prevent osteoporosis.

102. **(1)** The diaphragm predisposes many women to urinary tract infections. Some women are sensitive to the contraceptive creme/jelly. The diaphragm has been associated with toxic shock syndrome, hence its use should be avoided during menses and not left in place any longer than 24 hours.

103. **(3)** The primary mechanism of action of oral contraceptives is suppression of ovulation. Ovulation is suppressed in 95–98% of clients. Should ovulation occur, the other event likely to prevent conception is thickening of cervical mucous, causing the endometrium to become atrophic, making the uterine environment unfavorable for implantation.

104. **(2)** Though still unproved conclusively, it is believed that the IUD probably causes inflammation of the endometrium, effectively preventing implantation.

105. **(3)** A progesterone-releasing IUD acts to decrease blood loss and cramping.

106. **(2)** The client no longer requires the use of Provera to protect the endometrium from the potential effects of estrogen; therefore, the progestin can be discontinued and the client given continuous estrogen therapy without concern. The other dosage regimens listed are appropriate for a client with an intact uterus on HRT.

107. **(3)** The progestin only pill does not consistently suppress ovulation. This suppression occurs in only 40–60% of cycles. This makes the progestin only pill less effective than combined contraceptive pills. The mechanism of action that contributes to the progestin only pill's effectiveness is creating an atrophic endometrium and possibly altering tubal physiology by decreasing ovum transport. Progestin only pills contain no estrogen and are a good choice for the breast-feeding woman.

108. **(1)** Informed consent is essential. The pros and cons of HRT should be explained, but the choice is up to the client.

109. **(3)** Depo-Provera is frequently associated with menstrual cycle changes. In fact, this irregular bleeding is the most commonly cited reason for discontinuation. These menstrual cycle changes range from heavy, irregular bleeding to spotting bleeding and even amenorrhea. Nausea and acne are usually effects of estrogen and are not seen with Depo-Provera.

110. **(3)** Repeated studies have demonstrated an increase in HDL and a decrease in LDL levels associated with postmenopausal administration of oral estrogens. This alteration in lipoprotein fractions has a beneficial effect on coronary artery disease and stroke.

111. **(4)** Clients taking alendronate (Fosamax) are instructed to take the medication upon arising, 30 minutes prior to eating, with a full glass of water. Clients should be instructed to remain erect after taking the medication to prevent esophageal irritation. Taking medication with food (reduces bioavailability by 40%), coffee or orange juice (decreases bioavailability by 60%), or after eating significantly reduces absorption.

112. **(1)** Women with a uterus taking unopposed exogenous estrogen have an increased risk of endometrial cancer. The addition of progesterone decreases this risk. The addition of progesterone may prompt bleeding, which many women view unfavorably. Progesterone does not affect cervical cancer, breast cancer, or gallbladder disease.

113. **(3)** Metronidazole (Flagyl) in a single 2-gm dose is the treatment of choice for trichomoniasis. An alternative is dividing the 2 gm into divided doses given the same day. This regimen has less nausea and may improve compliance.

114. **(4)** Metronidazole (Flagyl) is the treatment of choice for bacterial vaginosis. However, pregnancy should be ruled out prior to beginning treatment because metronidazole should not be used if there is any possibility the woman is pregnant. The sexual partners do not have to be treated, and doxycycline is not the drug of choice.

115. **(3)** She requires added protection through this cycle because of the low-dose OC. Dilantin may also decrease effectiveness of OCs, especially low dose.

116. **(1)** Because of homeless status, the nurse practitioner needs to use a single-dose treatment. Erythromycin, though correct medication, is a poor dosing choice for her.

117. **(3)** The most common cause of PID in sexually active women is gonococcal infections. Gonococcal infections are often accompanied by chlamydia and they are usually both treated.

118. **(3)** The American College of Physicians recommends HRT be considered for all women, as it is believed that it reduces the levels of LDLs while increasing the levels of HDLs.

Prenatal Care

Diagnostic Tests

1. Which test is recommended to be performed in the last trimester of pregnancy?

   1. Papanicolaou smear.

   2. Chorionic villus sampling.

   3. Vaginal culture for Group B *Streptococcus*.

   4. Fasting blood glucose.

2. The nurse practitioner schedules a 38-year-old primigravida for an amniocentesis at 16 weeks' gestation. The nurse practitioner's explanation of the purpose of this procedure would be to:

   1. Assess for the possibility of twins.

   2. Determine the bilirubin level.

   3. Perform genetic studies.

   4. Assess lecithin-sphingomyelin (L/S) ratio.

3. Management of a client after an amniocentesis includes assessing for:

   1. Increased fetal activity.

   2. Elevated temperature.

   3. Spontaneous rupture of the membranes.

   4. Abnormal lung sounds.

4. During the first trimester, the nurse practitioner is discussing the monitoring of the growth of twins during the pregnancy. She would explain which test to the client?

   1. Nonstress test.

   2. Sonogram.

   3. L/S ratio.

   4. Amniocentesis.

5. Screening for gestational diabetes mellitus (GDM) during pregnancy includes:

   1. 1-hour postprandial 100-gm glucose screen for all women between 24 and 28 weeks.

   2. 3-hour 100-gm GTT at initial visit for all women with history of GDM.

   3. 1-hour postprandial 50-gm glucose screen at initial visit for women at risk.

   4. Glycosylated hemoglobin A_{1C} (HgbA$_{1C}$) for all women between 24 and 28 weeks.

6. A 23-year-old G3 P0 has a 1-hour post–50-gm glucose screen result of 210 mg/dl. What is the next appropriate step to take?

 1. Order a 3-hour 100-gm GTT.

 2. Order a fasting blood sugar (FBS).

 3. Order an HgbA$_{1C}$.

 4. Refer immediately for diabetic treatment.

7. A teenager returns to the clinic for contraceptive follow-up after being on a low-dose oral contraceptive (OC) for 3 months. She complains of amenorrhea × 2 months, urinary frequency, and leukorrhea. Vaginal exam reveals uterus about 6 cm and the presence of Chadwick's sign. The first diagnostic test indicated should be:

 1. Pregnancy test.

 2. Complete blood count (CBC).

 3. Microscopic urinalysis.

 4. Culture for gonorrhea and chlamydia.

8. At an initial prenatal visit occurring in the first trimester, which blood test is not recommended?

 1. Antibody screen.

 2. Rubella titer.

 3. Maternal serum α-fetoprotein (MSAFP).

 4. Hepatitis B surface antigen.

9. Which laboratory finding remains unchanged during pregnancy?

 1. White blood cell (WBC) count.

 2. Red blood cell (RBC) volume.

 3. Fibrinogen level.

 4. Prothrombin level.

10. The nurse practitioner managing a pregnant client with sickle cell trait would include in the plan which information?

 1. CBC each trimester.

 2. Weekly nonstress test.

 3. Urine cultures each trimester.

 4. Frequent ultrasounds for growth.

Physiology of Pregnancy

11. Normal cardiovascular physiologic responses to pregnancy include:

 1. Increased heart rate, increased cardiac output, decreased blood volume, and systolic murmur.

 2. Increased heart rate, decreased cardiac output, increased blood volume, and systolic murmur.

 3. Increased heart rate, increased cardiac output, increased blood volume, and systolic murmur.

 4. Decreased heart rate, increased cardiac output, increased blood volume, and diastolic murmur.

12. How does progesterone affect the gastrointestinal system during pregnancy?

 1. Causes nausea and vomiting early in pregnancy.

 2. Causes hypertrophy and bleeding of gums.

 3. Delays gastric emptying time and decreases intestinal peristalsis.

 4. Causes diarrhea due to increased intestinal peristalsis.

13. A pregnant client has a hemoglobin of 11.7 gm/dl. Which factor explains this finding?

 1. Presence of iron deficiency anemia.

 2. The trimester of pregnancy.

 3. Physiologic anemia of pregnancy.

 4. Anemia of chronic disease.

14. Several physiologic changes in pregnancy may mimic heart disease. Which of the following is an abnormal finding in pregnancy?

 1. Third heart sound (S$_3$).

 2. Leg edema.

 3. Systolic murmur.

 4. Diastolic murmur.

15. Which of the following is **not** a common urinary system finding during pregnancy?

    1. Physiologic hydronephrosis.

    2. Increased glomerular filtration rate.

    3. Increased urinary frequency.

    4. Proteinuria.

16. At 20 weeks' gestation, the nurse practitioner would expect to palpate the fundus at:

    1. The symphysis pubis.

    2. The umbilicus.

    3. Halfway between the symphysis pubis and umbilicus.

    4. The xiphoid.

17. During pregnancy, estrogen is responsible for:

    1. Hyperpigmentation.

    2. Facilitating implantation.

    3. Reducing smooth muscle tone.

    4. Decreased uterine contractility.

18. Which is **not** a placental hormone?

    1. Human chorionic gonadotropin (hCG).

    2. Estrogen.

    3. Relaxin.

    4. Cortisol.

19. What is the function of the placental hormone relaxin?

    1. Causes changes in the endometrium and relaxes smooth muscle.

    2. Stimulates the development of the ductal system of the breasts and causes hypertrophy and hyperplasia of the uterus.

    3. Aids in softening smooth muscle and connective tissue.

    4. Involved with metabolizing certain nutrients and aids in the growth of breasts and other maternal tissues.

20. The nurse practitioner understands that at 12 weeks of fetal development:

    1. Quickening is felt.

    2. Fetal heart tones should be heard with Doppler.

    3. Fetal heart tones should be heard with stethoscope.

    4. Respiratory movements occur.

21. A positive sign of pregnancy is:

    1. Softening of the cervix.

    2. Fetal heart beat.

    3. Enlargement of uterus and abdomen.

    4. Mother's perception of fetal movement.

22. The bluish discoloration of the cervix and vagina is known as:

    1. Goodell's sign.

    2. Chadwick's sign.

    3. Hegar's sign.

    4. Braxton Hicks' sign.

23. Which is **not** a normal cervical finding in the second trimester?

    1. Cervix firm.

    2. Cervical dilation.

    3. Cervix 2 cm long.

    4. Cervix posterior.

24. A woman who has missed her period for 5 weeks states that she has been having nausea with some vomiting in the morning hours. The woman also states that she may have a urinary tract infection due to frequency and fatigue. The nurse practitioner would recognize these symptoms to be:

    1. A possible systemic infection.

    2. Positive signs of pregnancy.

    3. Presumptive signs of pregnancy.

    4. Probable signs of pregnancy.

Prenatal Care

25. Dietary changes to reduce nausea and vomiting in pregnancy include:

    1. Eat small, frequent, low-fat meals and avoid spicy foods.
    2. Avoid carbonated beverages.
    3. Avoid eating first thing in the morning.
    4. Increase iron and prenatal vitamins to twice daily.

26. The average extra calories per day required for pregnancy are:

    1. 100 calories.
    2. 300 calories.
    3. 500 calories.
    4. 800 calories.

27. A 22-week-pregnant client is planning a prolonged car trip. The nurse practitioner's recommendations would **not** include:

    1. Support stockings.
    2. Frequent (every 1–2 hours) walking.
    3. Wearing a seat belt.
    4. Knee-high stockings.

28. The recommended visits for a low-risk client at 28 weeks of pregnancy is every:

    1. 4 weeks.
    2. Week.
    3. 2 weeks.
    4. 6 weeks.

29. The most common indication for genetic counseling is:

    1. Maternal age.
    2. Drug exposure during the first trimester.
    3. Increased MSAFP.
    4. History of previous stillbirth.

30. Clients at highest risk for having a child with Tay-Sachs disease are:

    1. Black.
    2. Jewish.
    3. Oriental.
    4. 35 years or older at conception.

31. The nurse practitioner teaches a prenatal client that a significant source of toxoplasmosis is:

    1. Rare hamburger.
    2. Fresh fruits.
    3. Raw oysters.
    4. Raw vegetables.

32. A pregnant diabetic client is in the clinic for a prenatal visit; she is at 34 weeks' gestation. She was last seen in the clinic 1 month ago and her dose of insulin had not changed from the previous month. This month her blood sugar remains in control with the same amount of insulin. The nurse practitioner would interpret this information as:

    1. This is normal and indicates the woman has been on her diet and her insulin needs are stable.
    2. The infant is developing well and his pancreas is helping to control the increased blood sugar from the mother.
    3. With the developing fetus, there should be an increase in the serum glucose for increased nourishment.
    4. The mother may be developing problems with placental insufficiency and should be thoroughly evaluated.

33. What would be appropriate management for a primigravida at term who experiences rupture of the membranes?

    1. Begin timing contractions.
    2. Begin pushing.
    3. Take a warm bath.
    4. Refrain from sexual intercourse.

34. An adult female presents with her spouse for a prenatal visit. During the exam, you notice bruising of the abdomen and back. You also note that the spouse does most of the talking during the history. The best approach to this situation is:

    1. Ask the spouse to leave the room so you can do a pelvic exam.

    2. Ask the client to accompany you to the lab for blood work, then ask about bruises.

    3. Ask the client about the bruises during the exam.

    4. Do nothing; domestic violence is beyond the scope of your practice.

35. A client at 20 weeks' gestation calls the nurse practitioner to ask if she can sit in a hot tub to help her relax. What is the best response to this question?

    1. A hot tub is encouraged; however, she should not sit in it longer than 30 minutes.

    2. She may use the hot tub; however, she should always have someone with her while she is in the tub.

    3. Hot tubs are not recommended due to the increase in vaginal infections during pregnancy.

    4. She should not use a hot tub during pregnancy, since the increase in body temperature is not considered safe.

36. Which statement is true about smoking during pregnancy?

    1. The rate of spontaneous abortions among smokers is the same as in nonsmokers.

    2. Risks of complications increase with the number of cigarettes smoked.

    3. Discontinuation of smoking during pregnancy has no effect on pregnancy outcome.

    4. There is not a relationship between smoking and sudden infant death syndrome (SIDS).

37. Chlamydia infections during pregnancy may be associated with:

    1. Transplacental transmission to fetus.

    2. Congenital anomalies of the eyes.

    3. Premature rupture of membranes.

    4. Fetal hydrops.

38. A primigravida at 38 weeks' gestation comes into the office for evaluation of her abdominal cramping. The nurse practitioner observes contractions that produce a very taunt abdomen and are irregular in occurrence. The woman states the contractions get stronger, then decrease. There is no vaginal discharge, and her cervix is dilated to 2 cm. What is the best interpretation and action for the nurse practitioner to take at this time?

    1. The woman is in early stages of labor, and due to her gestational level she should go to the hospital at this time.

    2. These are probably Braxton Hicks' contractions; send the woman home and have her notify the office if contractions become stronger or different.

    3. Order a sonogram and retain the woman in the office to evaluate the progress of the contractions.

    4. Draw blood for hCG levels, obtain urine sample for evaluation of infection, and monitor progress of contractions for next 4 hours.

39. During pregnancy, sexual relations are contraindicated:

    1. During the first trimester, when there is a history of spontaneous abortion.

    2. After 36 weeks' gestation.

    3. With the diagnosis of placenta previa.

    4. With excessive maternal weight gain.

40. The nurse practitioner is assessing a client who has a positive pregnancy test. The laboratory data indicate that the mother's blood group is O-positive and the father's is AB-negative. What risk is there for this pregnancy?

    1. The mother may build up antibodies to the infant's blood if the infant is type B-positive, which will be significant in future pregnancies.

    2. The mother is RH-positive; therefore, if the infant is Rh-negative there is an increased incidence of the infant building up Rh antibodies.

    3. Since the mother is O and the father is AB, there is an increased risk for the development of an ABO incompatibility.

    4. Type O blood is the dominant characteristic; the infant's blood will be in the O group and there will be no complications.

41. A 23-year-old client, who is in her twelfth week of pregnancy, comes to the clinic for her regular checkup. She has no history of complications or bleeding. The client is concerned regarding sexual activity and her pregnancy. What guidelines would the practitioner offer to this client?

    1. Normal sexual activity is permissible; it is normal if she experiences some abdominal cramping with orgasm.

    2. Her partner should wear a condom to prevent transmission of infection at the cervical os.

    3. Sexual intercourse should be limited to twice a week to prevent excessive stimulation of uterine contractions.

    4. Normal intercourse is permissible; however, she should not experiment with various positions.

42. The nurse practitioner is preparing to teach childbirth classes. The birthing center encourages the use of the Bradley method. What are the characteristics of this childbirth method?

    1. It is a partner-coached method with no medication during labor and delivery.

    2. The focus is on the mother's breathing and relaxation exercises.

3. It increases utilization of psychoprophylaxis, with focus on chest breathing and abdominal release.

4. The focus is on the use of an epidural after 6-cm dilatation, partner-coached breathing, and relaxation.

43. The pregnant client wishes to have further information regarding exercise guidelines. She runs on the treadmill 4 mph for 30 minutes daily, then does 30 additional minutes of free weights and lower leg machines at the gym. General guidelines should include all **except**:

    1. Keep the heart rate below 140 bpm.

    2. Limit free weight for upper body to <10 lb each.

    3. Limit exercise time to 30 minutes total.

    4. Avoid breathlessness and excessive heat.

Prenatal Complications

44. In performing a prenatal evaluation of a client who is 8 weeks pregnant, there are no identifiable factors in her history regarding complications with this pregnancy. What factors would the nurse practitioner identify as a potential problem for this pregnancy?

    1. Lower midabdominal pain accompanied by dizziness and shoulder pain.

    2. Nausea and vomiting each morning, increased fatigue, urine is negative for ketones.

    3. Increased urinary frequency, nocturia, and occasional afternoon headaches.

    4. Menstrual-like cramping, increased breast tenderness around the areola, and enlarged Montgomery's tubercles.

45. Which is not a treatment for the client with mild pregnancy-induced hypertension (PIH)?

    1. Modified bed rest.

    2. Monitor blood pressure (BP), weight, and urinary protein.

    3. Methyldopa (Aldomet) 250 mg PO tid.

4. Diet and nutritional counseling to increase water and protein intake, and decrease salt intake to <2 gm/day.

46. The nurse practitioner would note which finding as a possible sign of PIH?

    1. Urgency to urinate at night.

    2. Edema in the extremities and puffy face.

    3. Stomach cramps.

    4. Clear fluid discharge from the nipple.

47. Which is an **abnormal** complaint of the third trimester of pregnancy?

    1. Leukorrhea.

    2. Headache with blurred vision.

    3. Urinary frequency.

    4. Uterine contractions.

48. Which finding would the nurse practitioner assess in a client with a ruptured tubal pregnancy?

    1. Sharp, stabbing pain localizing to left quadrant with BP of 90/58.

    2. Board-like rigidity of the uterus with abdominal distention.

    3. Dilatation of the cervix and rapidly falling BP and pulse.

    4. Serosanguineous vaginal fluid with grape-like vesicles.

49. A prenatal client has a diagnosis of abruptio placentae. In order to detect complications, the nurse practitioner would:

    1. Check blood sugar q2h.

    2. Assess vital signs hourly.

    3. Position client in right lateral position.

    4. Monitor fibrinogen and coagulation studies.

50. Which is **not** an expected complication of the pregnant client 35 years or older?

    1. Spontaneous abortion (SAB).

    2. Pregnancy-induced hypertension.

3. Gestational diabetes.

4. Anemia.

51. What would be **incorrect** advice to the nonlaboring pregnant client upon the second-trimester diagnosis of a placenta previa?

    1. Pelvic rest.

    2. Report any bright red bleeding.

    3. Planned cesarean section.

    4. Follow-up ultrasound at 32 weeks' gestation.

52. A client at 32 weeks' gestation comes for her regular prenatal checkup. The client states that she has noticed an increase in discharge, which is clear with no particular odor and seems to be increased when she gets up in the morning. What should the nurse practitioner order or check at this time?

    1. Determine presence of frequency and urgency and get a urine sample.

    2. With a sterile speculum, obtain fluid sample from cervical area and perform a fern test.

    3. Draw a serum hCG level and perform a urine dipstick test.

    4. Perform a vaginal exam to determine level of dilatation and status of amniotic membrane.

53. Testing for gestational diabetes should be done:

    1. When a client has a history of a previous macrosomatia infant.

    2. If the client is obese.

    3. On all pregnant women.

    4. When the client has glycosuria.

54. Which is **not** a predisposing factor of PIH?

    1. Primigravida.

    2. Age >35.

    3. Multiple gestation.

    4. Hyperthyroidism.

55. For a pregnant client at 32 weeks' gestation with a BP of 140/92, weight gain the past 2 weeks of 4 lb, trace protein on urine dipstick, 1+ pitting edema in the feet, and 2+ reflexes, the probable diagnosis would be:

    1. Mild pregnancy-induced hypertension.

    2. Severe pregnancy-induced hypertension.

    3. Eclampsia.

    4. Hemolysis, elevated liver enzymes, low platelets (HELLP) syndrome.

56. Which is **not** an expected complication of the pregnant teen who is age 17 or younger.

    1. Premature labor and birth.

    2. Anemia.

    3. Gestational diabetes.

    4. Pregnancy-induced hypertension.

57. Which is least likely to be found in a client presenting with an ectopic pregnancy?

    1. Pain.

    2. Missed menses.

    3. Vaginal bleeding.

    4. Abdominal mass.

58. Which is **not** true about an ectopic pregnancy?

    1. 90% occur in the fallopian tube.

    2. Account for approximately 10% of maternal deaths.

    3. Prior history of pelvic inflammatory disease (PID) is reported in 50% of clients with ectopics.

    4. Previous ectopic pregnancy does not increase risk of another ectopic pregnancy.

59. A client presents to the clinic with a diagnosis of threatened abortion. The nurse practitioner describes this as:

    1. Vaginal bleeding with or without cramping and no cervical change.

    2. Vaginal bleeding with cramping and cervical change.

3. Loss of pregnancy symptoms, decrease in uterine size, and cervix closed and firm.

4. Cramping, bleeding, and incomplete expulsion of products of conception.

60. Which is an **abnormal** complaint in the first trimester of pregnancy?

    1. Nausea and vomiting.

    2. Fatigue.

    3. Vaginal bleeding.

    4. Low backache.

61. Ten weeks into a client's pregnancy, she begins to experience vaginal bleeding. The client's hCG levels remain elevated. The nurse practitioner would instruct the client to call the clinic with signs of:

    1. Nausea and vomiting.

    2. Abdominal pain or cramping.

    3. Urinary frequency.

    4. Fatigue and tiredness.

62. Which statement is true regarding the course of pruritic urticaria, papules, and plaques of pregnancy (PUPPP)?

    1. Perinatal mortality is increased.

    2. Pruritis is increased postpartum.

    3. Lesions first appear on abdomen.

    4. Onset is usually in the first trimester.

63. Cocaine use during pregnancy is associated with:

    1. Abruptio placentae.

    2. Postdate pregnancy.

    3. Macrosomatia infant.

    4. Maternal hypotension.

64. A pregnant employee who works at a day-care center is concerned about a recent outbreak of "fifth disease." The nurse practitioner understands that:

    1. Most parvovirus B19 infections in utero are associated with an increased number of congenital anomalies.

2. There are no isoimmunization-associated problems for the mother exposed to a young child with fifth disease.

3. Parvovirus B19 has caused hydrops fetalis and death in some fetuses who have been infected in utero.

4. The mortality risk for a fetus is extremely high, especially if the mother has never had fifth disease.

65. A young adult client, G2 P1 A0 L1, 10 weeks' gestation intrauterine pregnancy (IUP) is seen for her first obstetric intake history and physical. She knows when she conceived, and denies any vaginal bleeding or abdominal pain. The client has a soft, nontender fundus that measures 14 cm, the adnexal exam is negative for mass or tenderness, and no fetal heart tones (FHTs) are audible with the doptone. The most likely diagnosis seen on ultrasound is:

1. Multiple gestation.
2. Fibroid uterus.
3. Ectopic pregnancy.
4. 14-week viable IUP.

66. Which is an **abnormal** complaint in the second trimester or pregnancy?

1. Frequent uterine contractions.
2. Frequent fetal movement
3. Calf cramps.
4. Heartburn.

Pharmacology

67. Which immunization is contraindicated in pregnancy?

1. Polio vaccine.
2. Hepatitis B vaccine.
3. Measles-mumps-rubella (MMR).
4. Tetanus.

68. If studies in animals or pregnant women demonstrate evidence of fetal abnormality or risk, or if the potential for fetal risk clearly outweighs the possible benefit of the drug, the Food and Drug Administration (FDA) category for this drug is:

1. B.
2. C.
3. D.
4. X.

69. The nurse practitioner is aware that fetal exposure to tetracycline causes:

1. Blindness.
2. Hearing loss.
3. Tooth discoloration.
4. Limb deformities.

70. Which of the following may reduce the risk of neural tube defect when taken prior to conception?

1. Vitamin A.
2. Pyroxidine.
3. Folic acid.
4. Vitamin C.

71. The current recommendation for antepartum treatment of Rh-negative pregnant women, when Rh status of the partner is unknown, with Rh immune globulin (RhoGAM) includes:

1. Administration of 300 μg at 28 weeks and 36 weeks of pregnancy.
2. Administration of 300 μg at 28 weeks of pregnancy to all Rh-negative women.
3. Administration of 300 μg in each trimester.
4. No administration is needed until postpartum.

72. A woman who is 24 weeks pregnant calls the clinic to see if she can take famotidine (Pepsid) for her indigestion. What is the best response by the nurse practitioner?

    1. Do not take the medication; try aluminum hydroxide (Maalox).

    2. It is OK to take it, but do not take over two doses of 10 mg each per day.

    3. Rather than taking famotidine (Pepsid), take ranitidine (Zantac), as it is more effective.

    4. Have her make an appointment to more thoroughly investigate the cause of the indigestion.

73. Medication recommendations for pregnancy are categorized by the FDA regarding administration during pregnancy. What is the best description of a Category C drug?

    1. No studies are available in animals and humans; definitive evidence of risk to the human fetus exists.

    2. Animal studies do not indicate a risk to the fetus, but there are no controlled studies in humans.

    3. Controlled studies in women fail to demonstrate a risk to the fetus in the first trimester.

    4. Studies in animals or humans have demonstrated fetal abnormalities and there is evidence of fetal risk.

16   Answers & Rationales

Diagnostic Tests

1. **(3)** It is recommended to have a culture of the lower vaginal tract for Group B *Streptococcus* in late pregnancy, usually at or after the 36th week. If the mother is positive, she can be treated prior to delivery, thus decreasing the risk of group B strep infection in the newborn. The Pap smear is to be collected during the first prenatal visit, unless the mother has recent results available. Chorionic villus sampling is usually done around 9–11 weeks. Fasting blood glucose is usually obtained around 28 weeks gestation.

2. **(3)** The woman's age places her at risk for a Down's syndrome baby. The L/S ratio is tested in the third trimester for fetal lung maturity.

3. **(3)** Damage to the membranes is a possibility and a high-priority situation. Fever would not be an immediate problem. Fetal heart rate is monitored, not activity.

4. **(2)** The ultrasound test (sonogram) is used to assess growth of the fetus, position of the placenta, and position of the fetus. The nonstress test (NST) is used to observe the response of the fetal heart rate to the stress of activity. The L/S ratio determines if there is sufficient surfactant. An amniocentesis is performed to obtain amniotic fluid for analysis at a later date in the pregnancy, if indicated.

5. **(3)** This is standard screen for women at risk. It should also be done for all other pregnant women between 24 and 28 weeks' gestation. If the result of this test is 140 or above, then a 3-hour GTT is done.

6. **(2)** This is standard diagnostic decision tree for a screen >200 mg. If FBS is >130 mg, refer to and/or consult with physician for treatment plan.

7. **(1)** This is a clinical picture highly indicative of pregnancy.

8. **(3)** Routine prenatal labs include CBC, blood type and Rh status, antibody screen, hepatitis B surface antigen, syphilis screen, and rubella immune status. The MSAFP is done between 15 and 20 weeks, before which very little AFP is produced by the fetus, and results would be inaccurate.

9. **(4)** Red blood cell volume increases approximately 30%, and white blood cells increase 5000–12,000/mm^3. Fibrin, fibrinogen, and plasma levels of factors VII, IX, and X are also increased. Prothrombin levels remain unchanged.

10. **(3)** Sickle cell trait occurs in 8% of American blacks. These women are asymptomatic, not anemic, and usually have no problems except under conditions of hypoxia. There is no difference in perinatal outcome and these women do not require frequent ultrasounds or nonstress testing. They are at increased risk for asymptomatic bacteriuria and require a urine culture each trimester.

Physiology of Pregnancy

11. **(3)** In pregnancy, a hyperdynamic state is caused by an increase in blood volume, which results in a slightly increased heart rate and increased cardiac output. Systolic ejection murmurs are common and caused by increased flow across the pulmonic and aortic valves. Diastolic murmurs are abnormal and require referral.

12. **(3)** Progesterone affects the gastrointestinal system by decreasing smooth muscle tone, delaying gastric emptying, and decreasing intestinal peristalsis. Human chorionic gonadotropin is associated with nausea and vomiting early in pregnancy. Estrogen causes the gums to become hyperemic, soft, and swollen, with a tendency to bleed.

13. **(3)** The increase in plasma volume combined with a slower rise in RBC production produces a dilutional anemia. Hemoglobin and hematocrit decrease in relation to plasma volume. True anemia occurs with a hemoglobin <11 gm/dl and hematocrit <35%.

14. **(4)** Leg edema is due to increased venous pressure in the legs. Both components of the first heart sound become louder and there is an exaggerated splitting, and an S_3 gallop is common after midpregnancy. Systolic ejection murmurs are common and are due to the increased flow across the aortic and pulmonic valves. Diastolic murmurs are an abnormal finding.

15. **(4)** Changes in renal structure are influenced by estrogen, progesterone, increased blood volume, and uterine pressure. Changes in the collection system, such as dilatation of renal pelvis and ureters, cause a physiologic hydronephrosis. The glomerular filtration rate does increase during pregnancy. Increased urinary frequency is related to the increasing size of the uterus and its pressure on the bladder. Proteinuria is abnormal except in very concentrated urine or in the first voided specimen upon arising. Proteinuria is a warning of impaired kidney function or PIH.

16. **(2)** The expected fundal height at 20 weeks is at the umbilicus. At 12 weeks, the fundus can be palpated just above the symphysis, and at 16 weeks between the symphysis and umbilicus. The fundus is palpated at the xiphoid at approximately 36 weeks.

17. **(1)** During pregnancy, estrogen is responsible for stimulation of melanin-stimulating hormone, thus resulting in hyperpigmentation. Progesterone from the corpus luteum and later the placenta is responsible for facilitating implantation, decreasing uterine contractility, and reducing smooth muscle tone.

18. **(4)** There are five placental hormones: hCG, estrogen, progesterone, human placental lactogen, and relaxin. Cortisol is not a placental hormone.

19. **(3)** Relaxin aids in softening smooth muscle and connective tissue in preparation for labor and delivery. Progesterone relaxes smooth muscle and causes changes in the endometrium. Estrogen stimulates the development of the ductal system of the breasts and causes hypertrophy and hyperplasia of the uterus. Human placental lactogen is involved with metabolism of glucose, fatty acids, and amino acids. It also aids in the growth of the breasts and other maternal tissues.

20. **(2)** Fetal heart tones should be heard by 12 weeks and may be heard as early as 10 weeks. Quickening is felt at 16–20 weeks. Fetal heart tones can be heard by stethoscope at 20 weeks. Respiratory movements occur later in fetal development, at approximately 24 weeks.

21. **(2)** Positive evidence of pregnancy are fetal heartbeat, palpation of fetal movement by examiner, and visualization of the fetus (ultrasonography). Amenorrhea, nausea, emesis, urinary frequency, fatigue, skin changes, and mother's perception of fetal movement are presumptive evidence of pregnancy. Probable evidence of pregnancy includes softening of the cervix, softening of the lower uterine segment, cyanosis of cervix and vagina, Braxton Hicks' contractions, ballottement, palpation of fetal outline by examiner, and pregnancy tests.

22. **(2)** Chadwick's sign occurs at 6–8 weeks' gestation and is the bluish discoloration of the cervix and vagina. Goodell's sign is the

softening of the cervix that is seen as early as 4 weeks' gestation. Hegar's sign is the softening of the lower uterine segment. Braxton Hicks' are contractions of the uterus that can occur as early as 16 weeks' gestation.

23. **(2)** It is considered neither normal nor expected for one to have a dilated cervix at any time in the second trimester of pregnancy. The cervix will typically be firm, 2 cm long and posterior, as well as closed.

24. **(3)** Missed menstrual periods, nausea, vomiting, frequency, and fatigue are presumptive signs (subjective) of pregnancy. Probable signs of pregnancy are objective, such as Chadwick's sign, ballottement, and a positive pregnancy test. Positive signs of pregnancy are fetal heart rate or sonogram.

Prenatal Care

25. **(1)** Clients should eat frequent small meals to keep some food in the stomach at all times and avoid stomach distention. Sipping on carbonated beverages may be helpful. Having crackers at the bedside to take before rising in the morning may be a successful preventative measure.

26. **(2)** The pregnant woman requires approximately 15% more calories per day than nonpregnant women. This is approximately 300 calories per day and depends on the client's weight and activity level.

27. **(4)** Venous stasis occurs with prolonged sitting and may be a risk factor for thrombophlebitis. Support stockings and frequent walking should be encouraged. Knee-high stockings have elastic around the calf that may act as a tourniquet and should be avoided during pregnancy. Seat belts are recommended.

28. **(3)** The American College of Obstetricians and Gynecologists (ACOG) recommends visits every 2 weeks starting at 28 weeks until 36 weeks. At 36 weeks, visits are weekly until delivery.

29. **(1)** The largest group of women who potentially benefit from genetic counseling are those 35 and older. The number of births to women between 35 and 40 years old has increased by approximately 35% in the 1990s. The primary cause of congenital abnormalities in women older than 35 years is chromosomal abnormalities. The other answers are all reasons for genetic counseling, but to a much lesser degree.

30. **(2)** The incidence of the Tay-Sachs gene in the Jewish population is 1 in 30 as compared to 1 in 300 for the non-Jewish population.

31. **(1)** Undercooked red meat is a major source of toxoplasmosis. Pregnant women should be cautioned against eating undercooked meats. Cats are also shown to be hosts. Toxoplasmosis is spread through cat faces. Pregnant women should be warned about cleaning the litter box and contaminated soil.

32. **(4)** In the last two trimesters of pregnancy, the insulin needs should steadily increase due to the insulin antagonism from the placenta, as well as from the fetus. By not increasing her need for insulin, she could be showing signs of placental insufficiency.

33. **(4)** Without the protective barrier of the amniotic membrane, the mother and the baby are susceptible to infection. The client should refrain from sexual intercourse due to the possibility of introduction of pathogens. Bathing would also be a hazard due to the possibility of contracting an infection from the bath water.

34. **(2)** While Option #1 may work, it may also serve to arouse the spouse's suspicion and create a situation where you must then insist he leave or drop the request. Option #2 is best, as it gives a legitimate reason to quickly move the client from the room, provides a moment of privacy to inquire about the bruises, and provides an opportunity to move the client to a safe place if needed without creating confrontation.

35. **(4)** Hot tubs, saunas, or whirlpools are not recommended during pregnancy due to the substantial increase in body temperature. The increase in temperature is not considered safe, nor is the increase in syncope due to peripheral dilatation.

36. **(2)** The risk of complications and perinatal loss increases with the number of cigarettes smoked. Discontinuation or decrease in the amount of cigarettes smoked during pregnancy can reduce the risk of complications, especially for high-risk women.

37. **(3)** Premature rupture of membranes may be associated with chlamydia infections. Intrauterine transmission of *Chlamydia trachomatis* to the fetus has not been demonstrated. There is no evidence of fetal eye anomalies; however, without prophylaxis, conjunctivitis will develop in 30–50% of infants 7–15 days after birth.

38. **(2)** The symptoms presented are classic for false labor or Braxton Hicks' contractions. The characteristics of these contractions are that they occur high on the abdomen and "out front," and they may increase in intensity but then decrease with activity. They are not regular and do not precipitate any cervical dilatation. Cervical dilatation, leakage or rupture of membranes, and contractions 3–5 minutes apart are characteristic of labor contractions and an indication for the client to go to the hospital.

39. **(3)** In placenta previa, the placenta is improperly positioned in the lower uterine segment, covering all or part of the cervical os. There is an increased risk of bleeding. Management includes bed rest, no intercourse, no vaginal exams, instruction on what to do if bleeding occurs, and close fetal surveillance.

40. **(3)** There is increased incidence of ABO incompatibility if the mother is blood group O and the infant is either blood group A or B. Rh incompatibility occurs only when the mother is Rh-negative and is carrying an Rh-positive infant. In the most common cases of ABO incompatibility there is a production of maternal antibodies against the A cells or the B cells.

41. **(1)** Normal sexual activity is encouraged, and some cramping with orgasm is normal. Condoms are not necessary and there is no reason to limit sexual activity. Experimenting with various positions is encouraged to find a position of comfort.

42. **(1)** The classic description of this method is that the training is focused on the father or the partner (coach) rather than on the mother. The delivery is completely unmedicated. The Lamaze and Read methods focus on teaching the mother breathing and relaxation techniques. Psychoprophylaxis is a term associated with the Lamaze method.

43. **(3)** There is no reason to limit the amount of time for exercise, provided the client is feeling well. By keeping the heart rate below 140 bpm there is less chance for internal overheating and exhaustion. The ACOG suggests limiting the free weight use to <10 lb to avoid undue stress and strain on muscles and ligaments. Avoidance of breathlessness and excessive heat will allow for better circulation to the fetus.

Prenatal Complications

44. **(1)** Lower abdominal pain with referred shoulder pain and dizziness may be indications of bleeding. Referred shoulder pain is caused by irritation to the diaphragm, which may be air or blood. Other options presented are common discomforts of the first trimester of pregnancy and do not require immediate intervention; however, discomforts should be monitored.

45. **(3)** The use of medication is no longer felt to be useful in the treatment of mild PIH and, in fact, could be hazardous. The client is best treated conservatively with modified bed rest on the left side and dietary counseling, along with close monitoring of the BP, weight, and urinary protein. Close follow-up with examination for edema or symptomatic change and monitoring of the fetus are also performed.

46. **(2)** Classic signs of PIH are generalized edema of the extremities and around the face, proteinuria, and hypertension. Stomach cramps could be an indication of early labor or gastrointestinal upset. Clear nipple fluid would be an early sign of colostrum.

47. **(2)** Headache associated with blurred vision could represent early symptoms of mild pre-eclampsia or PIH and warrants further work-up to rule out a problem. The other symptoms are not of concern if they are not associated with other symptoms as well.

48. **(1)** The ruptured fallopian tube causes a sharp, sudden, stabbing pain. Symptoms of shock (decreased BP, increased pulse and respirations) occur, as the client quickly becomes a surgical emergency. Board-like abdominal rigidity is often noted with abruptio placentae. Grape-like vesicles are associated with hydatidiform mole.

49. **(4)** Prenatal clients with abruptio placentae are prone to the development of disseminated intravascular coagulation (DIC), which is characterized by abnormal fibrinogen and coagulation studies.

50. **(4)** The risk for anemia in pregnancy does not increase with age. The risks for SAB, PIH, and gestational diabetes do increase with maternal age.

51. **(3)** There is no reason to plan a cesarean section upon diagnosis of the placenta previa at this stage of the pregnancy, because the lower segment of the uterus goes through its final maturation between 28 and 32 weeks' gestation. There is an excellent chance that the placenta will migrate by the third trimester, thus allowing for vaginal birth, barring any other unforeseen factors.

52. **(2)** The client may be experiencing a leak in the amniotic fluid sac. A sterile speculum should be used for the examination to decrease the incidence of amnionitis. The "fern test" discriminates between vaginal discharge and amniotic fluid. Amniotic fluid forms a fern-like pattern on the slide and can be easily identified under a microscope. Another test to determine amniotic fluid is the nitrazine test; if the pH is 7, it is likely to be amniotic fluid. The normal pH of vaginal fluid is 3.5–5.

53. **(3)** Over one half of pregnant women who exhibit gestational diabetes lack the classic risk factors of family history of diabetes, unexpected stillbirth, prior macrosomatia infant, obesity, advanced maternal age, or glycosuria. The best answer is that all women should be screened for gestational diabetes.

54. **(4)** Predisposing factors in PIH include primigravida, <20 years or >35 years of age, women with vascular diseases (hypertension, systemic lupus erythematosis, diabetes mellitus, renal disease), family history, previous history of pre-eclampsia, and multiple gestation. Hyperthyroidism does not predispose to PIH.

55. **(1)** Mild PIH (pre-eclampsia) is consistent with a systolic BP ≥140 mm Hg or systolic rise ≥30 mm Hg, and/or diastolic BP ≥90 or diastolic rise ≥15 mm Hg, weight gain >2 lb/week, nondepenedent edema ≥1+ with normal reflexes. Severe pre-eclampsia symptoms include BP ≥160/100, weight gain >2 lb/week, generalized edema, proteinuria ≥3+, decreased urine output, and hyperreflexia. Eclampsia includes the above plus seizures. HELLP syndrome includes signs and symptoms of severe pre-eclampsia, enlarged and firm liver, epigastric or right upper quadrant pain and, frequently, jaundice.

56. **(3)** The pregnant teen is at increased risk for premature labor, anemia, and PIH. There is no documentation that the pregnant teen is at greater risk of gestational diabetes.

57. **(4)** Greater than 90% of clients presenting with ectopic pregnancies will complain of pain and will report a missed period. Approximately 80% will describe vaginal bleeding; however, only 50% will have a palpable abdominal mass.

58. **(4)** It is true that 90% of ectopic pregnancies are found in the fallopian tubes. Clients with PID have a sevenfold increase in the rate of ectopic pregnancy. A previous ectopic pregnancy is a risk factor and does increase the risk of subsequent ectopic pregnancy.

59. **(1)** A threatened abortion progresses to complete spontaneous abortion 50% of the time. Clinical findings are vaginal bleeding with or without cramping and no cervical change. Vaginal bleeding with cramping and cervical change is an inevitable abortion. An incomplete abortion is demonstrated by vaginal bleeding, cramping, and incomplete expulsion of products of conception. A missed abortion is diagnosed when products of conception are retained after fetal death. There is a decrease in uterine size, there is a loss of pregnancy symptoms, and the cervix is often closed and firm.

60. **(3)** Vaginal bleeding could represent a potential problem in the pregnancy during the first trimester. The other symptoms listed are important as well and warrant further discussion to rule out a problem.

61. **2)** Contractions, cramping, or continued bleeding may indicate a spontaneous abortion. The other symptoms are common in the first trimester.

62. **(3)** Lesions typically start on the abdomen, and spread to the thighs and possibly the buttocks. Onset of lesions is usually in the third trimester and usually resolves postpartum. There is no associated adverse perinatal outcome.

63. **(1)** Use of cocaine during pregnancy is associated with placental abruption, spontaneous abortion, and preterm labor. Maternal blood pressure and heart rate are increased. The fetus is at risk for intrauterine growth retardation, fetal distress, seizures, and death.

64. **(3)** Most fetuses are not affected; however, some undergo isoimmunization, which leads to hydrops fetalis and death. The mortality risk is actually low and there are usually no associated congenital anomalies.

65. **(1)** Multiple gestation will cause the uterus to enlarge faster than normal. It is not uncommon to have inaudible FHTs with the doptone at 10 weeks' gestation. A fibroid could cause the uterus to enlarge; however, it is generally accompanied by firmness to palpation of the uterus. Ectopic pregnancy could be the cause of inaudible FHTs but is usually accompanied by adnexal tenderness, mass, or vaginal bleeding. A 14-week viable IUP should have audible FHTs with the doptone.

66. **(1)** Contractions could represent early premature labor and should be monitored to rule out early cervical change. Not all contractions are "Braxton Hicks' contractions," and they need to be taken seriously. The other symptoms listed are important to discuss and rule out other associated symptomatology as well.

Pharmacology

67. **(3)** The MMR is a live virus and is contraindicated in pregnancy. Polio, tetanus, and hepatitis B vaccine are inactivated bacterial or DNA-based vaccines and are safe when indicated.

68. **(4)** The FDA has five pregnancy risk categories for drugs. Category X indicates fetal risk outweighs any benefit and use in pregnancy is contraindicated. Category B drugs show no evidence of fetal abnormalities and risk to the fetus is relatively unlikely. Category C drugs have potential for animal fetal abnormalities and/or no adequate well-controlled studies available in pregnant women, but benefits of drugs are thought to justify risks to the fetus. Drugs classified as Category D demonstrate positive evidence of human fetal risk and should be used only in serious disease or life-threatening situations where safer drugs are ineffective.

69. **(3)** Tetracycline binds with developing enamel and discolors the deciduous teeth between 26 weeks' gestation and 6 months of infancy.

70. **(3)** Recent studies have confirmed that folic acid taken prior to conception can reduce the risk of neural tube defect.

71. **(2)** Current recommendations for Rh immune globulin (RhoGAM) is administration of 300 µg to all Rh-negative women at 28 weeks of pregnancy. This is

considered protective for the remainder of the pregnancy.

72. **(1)** All histamine receptor blockers (Tagamet, Zantac, Pepsid) medications are Category B drugs for pregnancy and should not be taken. She should try another type of relief, and if the antiacid does not relieve the problem, then perhaps it should be more thoroughly investigated.

73. **(1)** This option best describes the Category C drug. Option #1 is Category A, Option #3 is Category B, and Option #4 is Category X.

Labor & Postpartum

Physical Examination & Diagnostic Tests

1. The most important obstetric measurement is the:

   1. Obstetrical conjugate.

   2. Diagonal conjugate.

   3. Midpelvis conjugate.

   4. Biparietal conjugate.

2. A 28-year-old female client is seen by the nurse practitioner for an office visit. Her last menstrual period (LMP) was 8 weeks ago; she is complaining of left lower quadrant abdominal pain, spotting, and fatigue. Her pelvic exam reveals cervical os closed, minimal blood in vaginal vault, uterus minimally enlarged, mild cervical motion tenderness (CMT), left adnexal fullness and tenderness, right adnexal within normal limits (WNL). Vital signs are stable. The serum pregnancy test is positive. What is the most cost-effective and useful test for the nurse practitioner to order?

   1. Computed tomography (CT) scan of the abdomen/pelvis.

   2. Barium enema.

   3. Pelvic ultrasound.

   4. Flat plate of the abdomen.

3. The biophysical profile includes which of the following parameters?

   1. Fetal breathing movements.

   2. Fetal tone.

   3. Fetal amniotic volume.

   4. All of the above.

4. In discussing the timing of contractions with a client, the nurse practitioner explains "frequency" as the interval from the:

   1. Beginning of one contraction to the beginning of the next.

   2. Beginning of one contraction to end of that contraction.

   3. End of one contraction to the start of the next contraction.

   4. End of one contraction to end of the next contraction.

5. The most common reason for a nonreactive nonstress test (NST) is:

   1. Fetal hypoxia.

   2. Maternal drug use.

   3. Fetal inactivity or sleep.

   4. Congenital heart defect.

6. In evaluating the pelvis of a pregnant woman, the nurse practitioner notes that the ischial spines are prominent, the diameter between the ischial spines is 8 cm, and there is a narrow sacrosciatic notch. What do these findings suggest?

   1. Anthropoid pelvis.

   2. Gynecoid pelvis.

   3. Wide pelvic inclination.

   4. Midpelvic contracture.

Labor & Postpartum Care

7. During a postpartum assessment, the nurse practitioner notes a cluster of external hemorrhoids. Which statement made by the client indicates a need for additional teaching?

   1. "I can give myself an enema every other day to reduce constipation."

   2. "I can take sitz baths for pain."

   3. "I can decrease the swelling by using a topical hydrocortisone cream."

   4. "I can take a stool softener to decrease the pain of a BM."

8. Ten days after delivery, a client is diagnosed with mastitis. The nurse practitioner would expect to find on the physical exam:

   1. Tender, hard, reddened breast.

   2. Dimpled skin on breasts.

   3. Lack of milk production.

   4. Nipple burning during feeding.

9. A predisposing factor in preterm labor is:

   1. Obesity.

   2. Previous spontaneous abortions.

   3. Prior preterm delivery.

   4. White race.

10. The ability of amniotic fluid to produce a ferning pattern when dried may be altered by:

    1. Meconium.

    2. Changes in vaginal pH.

    3. Presence of cervical mucus.

    4. Heavy contamination with blood.

11. Two to 4 months after delivery, an increase in scalp hair loss results from:

    1. Increased number of hairs in telogen.

    2. Hyperthyroidism.

    3. Fatigue.

    4. Sudden postpartum cardiovascular changes.

12. In a breast-feeding client having difficulty with milk production, the nurse practitioner understands that milk production will be increased by:

    1. More frequent suckling of infant.

    2. Longer duration of suckling.

    3. Cessation of suckling for 24 hours.

    4. Cold compresses to the breast.

13. During a breast exam on a lactating woman, which finding is cause for concern?

    1. Leaking of "watery" fluid from left breast.

    2. Cracked nipples that are tender to touch.

    3. Bilateral warm breasts that are distended.

    4. Inverted left nipple, flat right nipple.

14. A new first-time mother is being evaluated for a complaint of breast pain. Her infant is 3 weeks old and she is breast-feeding. The infant is gaining weight and seems satisfied after feeding. On exam the nurse practitioner finds a red, irritated nipple on one breast but no masses or tenderness to

the breast itself. An important part of the nurse practitioner's evaluation is:

1. A mammogram of the breast.

2. Examination of the infant's mouth.

3. A stat complete blood count (CBC).

4. An analysis of the milk.

15. A client delivers a healthy newborn with a cleft lip and cleft palate during a home delivery. The new mother and baby visit the rural outreach clinic the next morning. What actions would promote maternal–infant bonding?

1. Point out the newborn's normal characteristics.

2. Explain to the mother how the problem is not significant.

3. Have the mother begin taking care of the newborn immediately after delivery.

4. Explain to the mother that orofacial surgery will completely correct the defect.

16. A woman is discharged 48 hours after an uncomplicated delivery of a normal infant. She has a lateral episiotomy and was voiding easily on discharge. The next day she calls the nurse practitioner regarding increased pain in her perineal area. She has taken ibuprofen (Advil) as directed and her perineal area is very tender and swollen and she is having increasing difficulty voiding. What instructions would the nurse practitioner give the client?

1. Apply ice pack to the area to decrease swelling and discomfort.

2. Come into the clinic for evaluation of the episiotomy for a hematoma.

3. Have her place a warm heating pad on the perineal area.

4. Increase her fluid intake and decrease the amount of time she is standing up.

17. A woman comes to the clinic for a pregnancy test. The examination and test are positive for pregnancy and reveal she is about 6 weeks pregnant. She states that she had a cesarean birth with her first child due to her impaired cardiac status. She would

like to have a vaginal delivery this time. What is the best response by the nurse practitioner?

1. A cesarean delivery will most likely be the safest delivery method for her and her infant.

2. The type of delivery will be based on the progress of the pregnancy and the size of the infant.

3. If the infant size does not exceed the cephalopelvic dimensions, there is a good possibility of a normal vaginal delivery.

4. Her previous pregnancy and family history will have to be carefully evaluated before that decision can be made.

18. A young woman delivers a neonate with multiple congenital anomalies. Within 4 hours of delivery, the neonate dies. What anticipatory bereavement guidance might the nurse practitioner initiate:

1. Provide information about grief symptoms and the cyclic nature of the grief reaction.

2. Encourage the new mother to get pregnant as soon as possible.

3. Explain to her the importance of making major changes and decisions in her life to gain a sense of control over her circumstances.

4. Encourage her to "feel her feelings" and not take any antidepressants or antianxiety medications to relieve the grief symptoms that she may experience.

19. Which physical finding would make the nurse practitioner suspicious that her client had a postpartum infection?

1. Temperature 37.2°C (99°F) during first 24 hours postpartum.

2. Hemoglobin 11 gm, hematocrit 37%, white blood cell (WBC) count 9800/μl.

3. Urinalysis—hazy, occasional WBC, rare cast.

4. Lochia rubra, approximately 100 ml/pad.

20. The nurse practitioner is evaluating the involution of the uterus in a woman who is 1 day postpartum. What is the expected finding in this woman?

    1. The uterus is at the level of the umbilicus.

    2. The uterus is between the umbilicus and the symphysis pubis.

    3. The uterus is two finger-breadths above the level of the umbilicus.

    4. The uterus is palpable at the level of the symphysis pubis.

21. A woman is 1 month postpartum and is breast-feeding. She is concerned about getting pregnant again. What birth control measures would the nurse practitioner suggest for this client?

    1. Use a condom or progestin only birth control pills.

    2. If she does not menstruate, she will not get pregnant.

    3. Abstinence is the best method of birth control at this time.

    4. She should be fitted for a diaphragm.

22. A woman comes into the office concerned about the increasing tenderness and redness of an area in her left breast. Her infant is 3 weeks old and she is breast-feeding. She is diagnosed with mastitis. What is the best treatment for this woman?

    1. Culture the breast milk to determine the organism and the appropriate antibiotic.

    2. Stop nursing on the affected side until the infection is cleared, use ibuprofen (Advil) 400 mg q4h prn for discomfort.

    3. Trimethoprim-sulfamethoxazole (Bactrim) 2 tablets q12h × 5 days.

    4. Dicloxacillin (Dynapen) 500 mg PO q6h × 10 days, acetaminophen 325 mg 1–2 tablets q4h prn.

23. A woman returns to the clinic for her checkup 1 week postpartum. This was her first baby and she had a normal delivery with no complications. At this time, she is concerned that she is still experiencing a bloody discharge. What is the best action for the nurse practitioner to take?

    1. Discuss with the woman that this is normal and should go away in 10–14 days.

    2. Perform a pelvic exam and culture the fluid at the cervix.

    3. Obtain a specimen from the cervix to evaluate for the presence of chlamydia.

    4. Determine if the woman is using a pad or tampons for the discharge.

24. The nurse practitioner identifies what factors as being a contraindication to breast-feeding?

    1. Breast cancer.

    2. Breast abscess.

    3. Tuberculosis with negative sputum culture.

    4. Mother wants to take birth control pills.

25. A woman is breast-feeding her 3-week-old infant. She calls the clinic regarding one breast being very engorged with milk and the infant does not appear to be interested in nursing. What is the best recommendation for this woman?

    1. Use a large elastic bandage and wrap her chest to compress the engorged breast.

    2. Apply an ice pack between feedings and cover the breast with a warm, moist towel prior to feeding to increase the let down.

    3. Encourage the mother to wear a good supporting bra to promote comfort to the breast.

    4. Utilize a breast pump to relieve the immediate discomfort; advise her to feed the infant every 3–4 hours, and to utilize the fullest breast.

26. A client who is 2 weeks postpartum calls the clinic with complaints of increased tenderness in the lower abdomen and increasing problems with back pain not relieved by acetaminophen. Her vaginal discharge is bloody, but not excessive. What

is the best response by the nurse practitioner to this client?

1. Have the client come to the clinic/hospital immediately to check for late postpartum bleeding.

2. Increase her fluid intake, have her bring in a urine sample, and begin on trimethoprim-sulfamethoxazole (Bactrim).

3. Determine if her bowel movements are regular, if she has excessive flatus, and if she has any problem with constipation.

4. Evaluate her physical activity for excessive lifting, and determine if there is any difficulty with voiding.

27. Which statement is correct concerning postpartum thyroiditis?

1. It rarely occurs and may be immunologic in origin; hormone therapy is usually not indicated.

2. It usually presents with mild transient hyperthyroidism 1–2 weeks postpartum.

3. Mild hyperthyroidism symptoms occur 1–3 months postpartum, followed by a mild transient hypothyroidism.

4. Most women never recover and need to have a subtotal thyroidectomy.

Pharmacology

28. Which medication would be considered safe for use after the first trimester of pregnancy?

1. Metronidazole (Flagyl).

2. Tetracycline (Achromycin).

3. Isotretinoin (Accutane).

4. Angiotensin converting enzyme (ACE) inhibitors.

29. For the client who wishes to breast-feed and take oral contraception, the pill of choice is:

1. A 1/35 preparation.

2. A triphasic preparation.

3. A progestin only preparation.

4. A 1/50 preparation.

30. A pregnant client in the last trimester complains of a constant backache that is especially aggravated by walking, moving, and bending. There is no radiation to either leg. In addition to rest, massage, and physiotherapy, what would be appropriate to prescribe?

1. Acetaminophen (Tylenol).

2. Codeine.

3. Napoxyn (Anaprox).

4. Aspirin.

31. What is the antibiotic of choice for a mother who is breast-feeding and has mastitis?

1. Cloxacillin (Tegopen)

2. Tetracycline (Achromycin)

3. Gentamicin (Garamycin).

4. Amoxicillin (Amoxil).

32. What is the antibiotic of choice for a postpartum endometritis?

1. Erythromycin.

2. Penicillin.

3. Clindamycin (Cleocin) and gentamicin (Garamycin).

4. Trimethoprim-sulfamethoxazole (Bactrim).

17 Answers & Rationales

Physical Examination & Diagnostic Tests

1. **(2)** The diagonal conjugate is the most important, as it is the distance from the sacral promontory to the lower margin of the symphysis pubis. It determines the size of the pelvic inlet (≥11.5 cm is adequate size). The obstetrical conjugate is determined by adding 1.5–2.0 cm to the diagonal conjugate.

2. **(3)** This easy, inexpensive and relatively noninvasive test will help the nurse practitioner with confirming the diagnosis of ectopic pregnancy. It can be obtained quickly and is often rapidly available. The CT scan of the abdomen/pelvis will also show an ectopic, but it is neither cost-effective nor noninvasive. Neither barium enema nor a flat plate of the abdomen are of assistance in this case.

3. **(4)** The biophysical profile includes observation of fetal respiratory movement, fetal tone, gross fetal movements, measurements of amniotic fluid volume, and fetal heart reactivity. Each parameter is given a score of 2 if present; normal is 8–10.

4. **(1)** Frequency of contractions should be timed from the beginning of one contraction to the beginning of the next contraction.

5. **(3)** The most common reason for a nonreactive NST is fetal sleep or inactivity. The fetal sleep–wake cycle ranges from 20–40 minutes. If reactivity is not demonstrated in 20 minutes, continuing to 40 minutes usually accommodates the sleep–wake cycles. Fetal hypoxia and maternal smoking and drug use certainly affect fetal heart rate but are not the most common causes. Infants with a congenital heart defect do not exhibit a significant incidence of nonreactive NSTs.

6. **(4)** Midpelvic contracture is suggested by prominent ischial spines, the diameter between the ischial spines is <9.5 cm, there is a narrow sacrosciatic notch, and there are converging pelvic side walls. An anthropoid pelvis has narrow pelvic side walls, a backward sacrosciatic notch, and no prominence in the ischial spines. A gynecoid pelvis has straight side walls, a medium sacrosciatic notch, and no prominence in the ischial spines. A wide pelvic inclination is favorable for a satisfactory labor.

Labor & Postpartum Care

7. **(1)** An enema every other day to reduce constipation would negatively affect the normal bowel movement pattern and deplete the client's natural intestinal flora. Sitz baths, anti-inflammatory and analgesic topical ointments or sprays, along with stool softeners and increased bulk in the diet would be indicated in the management of the external hemorrhoids.

8. **(1)** Swelling, erythema, and pain are found in the upper, outer quadrant of the breast. Dimpled skin (orange peel appearance) is a potential sign of breast cancer. Nipple burning is related to positioning and inflation of the let-down reflex during feeding. Milk production starts about 4 days postpartum.

9. **(3)** The history of preterm birth is associated with 20–40% recurrence risk. Low prepregnancy weight and inadequate weight gain, not obesity, are associated with preterm labor. Maternal smoking, drug use (especially cocaine), low socioeconomic status, maternal age <17 and >35, and non-white race are all predisposing factors for preterm labor. Previous spontaneous or elective abortions are not risk factors.

10. **(4)** When air-dried, amniotic fluid produces a fern pattern. This microscopic arborization is accurate in confirming rupture of membranes in 90–95% of cases. Samples heavily contaminated with blood may not fern.

11. **(1)** Normally 15–20% of hairs are in telogen. In late pregnancy, this is reduced to <10%. After delivery, the percentage increases, and by 2 months postpartum, 20% of hairs are in telogen; therefore, there is a marked increase in hair loss at 2–4 months after delivery.

12. **(1)** More frequent suckling will increase production of milk more effectively than increasing the duration of suckling. Stopping or decreasing breast-feeding or applying cold compresses to the breasts will decrease milk production.

13. **(2)** Cracked nipples are a sign of irritation and may eventually cause skin breakdown with severe pain.

14. **(2)** Breast irritation in nursing mothers is often caused by *Candida albicans*. The source of the infection is most likely the infant's mouth (thrush).

15. **(1)** Initially after delivery, the mother needs an opportunity to accept the fact that her newborn has a congenital defect. Pointing out normal characteristics of the newborn will allow her to put the problem in perspective. Often, the mother will focus on the defect. Orofacial surgery will provide closure of the defect but will not completely correct it, as scarring will undoubtedly occur.

16. **(2)** The woman's complaints are characteristic of a hematoma formation; she should be evaluated. Warm moist heat (sitz baths, tub baths, etc), ibuprofen, and local anesthetics are recommended to decrease the discomfort of the episiotomy. When the pain is not relieved and there is difficulty voiding along with increased tenderness, she should be evaluated by the nurse practitioner.

17. **(1)** Since the first cesarean birth was done due to maternal health factors, it is highly likely that the second delivery will be cesarean also. If the first delivery had been due to infant distress of hemorrhagic problems, then there is the possibility of a vaginal second delivery providing the cesarean incision was a low transverse incision.

18. **(1)** Educating the new mother about the cyclical nature of grief and the importance of avoiding unnecessary lifestyle changes for 1–2 years is part of the anticipatory guidance the nurse practitioner gives to the bereaved young women. Short-term use of antidepressants (at a low-dose) or antianxiety agents (preferable to not use benzodiazepines due to their potential for addiction and overdose) are safe and effective for the treatment of insomnia and anxiety associated with the loss of the newborn.

19. **(2)** Leukocytosis (>10,000/µl), malaise, foul-smelling lochia, pyuria, abdominal tenderness, CMT, and temperature >38°C (100.4°F) are all symptoms of postpartum infection.

20. **(1)** The uterus rises to the level of the umbilicus within several hours to 2 days after delivery. After that time it will gradually descend into the pelvis. Anytime the uterus can be palpated above the umbilicus, the client should be evaluated for bladder distention or enlarged uterus.

21. **(1)** Nonestrogen birth control pills can be taken during breast-feeding, and there is no contraindication to condom use. If she does not menstruate, she is highly unlikely to get pregnant; however, she could become pregnant with the first ovulation prior to her period. A diaphragm cannot be properly fitted this soon after delivery, and abstinence is not a logical recommendation.

22. **(4)** An antibiotic should be started immediately and she should be encouraged to continue breast-feeding. Acetaminophen is recommended as an analgesic. Ibuprofen affects platelet aggregation and causes gastrointestinal disturbances. Sulfa-containing medications are not recommended if the woman is breast-feeding and the infant is <1 month old.

23. **(1)** This is within the range of normal physiologic changes expected at this time postpartum. There is no reason to culture the cervix and certainly not for a smear for chlamydia. She should not be using a tampon, but it is of no consideration when evaluating the discharge.

24. **(1)** There is considerable controversy regarding the role of breast-feeding and the progression of cancer. Considering the current controversy, it is considered a contraindication to breast-feeding. A breast abscess and tuberculosis with a negative sputum are not contraindications. The mother may take a birth control pill that is progestin only and does not contain estrogen.

25. **(2)** An ice bag is helpful between feedings. The warm towel will increase the let down when the infant is nursing. A breast pump only increases the production of milk in that breast, and the infant should be offered the breast every 2–2½ hours for 15–20 minutes per side.

26. **(1)** The back pain, low abdominal pain, and continuing to have bloody discharge are very suggestive of a late postpartum hemorrhage. She should be evaluated for a retained placental fragment or subinvolution of the uterus. The other options are not appropriate to this client presenting with these symptoms.

27. **(3)** This is a common problem that may occur 1–3 months postpartum, followed by a mild transient hypothryoidism. Suppression of hyperthyroid symptoms or temporary thyroid hormone supplementation may be necessary. Most women recover within 6–9 months; however, a significant number remain hypothyroid and need long-term thyroid hormone replacement.

Pharmacology

28. **(1)** Metronidazole is safe after the first trimester. The other listed medications, in addition to others, are all known teratogens and are therefore contraindicated in pregnancy.

29. **(3)** Estrogen inhibits milk production. Progestin only preparations are ideal for the breast-feeding client because they do not contain estrogen and, therefore, do not inhibit milk production. The other oral contraceptives listed contain estrogen in varying amounts.

30. **(1)** Acetaminophen can be prescribed to the pregnant client; aspirin should be avoided along with narcotics, such as codeine. Naproxyn (Anaprox) is contraindicated in the third trimester of pregnancy.

31. **(1)** Either cloxacillin or methicillin is appropriate, as both are effective against *Staphylococcus aureus* (including coagulase-positive *Staphylococcus*).

32. **(3)** First-line therapy is clindamycin (Cleocin) and gentamicin (Garamycin). Single-agent therapy with a second- or third-generation cephalosporin is an acceptable alternative. Ampicillin may be added to the regimen, especially if *Enterococcus* is suspected.

Mental Health

Psychosocial Examination & Diagnostic Tests

1. The mental status examination enables the nurse practitioner to identify:

   1. Intelligence quotient and reasoning.

   2. Abstract thinking and memory functioning.

   3. Reasoning and pyschomotor skills.

   4. Memory functioning and intelligence quotient.

2. A client with a history of psychiatric problems arrives at the clinic shouting that she is a messenger of God and knows the meaning of the prophecies in Revelations. This behavior is assessed as:

   1. A delusion.

   2. A hallucination.

   3. Magical thinking.

   4. An illusion.

3. An assessment of a client experiencing auditory hallucinations would most likely reveal:

   1. Client mumbling to self, tilted head, eyes darting back and forth.

   2. Performance of obsessive-compulsive rituals of turning off and on a radio, talking to self.

   3. Hyperactivity, expansive mood, easy distractibility.

   4. Cool, aloof, unapproachable, avoiding enclosed areas.

4. The MAST and the CAGE are screening instruments for which disease process?

   1. Glaucoma.

   2. Depression.

   3. Alcoholism.

   4. Diabetes.

5. When receiving the records from another agency, the nurse practitioner notes on the summary sheet that the client has a dual diagnosis. This means the client has:

   1. Both manic and depressive symptoms of bipolar affective disorder.

   2. Two closely related psychiatric disorders (e.g., panic disorder and bulimia nervosa.

   3. Coexistence of both a psychiatric disorder (e.g., depression) and a substance abuse disorder (e.g., alcohol dependence).

   4. Coexistence of a personality disorder (e.g., borderline personality) and a psychiatric disorder (e.g., panic disorder).

6. While completing the history on an older adult, the nurse practitioner understands that when a client "makes up stories or answers" to the questions, this is known as:

   1. Perseveration.

   2. Confabulation.

   3. Echolalia.

   4. Alcoholic encephalopathy.

7. In taking a history from a client with depression, which is the most important question for the nurse practitioner to ask?

   1. Have you ever experienced hallucinations, delusions, or illusions?

   2. Have you ever been hospitalized in a psychiatric facility?

   3. Do you regularly take antidepressants or other medications?

   4. Have you thought about or attempted suicide?

8. While taking a history, the nurse practitioner is aware that the following drug is the most commonly first used by an adolescent.

   1. Nicotine.

   2. Alcohol.

   3. Marijuana.

   4. Crystal methamphetamine.

9. A common laboratory finding associated with bulimia nervosa is:

   1. Hyperkalemia.

   2. Hypochloremia.

   3. Elevated liver enzymes.

   4. Platelet abnormalities.

10. Which statement is correct about mental health in the older adult and supports research findings in the literature?

    1. Self-esteem does not decline as a person ages.

    2. Older adults are consistently concerned about their physical appearance.

    3. Older adults have a negative self-image compared to younger adults.

    4. Learning ability is not maintained due to loss of short-term memory.

Psychiatric Disorders

11. A client calls the clinic and asks to speak to the nurse practitioner. When he/she answers the telephone, the client states that she is going to commit suicide. The priority goal is to:

    1. Refer the client to an appropriate treatment facility.

    2. Encourage ventilation of angry and depressed feelings.

    3. Assess the lethality of the suicide plan.

    4. Establish rapport with the client.

12. During an intake interview with a 26-year-old woman diagnosed with generalized anxiety disorder, the nurse practitioner might observe what type of behaviors?

    1. An inflated sense of self.

    2. Constantly relates to future events.

    3. Is unable to concentrate and is irritable when questioned.

    4. Appears nervous and frightened of the nurse during the interview.

13. The nurse practitioner understands the following about elder abuse:

    1. It is often reported by the victim.

    2. Abuse tends to de-escalate from the perpetrator.

    3. Midshaft fractures of the humerus or femur rarely indicate abuse.

    4. Bruises and lesions are often found on the inner aspects of extremities.

14. While talking with a client about her chemical dependency, the client states, "I wish I would have never used cocaine. It's ruined my life!" What would be the most appropriate response by the nurse practitioner?

    1. "You should think before you do something."

    2. "Things will work out, don't worry."

    3. "It sounds like you've thought a lot about your cocaine use."

    4. "You shouldn't be so hard on yourself. You can change."

15. The nurse practitioner would expect which symptoms in a client with a diagnosis of schizophrenia?

    1. High energy with varying sleep patterns and nonstop conversation.

    2. Extreme and frequent mood swings with hyperactivity and difficulty concentrating.

    3. Paranoia, delusions, hallucinations, and diminished self-care.

    4. Antisocial, manipulative, charismatic, and able to lie convincingly.

16. A middle-aged, upper-middle class, married female presents to your clinic for the third time in 2 months with a complaint of headache, gastrointestinal (GI) upset with abdominal pain, and difficulty sleeping. Past exams have been essentially negative. You suspect the client suffers from depression, but she has been reluctant to complete even the briefest of screenings. Today, the client requests "something for sleep," again stating she "doesn't have time to take a bunch of tests." Which diagnosis seems most likely?

    1. Hypochondriasis.

    2. Domestic violence.

    3. Addiction.

    4. Irritable bowel syndrome.

17. An elderly client was taken to the clinic in a confused state that began suddenly 24 hours ago. She fails to be oriented to person, time, or place. She was incontinent of urine due to her confusion. She looks apathetic and is drowsy. The nurse practitioner would suspect:

    1. Delirium.

    2. Dementia.

    3. Depression.

    4. A psychotic disorder.

18. An older client comes to your office with the complaint of confusion. The daughter is concerned that her mother is developing Alzheimer's disease. Which of these assessments would indicate this client is experiencing delirium instead of dementia?

    1. The confusion has been slowly developing.

    2. The confusion started after she began taking cimetidine (Tagamet).

    3. The client's attention span has not been affected.

    4. The client's memory has been impaired.

19. A 16-year-old adolescent is 54 inches in height. The nurse practitioner identifies the following as a positive effective coping behavior:

    1. Acts as the class clown.

    2. Has a rehearsed reply to teasing comments.

    3. Spends most of his free time watching television.

    4. Has predominantly friends that are short statured.

20. The nurse practitioner is examining an older adolescent who has been a long-term intravenous cocaine user. What other findings would alert the nurse practitioner to a frequent complication?

    1. Epistaxis and chronic rhinorrhea.

    2. Cardiac arrhythmias and hypertension.

    3. Chest congestion and wheezing.

    4. Hepatitis and cellulitis.

21. The nurse practitioner is comparing the typical signs of depression in the adolescent with the adult client. The depressed adolescent would present with:

    1. Lonely feelings.

    2. Sad, flat affect.

    3. Anger and acting out behavior.

    4. Feelings of powerlessness and anxiety.

22. While interviewing a teenager to determine her level of health, the nurse practitioner recognizes symptoms of anorexia nervosa. Which characteristic of anorexia nervosa would be noted in the initial assessment interview?

    1. Below to average intelligence.

    2. Increased libido.

    3. Vigorous daily exercise.

    4. Tachycardia.

23. A teenaged female client is brought to the nurse practitioner for evaluation by her grandmother with whom she lives. The teenager has been vomiting and her grandmother believes that she is becoming confused. The grandmother relates that the client has been upset lately over a breakup with her boyfriend. What will the nurse practitioner investigate as a possible cause for this teenager's symptoms?

    1. Appendicitis.

    2. Ectopic pregnancy.

    3. Drug overdose.

    4. Sexually transmitted disease.

24. An adult client has a history of irritability, loss of appetite, inability to concentrate, and feelings of depression and "burn out" at work. Recently, she relates missing several days at work, and she is doing and taking everything she can to relax. What would be an appropriate question to ask this client?

    1. "Do you drink alcohol or take drugs?"

    2. "Have you ever felt this way before?"

    3. "When you feel depressed, do you talk to your husband?"

    4. "Have you lost your job?"

25. A teenager comes to the office of the nurse practitioner and states that she was raped several hours ago by her boyfriend. The immediate action taken by the nurse practitioner is:

    1. Perform a pelvic examination to determine injuries to the client.

    2. Accompany her to the emergency department for an exam.

    3. Send her immediately for counseling to help her deal with this situation.

    4. Call the client's parents so they can be with her.

26. Physical findings of cocaine abuse include:

    1. Bradycardia, miosis, hypertension.

    2. Hypertension, tachycardia, tremor.

    3. Hypotension, bradycardia, abdominal cramps.

    4. Decreased level of consciousness, tachyardia, excessive salivation.

27. While interviewing an adolescent female presenting with her mother for birth control counseling and examination, you detect signs of family tension. During the physical exam, while the mother is out of the room, the daughter admits to frequent marijuana use and occasional drinking. What assessment information would most confirm the presence of actual or potential violence in the home?

    1. Signs of general neglect.

    2. Injuries at different stages of healing.

3. Client's response to a direct question.

4. Admitted fear of mother's boyfriend.

28. All of the following behaviors meet the criteria outlined in the *Diagnostic and Statistical Manual of Mental Disorders, Fourth Edition* (DSM-IV) for substance abuse, **except**:

    1. Repeated arrests for drunk driving.

    2. Multiple absences from work due to substance use.

    3. Chronic anxiety attacks.

    4. Recurrent arguments with spouse about his/her drinking behavior.

Pharmacology

29. A client has been receiving fluphenazine (Prolixin) for the past 3 weeks. The nurse practitioner's assessment notes the following: temperature elevated (41°C), marked muscle rigidity, agitation, and confusion. The nurse practitioner understands these findings are often associated with the diagnosis of:

    1. Acute dystonia.

    2. Tardive dyskinesia.

    3. Neuroleptic malignant syndrome.

    4. Extrapyramidal disorder.

30. Of the following antidepressants, which one has the most sedating side effects, making it a good sleeping agent?

    1. Fluoxetine (Prozac).

    2. Doxepin (Sinequan).

    3. Trazadone (Desyrel).

    4. Paroxetine (Paxil).

31. The nurse practitioner's physical exam on an adolescent is as follows: disheveled appearance, 5-lb weight loss since last visit 2 months ago, pulse strong and regular at 128, 4+ deep tendon reflexes, nasal mucosa erythematous and ulcerated. His mother relates that he has been getting in trouble at school, avoids the family, has no appetite, and is not sleeping much at night. The nurse practitioner suspects drug use of:

    1. Heroin.

    2. Marijuana.

    3. Lysergic acid diethylamide (LSD).

    4. Crack cocaine.

32. A client comes to the rural clinic having taken an undetermined amount of heroin. Prior to transferring the client to a psychiatric treatment facility, the nurse practitioner anticipates the drug of choice for an opioid overdose is:

    1. Clonidine (Catapres).

    2. Methadone (Dolophine).

    3. Naloxone (Narcan).

    4. Naltrexone HCl (Revia).

33. Benzodiazepines are useful in the treatment of all the disorders below, **except**:

    1. Alcohol withdrawal.

    2. Anxiety.

    3. Obsessive-compulsive disorder.

    4. Seizures.

34. When starting a psychotropic medication in the elderly, a good rule of thumb is:

    1. Start low, go slow.

    2. Higher doses are almost always needed.

    3. Side effects of psychotropic medications will usually not impact other medications.

    4. The same adult dosages can be used initially without any problems.

35. A client is a 20-year, two-pack-a-day smoker with a history of chronic bronchitis. What is the prescription to give to this client who wishes to stop smoking?

   1. Nicotine polacrilex (Nicorette) gum 2-mg piece, chew for 30 minutes, q1–2h × 6 weeks, then q2–4h × 3 weeks, then q4–8h × 3 weeks, then discontinue.

   2. Nicotine patch (Nicoderm) 21 mg/24 hr qd × 6 weeks, then 14 mg/24 hr qd × 2 weeks, then 7 mg/24 hr × 2 weeks, then discontinue.

   3. Bupropion HCl (Zyban) 150 mg qd × 3 days, then 150 mg bid for 7–12 weeks and to stop smoking when medication is started.

   4. Nicotine patch (Nicoderm) 14 mg/24 hr qd × 6 weeks, then 7 mg/24 hr qd × 6 weeks, then discontinue.

18 Answers & Rationales

Psychosocial Examination & Diagnostic Tests

1. **(2)** The mental status examination provides a basic assessment of the client's intellectual functioning (reasoning, abstract thinking, memory). The intelligence quotient (IQ) is determined by psychological testing. Psychomotor skills assessment is part of a neurologic examination.

2. **(1)** Delusions are false, fixed beliefs that can be of a persecutory or grandiose nature. In this instance, the client is experiencing a delusion of grandeur. A hallucination is a false sensory experience. An illusion is a misinterpretation of reality. Magical thinking is when the client feels that his thoughts or wishes can control other people.

3. **(1)** The client experiencing the auditory hallucination will often look out into space and act as if he is listening to someone talking. This is associated with behaviors such as tilting the head, mumbling, and eye movement.

4. **(3)** The Michigan Alcoholism Screening Test (MAST) and the CAGE (Cut down, Annoyed, Guilty, Eye opener) are used to alert providers to the possibility of alcoholism.

5. **(3)** Dual diagnosis involves both a psychiatric diagnosis and a substance abuse diagnosis.

6. **(2)** The fabrication of events or situations to fill in gaps in the memory, usually in a plausible way, is a classic definition of a client who is experiencing dementia due to chronic alcoholism. Clients with alcohol amnesic disorder or Korsakoff's syndrome may experience confabulation. Echolalia is the parroting or automatic, meaningless, repeating of another's words. Perseveration is the involuntary persistent repetition of an idea or response (i.e., client keeps repeating the same phrase over and over).

7. **(4)** Although the other questions are important to obtain during the initial history, it is most important to ascertain whether or not the client has contemplated suicide. In addition, determination of a specific plan and the means to do it are also involved in the questioning about suicidal ideation.

8. **(1)** Nicotine is known as the "gateway drug" and the drug most commonly used first by adolescents.

9. **(2)** The other abnormalities are not usually associated with bulimia. The hypochloremia is associated with the purging (self-induced vomiting).

10. **(1)** According to research, self-esteem along with attitude and morals are maintained as a client ages, and older adults tend to have a positive self-image when compared to younger adults. Learning ability is maintained, although more time is often needed for the early phases of the learning process. Retrieval of information in long-term memory is slower and short-term memory is diminished.

Psychiatric Disorders

11. **(4)** The nurse practitioner must first establish trust and rapport with the caller before an assessment can be made. If rapport is not established, the client will hang up the phone. The nurse practitioner understands that by keeping the client talking, she is prevented from acting out the suicidal threat.

12. **(3)** Impaired concentration and irritability are major characteristics of generalized anxiety disorder. Clients are more focused on the here and now and have low self-esteem.

13. **(4)** Bruising on the extensor surfaces of the arms is common and usually not considered abuse, while bruising on the inner surfaces of extremities and areas with different stages of resolution are often found in the elderly abused client.

14. **(3)** The nurse practitioner's statement acknowledges the client's feelings and is open-ended, which promotes open discussion and helps the client clarify her feelings and thoughts. Option #1 is condescending and punitive. Option #2 offers false reassurance. Option #4 tends to discount the client's feelings.

15. **(3)** The characteristics of schizophrenia are delusions, tangential thought, suspiciousness, disorganized behavior, and hallucinations.

16. **(2)** The indicators of domestic violence in this case are the multiple vague physical complaints without supporting objective data, the suspected depression, and the reluctance to wait around in the clinic for extended periods of time. This client is on the verge of disclosing, if a provider would only ask her about domestic violence.

17. **(1)** Due to the acute confusion state and the incontinence, she is experiencing delirium. This is most likely secondary to a urinary tract infection. Dementia is more insidious versus acute. Depression and psychosis are not consistent with the assessments. The major symptoms in depression would include loss in interest; loss of sleep; decreased appetite, concentration, and activity; increased guilt; decreased energy; or potential suicidal thoughts. Psychotic disorder includes thoughts and behavior where the client is not in touch with reality.

18. **(2)** A history of a new medication with an abrupt onset of confusion must be reviewed closely. An adverse reaction of cimetidine (Tagamet) is confusion in the elderly. Dementia results in confusion that slowly develops. The attention span and memory may be affected in each diagnosis.

19. **(2)** Role playing and planning a rehearsed reply to teasing comments about short stature are helpful tools to deal with this issue. Although humor can be effective, constantly clowning around for attention is not positive coping behavior. Withdrawal (i.e., watching television or reading) is not effective coping and may indicate depression. Spending time and associating only with younger adolescents who are the same height is not a positive coping behavior and may hinder normal maturation.

20. **(4)** More than 50% of intravenous cocaine users develop hepatitis, phlebitis, endocarditis, and acquired immunodeficiency syndrome (AIDS). Epistaxis, rhinorrhea, and nasal congestion are seen most often in intranasal users of cocaine. Chest congestion, wheezing, and eventual emphysema occur with chronic freebase (crack) smokers. Although cardiac arrhythmias, hypertension, and respiratory arrest can occur, they are not the common complications.

21. **(3)** Adults who are depressed typically display findings noted in Options #1, #2, and #4. Adolescents often act out in defense of trying to protect themselves from feelings of vulnerability and dependency. Noting signs of anger and frustration in the adolescent is important to evaluate, as the significance of the behavior may indicate symptoms of depression.

22. **(3)** People with anorexia nervosa will exercise up to 4 hours a day. They are of above average intelligence in most cases, suffer from bradycardia, and have decreased libido.

23. **(3)** In teenage girls, the most common form of suicide attempt is by drug overdose. The combination of vomiting and confusion suggest a drug overdose. The teenager should be evaluated immediately for life-threatening cardiac dysrhythmias.

24. **(1)** The nurse practitioner would suspect this client to have a diagnosis of substance-induced mood disorder. It would be appropriate to determine exactly how much, how long, and how often she consumes alcohol or any other drugs. The key points in the situation are the occupational burnout, depressive symptoms, and ineffective coping measures (taking and doing everything to relax, but with no relief).

25. **(2)** This client should be examined by emergency department personnel, many of whom are specially trained to collect the evidence needed to testify in court about the rape. The exam should not be done in the office unless the nurse practitioner has been trained in evidence collection and has a rape evidence collection kit. The exam must be done quickly before evidence is destroyed. The client decides who should be called for support. While she is encouraged to call her parents, she is also offered the support of rape crisis and other resources.

26. **(2)** Bradycardia and excessive salivation are not found with cocaine abuse. There are no drug antagonists that can be used for cocaine overdose, although naloxone is given to reduce the concurrent toxic effects of other narcotic drugs that may be in the client's body system.

27. **(4)** While all of the answers may contribute to a clinician's suspicion of family violence, the admission of genuine fear of a household member is considered and excellent indicator of actual or potential violence and the level of danger in a home.

28. **(3)** Chronic anxiety attacks are not part of the DSM-IV criteria.

Pharmacology

29. **(3)** The client is experiencing a rare problem called neuroleptic malignant syndrome. This client would require immediate referral and hospitalization. Acute dystonia, parkinsonism, and akathisia are associated with extrapyramidal disorder or acute movement disorder. Tardive dyskinesia occurs late in therapy and is often irreversible. Slow worm-like movements of the tongue are the earliest symptom, followed by grimacing, lip smacking, and involuntary limb movements.

30. **(3)** Trazadone (Desyrel) has sedation as a side effect, which has made it less popular as an antidepressant; however, it is commonly prescribed for insomnia.

31. **(4)** Often, some of the first indications of drug use in adolescents are related to a sudden change in behavior or school performance. Symptoms of heroin use are constricted pupils, respiratory depression, needle tracks, and poor nutrition. Symptoms of marijuana use are slow reflexes, tachycardia, conjunctival injection, nasal congestion, and increased appetite. Symptoms of LSD use are dilated pupils, reddened eyes, hypertension, increased appetite, and hallucinations. The use of central nervous system stimulants, like crack cocaine, leads to hypertension, weight loss, anorexia, insomnia, hyperreflexia, and a perforated or ulcerated nasal septum.

32. **(3)** Naloxone is a narcotic antagonist and is used for the reversal of narcotic depression, including respiratory depression. Clonidine (Catapres) is a central α-agonist and is indicated for treatment of hypertension. Methadone is used in the treatment of opoid addition. The Food and Drug Administration has placed methadone in a special drug category that allows medically supervised administration of the drug to addicts with chronic, intractable addiction to heroin. Naltrexone's therapeutic classification is "narcotic detoxification adjunct."

33. **(3)** Seizures, alcohol withdrawal, and anxiety are commonly treated with benzodiazepines. They are **not** the first drug of choice for obsessive-compulsive disorder, selective serotonin reuptake inhibitors are usually used.

34. **(1)** Dosages should be reduced by 30–50% to start therapy and gradually increased as necessary. Adverse effects are likely to occur because of slowed drug metabolism that occurs with aging. These include hypotension and arrhythmias, and sedative and anticholingeric effects.

35. **(2)** A highly-nicotine-dependent client benefits from intense counseling and prescription of alternative nicotine delivery during the smoking cessation process. Usually the nicotine patch is the preferred form of replacement, as the gum is noncontinuous and withdrawal symptoms may occur during nonchewing times. The nicotine patch delivers a fixed dose of nicotine on a continual basis, is applied once daily, and eliminates the GI upset that often occurs with the gum. If this client insisted on using the gum, the dose should be 4 mg, not 2 mg. Option #4 is too low of a dose to start on this client and is not the correct dosing schedule. Zyban (bupropion HCl) would be used in conjunction with the nicotine patch, and clients are to quit smoking 1–2 weeks after starting the Zyban, not immediately.

Emergencies

1. While visiting a rural public school, an adult was bitten on the hand by a raccoon. At the rural clinic, the nurse practitioner cleansed the wound. The next action is:

   1. Administer tetanus antitoxin.

   2. Contact local animal control authorities.

   3. Administer rabies immune globulin (RIG) and human diploid cell vaccine (HDCV).

   4. Teach the family how to do hourly soaks to the hand using normal saline and peroxide.

2. An adult is brought to the clinic with a history of an insect bite last evening. What presenting symptom would be associated with the bite of a brown recluse spider?

   1. Paresthesias in all extremities.

   2. Edematous, erythematous area with coalescing macules.

   3. Tissue sloughing in the bite area within 8–10 hours.

   4. Development of a central black eschar or "sinking infarct" in 6–12 hours.

3. The nurse practitioner understands that cat bites become infected more often than dog bites because:

   1. Dogs have "cleaner mouths" than cats.

   2. Cat bites are often deep puncture wounds.

   3. Dog bites are usually on the face, which makes them more susceptible to infection.

   4. Cat bites are usually associated with clawing and spreading of microorganisms.

4. When do bites due to insects, spiders, snakes, and bees most commonly occur?

   1. Fall.

   2. Spring to fall.

   3. Winter.

   4. Any time of the year.

5. An adult was bitten by a neighbor's dog 3 days ago. She has developed an infection in a large wound on her lower leg. What would be appropriate management of this client?

   1. Prescribe amoxicillin/clavulanate potassium (Augmentin) 250 mg PO tid × 14 days.

   2. Approximate the edges of the wound together with suture.

   3. Prescribe cephalexin (Keflex) 500 mg PO tid × 7 days.

   4. Have the client return to the clinic for follow-up in 2 weeks.

6. Medical management for a brown recluse spider bite includes:

   1. Warm, moist soaks to the area.

   2. Ice pack and elevate area.

   3. Active and passive range of motion to area.

   4. Avoid use of antihistamines.

7. An adult has been bitten by a black widow spider while doing yard work. She is having a severe reaction. The nurse practitioner expects:

   1. Hypotension and shock.

   2. Localized pain, erythema, and edema in the area.

   3. Black eschar of sloughing tissue within 4 hours of the bite.

   4. Abdominal rigidity, nausea, and headache.

19 Answers & Rationales

1. **(3)** Any type of animal bite that might be associated with an animal that may potentially harbor rabies (skunks, bats, raccoons, foxes, coyotes, rats) should be treated with both active and passive rabies immunization. Tetanus antitoxin would be indicated, if the child was not current on the immunization. Animal authorities would be called after the initial treatment to locate the animal and sacrifice it, so that the brain could be examined for rabies.

2. **(4)** Brown recluse spiders produce sharp pain at the instant of the bite with subsequent minor swelling and erythema. Tissue necrosis may occur within 4 hours. A blue-gray to black macular halo may surround the bite with eventual widening and sinking of the center of the lesion, leading to a "sinking infarct" that leaves a deep ulcer that takes weeks or months to heal.

3. **(2)** Deep puncture wounds are more likely to get infected with anaerobic organisms. Bites on the hand have the highest infection rate, while bites on the face have the lowest infection rate.

4. **(2)** Insects are more active, reproduce, and are in greater numbers in the warm months (i.e., spring to early fall).

5. **(1)** Amoxicillin clavulanate potassium (Augmentin) is an excellent choice for the empiric treatment of animal bites. Keflex is not indicated due to resistant strains of *Pasteurella multocida*, organism present in 25% of dog bites and 50% of cat bites. An infected bite should be followed up on a daily basis, until the infection clears. Open-wound management is indicated, not suturing.

6. **(2)** Heat application is contraindicated, ice packs are preferred, as is elevation to decrease the edema. The area should be immobilized. Tetanus toxoid may be given along with antihistamines to reduce swelling and relieve itching.

7. **(4)** In addition to these symptoms, bronchospasm, hypertension, seizures, and altered mental status may occur. Black eschar is associated with a brown recluse spider bite.

20

Research & Theory

Research

1. When designing a research project that will involve clients, from the options presented, the most important point to be included in the written consent to participate is:

   1. The directions regarding the use of a black pen.

   2. The anticipated date for publication of the completed research report.

   3. The assurance of privacy and confidentiality.

   4. The number of previously published research studies about this topic.

2. When determining whether to incorporate into your clinical practice a new procedure based on the findings of a recent study, which of the following should you consider?

   1. The statistical significance of the findings.

   2. The statistical relevance of the findings.

   3. The statistical software program used.

   4. The statistical background of the researcher.

3. The research process is similar to the processes nurse practitioners use to provide client care in that both are decision-making processes that include the steps (in the order presented here) of:

   1. Assessing, teaching, evaluating, and discussing.

   2. Defining, planning, implementing, and charting.

   3. Questioning, evaluating, diagnosing, and teaching.

   4. Assessing, planning, implementing, and evaluating.

4. Both descriptive and inferential statistics are used in research. However, their purposes are different in that:

   1. Inferential statistics are used for assigning participant code numbers.

   2. Descriptive statistics are used for assigning participant code numbers.

   3. Inferential statistics are used for hypothesis testing.

   4. Descriptive statistics are used for hypothesis testing.

5. In an ambulatory care setting, the nurse practitioner might find it difficult to utilize nursing research because:

   1. The demands of providing primary care leave little time for research utilization.

   2. Procedures for research utilization have not been well defined in the literature.

   3. Research published in professional journals is too difficult to access by clinicians.

   4. Ambulatory care settings have little in common with the settings used for most research.

6. While nursing theories vary greatly in their perspective of nursing care, all nursing theorists explicitly incorporate three key concepts. These three concepts, which are basic to nursing care, are:

   1. Individuals, families, and communities.

   2. Primary, secondary, and tertiary prevention.

   3. Past, present, and future well-being.

   4. Person, health, and environment.

7. The scientific method for conducting research uses the null hypothesis, which is statistically based. The correct format for the null hypothesis is:

   1. There are no significant differences between two groups.

   2. Group "A" is greater than group "B."

   3. Group "A" is less than group "B."

   4. There is a 95% probability that group "A" is different from group "B."

8. When evaluating claims made on advertisements, such as "Drug X has been used for 5 years with over 1 million doses administered in the United States, Canada, and Great Britain. Drug X stops heartburn, aids in digestion, and prevents esophageal reflux and is the 'treatment of choice' to relieve GERD," the nurse practitioner realizes that the claim is:

   1. Invalid, as there is no control or comparison group or statistics stated.

   2. Valid, as there are sufficient numbers of users who have had success.

   3. Invalid, because the level of significance is not mentioned to be at the 0.05 level.

   4. Valid, as the cohort and Hawthorne effect are operating.

9. The utilization of research in nursing practice can be equated with:

   1. The nursing process.

   2. The change process.

   3. Discharge planning.

   4. Family planning.

10. You are compiling monthly statistics for your practice, and one of the elements of your analysis is the cultural background of your clients. What level of data is "cultural background"?

    1. Nominal level data.

    2. Ordinal level data.

    3. Interval level data.

    4. Ratio level data.

11. A nurse practitioner practicing with a physician in general practice is compiling the practice statistics at the end of the month. The clients who received care range from infants to the elderly. Of the following data from the monthly report, which is most likely to be normally distributed?

    1. The lab tests scheduled for the clients.

    2. The gender of the clients.

    3. The primary diagnosis of the clients.

    4. The age of the clients.

12. A nurse practitioner practicing with a physician in general practice is compiling the practice statistics at the end of the month. The clients who received care range from infants to the elderly. The nurse practitioner and the physician want to know the average monthly income of their clients. Which would be the most appropriate statistical measure of the "average income" assuming income was exact in dollars and cents?

    1. The mean.

    2. The median.

    3. The mode.

    4. The range.

13. A nurse practitioner is evaluating research articles for a utilization project. The majority of the articles report that either random selection or random assignment was used to select the sample for that study. Because certain procedures in research are used across disciplines, what can be assumed for studies where randomization has been used?

    1. The ages of the research subjects in these studies will be negatively skewed.

    2. The research subjects in these studies will automatically be half male and half female.

    3. The ages of the research subjects in these studies will be positively skewed.

    4. The researchers were attempting to obtain the most representative sample.

14. The ability to predict outcomes of care is desirable both in research and in practice. If a nurse practitioner wanted to create a theoretical model for a specific aspect of his/her practice to predict the client outcomes, which statistical analysis method would be used too analyze the clinical data?

    1. Descriptive statistics.

    2. Repeated measures t-test.

    3. Multiple regression.

    4. Chi-squared for independent samples.

15. Research articles are being evaluated for a utilization project. What can the nurse practitioner do if he/she does not understand the statistical procedures that were used for the analysis of data in an article?

    1. Assume that the correct procedure was used, and read about the method or consult a statistician for an explanation of the statistics.

    2. Assume that the article is beyond his/her ability to understand, so set that one aside and go on to the next article.

    3. Assume that the correct procedure was used and, instead of reading the results section, read the discussion of the findings section.

    4. Assume that the article is beyond his/her ability to understand and use someone else's critique of the reported study.

16. The nurse practitioner has determined that the office procedures for diagnosing and stabilizing new diabetics need to be evaluated and possibly changed. Which would be the best choice for the first phase of the evaluation?

    1. Design and conduct a double-blind clinical trial.

    2. Design and conduct a research utilization project.

    3. Design and conduct a research project comparing men and women.

    4. Design and conduct a study to test Callista Roy's theoretical model.

17. The nurse practitioner was reading a nursing research article in which there were no statistically significant findings. The most appropriate response would be:

    1. "Reading this article was a waste of my time."

    2. "Because of reading this article, there is no reason to conduct similar studies."

    3. "Reading this article raises new questions for my practice."

    4. "Because of reading this article, I will immediately change my practice."

18. The verification of the more abstract nursing theories (e.g., Martha Rogers) is often hampered by:

    1. The lack of adequate measures for the theoretical concepts.

    2. Prior studies that did not support the theory.

    3. The lack of adequate laboratory settings for conducting experiments.

    4. Prior studies that were conducted in other countries.

19. In a recently published study, the researcher reported "the statistical analysis used to identify the differences between the two variables was Pearson's correlation." Which most specifically tells what is wrong with this statement?

    1. Pearson's correlation can be used only with three or more variables.

    2. Pearson's correlation actually identifies the common factors between variables.

    3. Pearson's correlation can be used only when there is a single variable.

    4. Pearson's correlation actually identifies the relationship between variables.

20. Qualitative research studies are conducted by nurse researchers because:

    1. Qualitative studies help to identify and define nursing concepts.

    2. With qualitative methods, there are no concerns about the rights of research subjects.

    3. Qualitative approaches provide precise measures for statistical analysis.

    4. Nurse researchers find qualitative research designs easier to use.

21. The normal ranges of blood chemistry values are most like which statistical concept?

    1. The standard error.

    2. The mean.

    3. The standard deviation.

    4. The median.

22. The five major sequential steps of research utilization are:

    1. Establish a client relationship, assess the client's health, diagnose, devise a plan of care, evaluate the treatment.

    2. Identify the problem, assess published research, design the innovation, evaluate, decide whether to adopt the innovation.

    3. Review the popular literature, review the practice's clients, summarize the findings, evaluate, teach the client.

    4. Review the client's lab reports, complete a thorough health assessment, diagnose, implement the treatment, evaluate.

23. Both *qualitative* and *quantitative* research methods are used in nursing research because:

    1. Master's-prepared nurses conduct quantitative studies, while doctorally prepared nurses conduct quantitative studies.

    2. Master's-prepared nurses conduct qualitative studies, while doctorally prepared nurses conduct quantitative studies.

    3. They complement each other because they produce different types of findings about the same concepts.

    4. They complement each other because they produce the same types of findings about different concepts.

24. Nursing research subscribes to the scientific method for the design of research studies. The advantage of this is that:

    1. Nursing research is based on logically constructed arguments.

    2. Nursing research is designed to answer any research question.

    3. Nursing research findings are precise and need not be duplicated.

    4. Nursing research findings are generalizable to all client populations.

25. With the restructuring of health care delivery and a shift in the provision of nonacute care from the hospital to the ambulatory care settings and the home,

previous nursing research that was
conducted in hospitals:

1. Now becomes applicable to all in-hospital
providers of care.

2. Remains relevant in the new settings;
client care is unchanged.

3. Should be applied directly to client care
provided in the new settings.

4. May no longer be applicable to the
delivery of client care.

26. Nurse researchers strive to substantiate
causality so that client outcomes can be
consistently predicted. For the nurse
practitioner, the ability to predict the
outcomes for every client could mean that:

1. The appropriate treatment would be
prescribed for clients.

2. No further studies would need to be
conducted about treatments.

3. The client's individual qualities would
not need to be considered.

4. Treatments would not need to be
individualized for each client.

27. The reason that quantitative research
articles always have a section containing
descriptive findings is that descriptive data
analysis:

1. Provides the basis for making inferences
about the findings.

2. May yield statistically significant
findings that were unexpected.

3. Is conducted for predicting client
outcomes in nursing settings.

4. Organizes the data for clearer
understanding of subjects and variables.

28. The difference between univariate and
multivariate studies is:

1. The number of subjects in the sample.

2. The number of variables being studied.

3. The number of sites for collecting data.

4. The number of statistical hypotheses.

29. The theoretical basis for nursing practice is:

1. A relatively new approach to nursing
care.

2. Borrowed from other professions such as
medicine.

3. As old as formal nursing and began with
Florence Nightingale.

4. Unrelated to the conduct of nursing
research studies.

30. The independent variable and the
dependent variable of a research study
might be thought of as:

1. The cause (the independent variable) and
the effect (the dependent variable).

2. The median (the independent variable)
and the mode (the dependent variable).

3. The outcome (the independent variable)
and the treatment (the dependent
variable).

4. The sample (the independent variable)
and the population (the dependent
variable).

31. *Variance* is a key statistical concept. How
would our current research methods change
if there were no variance?

1. We would need to increase the sample
size in all of our research studies to 100
research subjects or greater.

2. Since our current research methods do
not depend on the presence of variance,
we would not need to change our current
methods.

3. We would need to decrease the sample
size of all our research studies to 15
research subjects.

4. Since our current research methods are
based on the presence of variance, we
would not be able to use our current
methods.

Theory

32. Nursing practice based on nursing theory contributes to the professionalization of nursing practice by:

    1. Adapting the medical model to nursing care.

    2. Limiting the choice of treatments for clients.

    3. Determining what type of clients will be seen by the nurse.

    4. Providing a consistent perspective for providing care to clients.

33. A nurse practitioner has decided to incorporate a nursing theoretical model into his/her practice. Which nursing model is most applicable to an ambulatory care setting?

    1. Orem's Model of Self-Care.

    2. Roy's Adaptation Model.

    3. Roger's Unitary Person Model.

    4. King's System Model.

34. Which nurse theorist is considered to have general systems theory as philosophical orientation to her model?

    1. Sister Callista Roy.

    2. Martha Rogers.

    3. Rosemarie Parse.

    4. Betty Neuman.

35. Which nurse theorist addresses nursing outcomes in terms of primary, secondary, and tertiary prevention?

    1. Sister Callista Roy.

    2. Betty Neuman.

    3. Imogene King.

    4. Jean Watson.

36. Which nursing theorist's model primarily addresses health promotion?

    1. Jean Watson.

    2. Betty Neuman.

    3. N. J. Pender.

    4. Sister Callista Roy.

20 Answers & Rationales

Research

1. **(3)** By federal law, clients must be assured of their privacy and confidentiality. The other information is interesting and may be included, but is not required by federal law.

2. **(1)** In published reports, of the choices listed, only the first choice is consistently reported by researchers. The clinical relevance is considered, not the statistical relevance. The specific program used does not make a difference, since all are based on the same statistical formulas. Researchers frequently work with statistical consultants, so that a researcher's background is not a limitation to a published study.

3. **(4)** Only the last choice contains those elements common to both processes, which are assessing, planning, implementing, and evaluating.

4. **(3)** Only Option #3 is true. Neither type of statistics is used to assign participant code numbers. Descriptive statistics are used to describe the sample.

5. **(1)** Inadequate time can be a barrier to research utilization in any setting. The process of research utilization is well delineated by researchers. With the ever-increasing availability of professional journals via the Internet, access is rarely a problem. There is a considerable body of research that has been conducted in ambulatory care settings.

6. **(4)** All current theories incorporate person, health, and environment. Other concepts may or may not be explicitly included in nursing theories.

7. **(1)** The correct format for the null hypothesis is "There are no significant differences between two groups." The alternate or research hypothesis may take the other forms.

8. **(1)** Even though the claims detail extensive use of Drug X, there must be statistical evidence as demonstrated through the use of control or comparison groups that will render a level of significance.

9. **(2)** Incorporating research findings into practice often results in a change in practice. The nursing process is most like conducting research.

10. **(1)** The variable of "cultural background" is categorical data or nominal level data.

11. **(4)** The gender and primary diagnosis are nominal level data, and the lab tests would be skewed, while the age would approximate the normal curve.

12. **(2)** The median income would be most representative of the average because the income of 50% of the clients is above and 50% is below the median. The mean could be influenced by one client with a very high or a very low income, and the mode only identifies the income that is reported most often. The range only identifies the lowest and the highest income and does not present an average.

13. **(4)** Randomization is a research technique used to increase the amount of control in any research design. The other three options are false; they do not occur because of randomization.

14. **(3)** Of the choices, only multiple regression examines the relationship between two or more variables in a way that permits prediction.

15. **(1)** In reviewing research, it is necessary to understand the statistical methods that the researcher used in order to determine the value of the study findings for the practice setting. The researcher's discussion may not provide the full extent of the findings, while someone else's critique may reflect a specific point of view that does not apply in every situation.

16. **(2)** As a first step, a research utilization project would provide a thorough review of the published literature on which to base a change. A full study may not be needed, and testing a theoretical model is not appropriate for this situation.

17. **(3)** The lack of significant findings is an important piece of information about the topic of the research, and definitely is not a waste of time. Particularly when findings are nonsignificant, more studies need to be conducted about this topic. Ideally, changes in practice are based on the findings of more than one study.

18. **(1)** The lack of adequate measures for theoretical concepts is a major roadblock in many areas of research, and particularly so with the more abstract theories. Prior studies always provide information about the theory, even when conducted in other countries. More abstract concepts tend not to be studies in lab settings.

19. **(4)** Correlations identify the relationships between variables. Two or more variables may be used. Factor analysis is used to identify common factors.

20. **(1)** The purpose of qualitative designs is to identify and define nursing concepts. Qualitative designs do not yield precise measures, are usually not analyzed statistically, are more difficult to use, and

carry the same concerns about the rights of subjects as all other research designs.

21. **(3)** The normal ranges of blood chemistry values are based on studies that identified the standard deviation for each blood chemical. The mean and the median are averages, and the standard error is not applicable to this situation.

22. **(2)** This option contains the published steps. All other options are nursing actions taken on behalf of the client (in no particular order).

23. **(3)** The two methods do complement each other because they produce different types of findings about the same concepts. The educational preparation of the researcher does not dictate the research method used.

24. **(1)** The scientific method is highly organized, and is based on logical reasoning. Findings are rarely precise and studies do need to be duplicated. Some questions are not answerable by our current research methods. Because of small samples and other limitations, many findings from nursing research are **not** generalizable.

25. **(4)** Such a drastic change in health care delivery may make previous studies no longer applicable to nursing care. Health care restructuring has changed the way client care is provided.

26. **(1)** The ability to always predict client outcomes would mean that every client would receive the exact treatment for that individual. Treatments would still have to be individualized and individual qualities would need to be considered. Because new treatments are always being devised, there would be a need for ongoing research.

27. **(4)** Descriptive data analysis does organize the data, and it facilitates understanding. Descriptive statistics cannot be used for significance testing or for making inferences; for this, inferential statistics are used. Predictions are made from studies that use inferential statistics.

28. **(2)** "Variate" refers to the number of variables in the study.

29. **(3)** The theoretical basis for nursing practice began with Florence Nightingale and has been used for practice and for research for over a century. Nursing theories are specifically developed for nursing.

30. **(1)** The independent variable may be considered the cause or the treatment, and the dependent variable may be considered the effect or the outcome. The median, mode, sample, and population are not designations for the independent or the dependent variables.

31. **(4)** All our current research and statistical analysis methods rely on the presence of variance or variation; so that if variance is no longer present, our current methods could no longer be used. If there is no variance, a sample of one would be adequate.

Theory

32. **(4)** Theory-based practice contributes the consistent perspective that permits the comparison of care across settings. Theory-based practice does not necessarily limit treatments or determine client types. Theory-based practice specifically eliminates reliance on the medical model.

33. **(1)** Orem's theory focuses on the client participating and being in control of his/her own health care. Roy's model is most appropriate for acute care settings, Roger's is most appropriate for holistic health settings, and King's is most appropriate for mental health settings.

34. **(4)** Betty Neuman's Health Care Systems Model, Imogene King's Systems Interaction Model, and Dorothy Johnson's Behavioral Systems are based on general systems theory. Roy's Adaptation Model is based on stress and adaptation as the framework. Martha Rogers's Science of Unitary Human Beings and Rosemarie Parse's Human Becoming Model are based on a humanistic developmental framework.

35. **(2)** Betty Neuman identified the need to implement nursing interventions through use of one or more of three prevention modalities (primary, secondary, tertiary prevention).

36. **(3)** Pender's Health Promotion Model is an excellent nursing model that readily fits into a nurse practitioner's scope of practice. The other theorist's models are Betty Neuman's Health Care Systems Model, Jean Watson's Human Science and Human Model of Caring, and Roy's Adaptation Model.

21

Issues & Trends

1. Considering the four advanced practice roles—clinical nurse specialist, nurse practitioner, certified nurse midwife, and nurse anesthetist—which role became accepted by and included into the practice arena without significant controversy?

    1. Clinical nurse specialist.

    2. Nurse practitioner.

    3. Certified nurse midwife.

    4. Nurse anesthetist.

2. Historically, who was one of the most outspoken opponents of the nurse practitioner role?

    1. Loretta Ford.

    2. Hildegard Peplau.

    3. Martha Rogers.

    4. Dorothea Orem.

3. Who started the first nurse practitioner program?

    1. Hildegard Peplau.

    2. Mary Breckenridge.

    3. Agnes McGee.

    4. Loretta Ford.

4. Which is the most important aspect in developing health policy skills in the nurse practitioner?

    1. Develop political allies in Congress.

    2. Work on a campaign.

    3. Support causes such as prevention of teen pregnancy or acquired immunodeficiency syndrome (AIDS).

    4. Write letters and editorials.

5. Which is the least important barrier to collaborative advanced nursing practice?

    1. Prescriptive authority.

    2. Reimbursement privileges.

    3. Legal scope of practice.

    4. Political activism.

6. For the nurse practitioner to obtain reimbursement, an understanding of which is important?

   1. Minimum Nursing Data Set (MNDS).

   2. *International Classification of Diseases, 9th ed.* (ICD-9)CM, Physician's Current Procedural Terminology (CPT), and *H*ealth *C*are Financing Administration *C*ommon *P*rocedure *C*oding System (HCPC).

   3. HCPC codes and NANDA diagnosis.

   4. Medicare and Medicaid number.

7. Steps of the change process according to Kurt Lewin are:

   1. Unsolving, mobilizing, recruiting, finalizing.

   2. Building relationships, acquiring resources, choosing solution, stabilizing.

   3. Unfreezing, moving, refreezing.

   4. Forming, storming, norming.

8. What was the major impetus for nurse practitioner development?

   1. Need for an expert nurse clinician.

   2. Shortage of primary care physicians.

   3. Trend for specialized nurses to diagnose and manage unstable acute and chronic clients.

   4. Movement of graduate nursing education to diagnosis and treatment of major illness.

9. The nurse practitioner understands that Medicare B provides:

   1. Hospitalization costs for the insured.

   2. Health insurance benefits for low-income families.

   3. Benefits that cover physicians, nurse practitioners, medical equipment, and outpatient services.

   4. Outpatient laboratory, radiography services, and skilled nursing care in appropriate facilities.

10. What is the impact of the Balanced Budget Act of 1997 on nurse practitioner practice?

    1. Authorizes all states to provide nurse practitioners prescriptive authority.

    2. Provides for only well visits and primary care services.

    3. Prevents a physician from billing 100% for a nurse practitioner's services.

    4. Allows direct Medicare payments to nurse practitioners in both rural and urban settings.

11. In the clinic, you have observed the following: one medical assistant is usually pleasant and helpful; the other is often abrasive and angry. The most important basic guideline to be observed by the nurse practitioner nurse who must resolve a conflict between two medical assistants is:

    1. Require the medical assistants to reach a compromise.

    2. Weigh the consequences of each possible solution.

    3. Encourage ventilation of anger and use humor to minimize the conflict.

    4. Deal with issues, not personalities.

12. A male nurse practitioner approaches another nurse practitioner who is his friend and tells him that one of the female physicians at the clinic often follows him into the supplies room and tells him how good looking he is. Yesterday, she patted his hand and said, "I wish we would get to know each other better. I would make it worth your while—better benefits at the clinic, more money." The male staff nurse asks his friend, "What do I do? I don't want to date her, but I don't want to lose my job. I just want her to leave me alone!" The best reply for the friend would be:

    1. "Tell her that her behavior makes you feel uncomfortable and that you want her to stop."

    2. "Go for it!! Date her and see if you get what she promises."

    3. "Go as soon as possible to the human relations office at the agency and relate to them the entire situation."

    4. "Contact your lawyer and get advice as soon as possible, in case she decides to turn the tables and accuse you of advances."

21 Answers & Rationales

1. **(1)** According to the National Commission on Nursing (1983) and the Task Force on Nursing Practice in Hospitals (1983), the clinical nurse specialist (CNS) role was accepted quite rapidly. The psychiatric clinical nurse specialist role is considered the oldest and most highly developed of the CNS specialities and helped initiate the growth of other CNS specialities.

2. **(3)** Martha Rogers argued that the development of the nurse practitioner role was a ploy to lure nurses out of nursing and into medicine, hence weakening and undermining nursing's unique role in health care. This led to a major division within nursing, which led to barriers in the establishment of nurse practitioner educational programs within the mainstream of graduate nursing education.

3. **(4)** Loretta Ford R.N., Ph.D. and Henry Silver, M.D. established the first pediatric nurse practitioner program at the University of Colorado. Mary Breckenridge established the Frontier Nursing Service in the depressed rural mountain area of Kentucky which led to training nurse midwives. Agnes McGee is credited with offering the first postgraduate program for the nurse anesthetist role at St. Vincent's Hospital in Portland, Oregon. Hildegard Peplau started the first psychiatric clinical nurse specialist program at Rutger's University.

4. **(1)** Although all of these activities are important for helping the nurse practitioner to develop policy skills, the most important is developing political allies. Having political allies in decision-making places (legislature) will enable the nurse practitioner to be active and informed regarding issues surrounding regulation, limitations on admitting privileges and prescriptive authority, and managed care.

5. **(4)** There are three major issues that are central to the expansion of the nurse practitioner role—prescriptive authority, reimbursement privileges, and legal scope of practice. Although political activism is important, it is not specific to collaborative practice.

6. **(2)** The ICD-9-CM codes are diagnostic codes that identify the condition, illness, or injury to be treated and are used for billing insurance carriers. CPT codes specify the procedure or medical service given (over 7000 terms). Medicare and state Medicaid carriers are required by law to use CPT codes. The HCFA HCPC is used for reporting supplies and medical equipment.

7. **(3)** Lewin described three processes of change: unfreezing—involves breaking the habit, disturbing the equilibrium; moving—development of new responses based on new information with a change in attitudes, feelings, behaviors, or values; and refreezing—reaching a new status quo, stabilizing and integrating new behaviors with appropriate support that is available to maintain the change. Forming, storming, and norming refer to the stages of group process development. Option #2 is Havelock's change theory steps.

8. **(2)** According to most sources, the nurse practitioner role developed due to a shortage of primary care physicians in the 1960s and 1970s, as medical specialization was the trend.

9. **(3)** Medicare is regulated by the federal government and includes the services described, plus out-patient laboratory and radiography. Hospitalization costs are covered under Medicare Part A.

10. **(4)** A crucial and significant piece of legislation that allows direct payments to nurse practitioners at "80% of the lesser of either the actual charge or 85% of the fee schedule amount of the same service if provided by a physician." This does not change the "incident to" rule, which allows a physician to bill for 100% for a nurse practitioner's services (i.e., provided the physician is in the suite at the time of the service and readily available to provide assistance).

11. **(4)** Conflict must be addressed directly by the nurse practitioner. The personal characteristics of each of the medical assistants must not enter into the conflict resolution process. Determine what the issue of conflict is and then work on possible solutions to resolve the issue. Compromise is just one method of conflict resolution, where both parties must be willing to give up something.

12. **(1)** There are two ways to deal with sexual harassment at work: informally and formally through a grievance procedure. Always start with the direct approach; ask the person to STOP! Tell the harasser in clear terms that the behavior makes you uncomfortable and that you want it to stop immediately.

22

Legal & Ethical Issues

1. An occurrence-form professional liability insurance policy is preferred because:

   1. The amount of insurance money available to pay a claim increases with each renewal of the policy.

   2. The policy proceeds are available to pay claims regardless of when the claim is reported to the carrier.

   3. The carrier will be notified of a potential claim during the policy period.

   4. The coverage is broader than that provided by a claims-made policy form.

2. Early reporting of a potential professional liability claim is advantageous because:

   1. Insurance carriers have a 10-day reporting window after which the coverage is canceled.

   2. Documents and witnesses needed to defend the claim are more likely to be available at the time of the event.

   3. Your insurance premiums will be reduced upon a good-faith showing of cooperation with the carrier.

   4. Risk management personnel require such reporting in order to comply with Joint Commission on the Accreditation of Healthcare Organizations (JCAHO) mandates.

3. Your nursing license may be in jeopardy if:

   1. You appropriately delegate medication administration to a trusted RN employee who administers a fatal dose.

   2. You delegate client assessment tasks to an LPN who has been floated to your outpatient clinic for the day.

   3. You provide nursing care services consistent with established standards of practice in your jurisdiction.

   4. The medical assistant in your supervising physician's office exceeds the scope of her authority, but you take prompt action to correct the problem.

4. Your client is a 46-year-old mentally retarded woman who has been diagnosed with colon cancer. Consent for her corrective surgery should be obtained from:

   1. The client herself.

   2. The client's 84-year-old mother, who is her closest relative.

   3. The client's court-appointed guardian.

   4. The administrator of the group home where the client lives.

5. Your client is a 75-year-old woman with metastatic cancer. Her affairs are in order; she has arranged all her finances and her own funeral rites. She has systematically secured enough barbiturates to successfully end her life; she asks you to mix the drugs for her in some pudding to make them palatable for ingestion. Your best course of action would be:

1. Mix the medications as requested and stay with her while she consumes the preparation.

2. Consult with her family and attending physician to warn them about the client's proposed course of action.

3. Seek an immediate order for an antidepressant.

4. Sit down with the client and conduct a physical and psychological needs assessment.

6. The Patient Self-Determination Act, passed by Congress in 1990, resulted in which of the following policy changes?

1. Hospitals are mandated to assist every client to create a "living will."

2. Federally funded managed care organizations (MCOs) are required to inform subscribers about their rights under state law to create advance directives.

3. Home health agencies are required to have "do-not-resuscitate" orders on file for all terminally ill clients.

4. Hospitalized clients are obligated to select a surrogate decision maker to make health care decisions for them if they become incapacitated.

7. Both the Food and Drug Administration (FDA) and the Department of Health and Human Services (DHHS) have regulations governing research activities on human subjects. The principal investigator is responsible for:

1. Securing a signed special research consent form.

2. Reporting back to the Institutional Review Board if a subject is injured during the course of the study.

3. Appearing before the Institutional Review Board to present the study and secure approval to proceed with subject recruitment at the facility.

4. All of the above.

8. If you are served with a summons and complaint (i.e., lawsuit documents), the first step you should take is:

1. Call the client to determine the basis for the action and what you allegedly did wrong.

2. Call the client's lawyer (listed on the first page of the lawsuit) to get more information about the case.

3. Call your insurance company for instructions on how to proceed.

4. Confer with your colleagues and review the chart to see if you need to clarify your notes.

9. As a nurse practitioner in an impoverished rural area, you frequently encounter female clients in situations of domestic violence with few community options for referral. Participating in community education forums and fundraising for a safe house is an example of applying the ethical principle of:

1. Autonomy.

2. Nonmaleficence.

3. Justice.

4. Veracity.

10. Nurses practicing in expanded roles should carry professional liability insurance for which of the following reasons?

1. Premiums are often modest and are a tax-deductible business expense.

2. Even if the employer insures the nurse practitioner, there may be situations of conflict between employer and nurse necessitating separate legal counsel, a covered benefit under the policy.

3. As roles expand, so does the liability potential.

4. All of the above.

11. The confidentiality of medical records is always a valid concern, especially in this age of computerization, "smart cards," and fax machines. Release of medical information to third parties is:

    1. Addressed mainly in state laws or statutes.

    2. Prohibited without the informed consent of the client.

    3. Automatic when the requesting party is a third-party payor or insurer.

    4. Disallowed if the records contain proof of a diagnosis of acquired immunodeficiency syndrome (AIDS).

12. Which categories of persons are **not** included in the definition of disability under the Americans with Disabilities Act?

    1. Profoundly deaf employees.

    2. Persons who are wheelchair bound.

    3. Current users of illegal drugs.

    4. Mentally retarded persons.

13. If your client is having a problem with a managed care plan, you can offer to assist in the following ways:

    1. Suggest that the client contact the customer service department (may be called "member services") at the plan to resolve the issue; a formal grievance filing may be necessary.

    2. Remind the client who is a member of the "senior" plan for Medicare recipients, that he/she may complain to the federal Office of Personnel Management (OPM).

    3. Remind the client that the state's insurance department also investigates complains against health plans.

    4. All of the above.

14. Health policy theorist Daniel Callahan believes that our health care system could be improved by:

    1. Making the care of the chronically ill our first priority, so that these individuals are not abandoned by the health care system.

    2. Making preventive care the first priority.

    3. Maintaining the current allocation of dollars to high-tech care.

    4. Leaving the system "as is" and let market forces determine the allocation of health care dollars.

15. If a piece of equipment malfunctions while being used on a hospitalized client, the risk manager would probably recommend the following course of action:

    1. Return the item to the manufacturer with a description of the problem and a request for analysis.

    2. Tag and sequester the item at the facility and defer analysis pending risk management review of the litigation potential.

    3. Send the item to the biomedical engineering department with a request for immediate equipment breakdown and troubleshooting.

    4. Repair the item, either in-house or by an outside contracted firm, and return it to service as soon as possible.

16. Nurse expert witnesses are essential in the adjudication of most professional negligence claims against nurses. The following criteria for nurse experts are sought by attorneys:

    1. Appropriate professional education, preferably at the technical level.

    2. Relevant and recent professional work experience.

    3. Ability to understand and articulate the legal issues involved in the claim.

    4. Published authorship of medical texts in the clinical subject areas.

17. Which federal law mandates the tracking of implantable medical devices?

    1. The Administrative Procedures Act (APA).

    2. The Patient Self-Determination Act (PSDA).

    3. The Safe Medical Devices Act (SMDA).

    4. The Omnibus Budget Reconciliation Act (OBRA) of 1987.

18. Which of the following are elements of a broad-based risk management program?

    1. A hazardous materials compliance program as part of a comprehensive safety and security system.

    2. An early-warning/incident reporting program to identify elements of risk.

    3. A system of contract review to avoid assuming liabilities that should be borne by others.

    4. All of the above.

19. The type of insurance coverage that is purchased (or self-insured) by an organization to handle employee job-related injuries is:

    1. Professional liability insurance.

    2. Business interruption insurance.

    3. Directors and officers insurance.

    4. Worker's compensation insurance.

20. While driving your personal vehicle on a job-related errand, you are struck by a semitrailer on the interstate. The car is totaled and you are severely injured. Which insurance policies will respond to these losses?

    1. Your personal auto policy and your employer's worker's compensation policy.

    2. The employer's business auto policy and worker's compensation policy.

    3. Your homeowner's policy.

    4. The semitrailer driver's personal auto policy.

21. Nurse practitioners with hospital privileges may be impacted by the part of the Health Care Quality Improvement Act known as the National Practitioner Data Bank. Which of the following statements about the Data Bank is **not** true?

    1. Professional liability insurance claims payments made on behalf of nurse practitioners must be reported to the Data Bank.

    2. The facility granting medical staff privileges must query the Data Bank before approving a practitioner's privileges.

    3. The purpose of the Data Bank is to have a national source of information about malpractice claims, licensure actions, and restrictions on privileges so that practitioners may not easily move from one jurisdiction to another to escape quality review.

    4. Insurance companies report all malpractice payments made on behalf of affected practitioners, regardless of the amount of the payment.

22. In 1985 Congress took action against a phenomenon known as "patient dumping" by enacting what was known at the time as the COBRA law, now referred to as EMTALA, the Emergency Medical Treatment and Active Labor Act. Which statement about EMTALA is **not** true?

    1. The original purpose of the statute was to prohibit the transfer of uninsured and untreated clients from the emergency department of one hospital to another (usually the county hospital).

    2. Subsequent rules and case law have expanded the statute so that almost any unauthorized transfer of a client from one facility to another is potentially problematic.

    3. In order to effect a proper transfer, the forwarding facility need neither notify nor secure the acquiescence of the receiving facility.

    4. The transferring facility must utilize appropriate transport methods and send copies of clients' medical records.

23. You are a nurse practitioner wishing to effect change in the state's laws regarding the dispensing of prescription medications by nurse practitioners. You would take your case to:

    1. The state legislature.

    2. The state board of nursing.

    3. The state board of pharmacy.

    4. The nursing specialty organization.

24. The common meaning of "gag clauses" or "gag orders" in the managed care arena is:

    1. The managed care organization (MCO) declines to publish, in its subscriber contracts, the treatments that are excluded from coverage under the plan.

    2. The MCO refuses to allow its member services personnel to answer certain subscriber questions about covered benefits.

    3. MCO contracts with providers disallow providers' offering treatment alternatives that the providers know are not covered by clients' plans.

    4. Providers are prohibited from offering experimental treatment to clients.

25. Under the Safe Medical Devices Act of 1990, the following health care providers or organizations are required to report the death of a client to the Food and Drug Administration (FDA) if the death is related to the use of a medical device:

    1. Physicians' office staff.

    2. Hospitals, home health agencies, and ambulance companies.

    3. Nurse family members treating clients without compensation.

    4. Physicians making home visits.

26. A client receives a medication that was intended for another person. An appropriate way to document this event in the medical record would be:

    1. "Client was given x mg of y drug in error."

    2. "x mg y drug administered to client. No adverse effects noted. Physician notified."

    3. "Client received wrong medication. Incident report filed. Practitioner disciplined."

    4. "Practitioner inadvertently administered y drug to wrong client. Supervisor notified. Family threatening litigation."

27. The one reason that clients offer, above all others, for suing practitioners for medical negligence is:

    1. The care they received was substandard.

2. The provider made an honest mistake.

3. The client was not "heard" when he/she attempted to communicate with the provider.

4. The client participated fully in all aspects of medical decision making, but the results were disappointing.

28. Informed consent is based upon the ethical principle of:

    1. Beneficence.

    2. Respect for persons.

    3. Nonmaleficence.

    4. Autonomy.

29. The four elements of a professional negligence claim are:

    1. Duty, fulfillment of duty, professional relationship, and wrongful act.

    2. Professional responsibility, fault, harm to the client, and wrongful act.

    3. Duty, breach of duty, causal connection between the act and the harm, and harm to the client.

    4. Professional relationship, intentional wrongful act, proximate cause, and damage to the client.

30. You are making an initial home health care visit to an elderly lady whose spouse tells you that she is often confused. He answers all your questions and dominates the discussion. You proceed to do your initial assessment; the wife does seem to be oriented to time, place, and person. Who is the proper party to sign the written form to request/consent for services?

    1. The husband.

    2. The wife/client.

    3. The attending physician.

    4. The home health aide who will be providing continuing care.

31. An expert witness is usually required in a nursing negligence case because:

    1. Knowledge of medical or nursing facts is not considered intuitive to a lay jury.

    2. Jurors are allowed to use their "sixth sense" regarding the facts presented to them.

    3. Fact witnesses are not able to present an unbiased account of the circumstances in dispute.

    4. Appropriately credentialed experts have more credibility in the eyes of lay jurors.

32. The standard of care for a nurse practitioner, in a trial, will be established by expert witness(es). The expert opinion will be based upon:

    1. National norms for the specialty.

    2. Facility policies and procedures.

    3. Professional literature.

    4. All of the above.

33. Alternative Dispute Resolution (ADR) is a process where the parties to a dispute resolve their differences outside of a court trial. Advantages to this system of problem solving include all of the following **except**:

    1. The parties usually prefer the process because they have their opportunity to be heard in a less formal and less intimidating environment.

    2. The process is often less time consuming and less costly than traditional litigation.

    3. Damage awards are less likely to include nonfinancial compensation.

    4. Insurers are amenable to working with mediators with a track record of fairness and successful case resolution.

34. The statute of limitations is:

    1. The state law that prescribes the time frames within which a nursing negligence action may be filed.

    2. The law that states that minors have no legal authority to sue nurses for malpractice.

    3. The law that limits the right of clients to sue nurse practitioners for negligent acts.

    4. The federal law that limits a nurse practitioner's right to countersue a client for malicious prosecution.

35. You are a family nurse practitioner driving along the interstate on your way to a nursing seminar. You observe a head-on collision and decide to stop to render aid. Which statement is **false** with respect to your potential liability for malpractice?

    1. You had no legal obligation to stop to render assistance; if you had driven by the accident, there would be no liability on your part.

    2. If you provide appropriate nursing care, gratuitously, you will be protected from liability under your state's Good Samaritan law.

    3. Even if you act in a grossly negligent manner, the Good Samaritan law will shield you from liability.

    4. The protections afforded by the Good Samaritan law may differ from state to state; you should research your state's law on the subject.

36. If you are subpoenaed to appear for a deposition in a nursing negligence case, appropriate preparation is prudent. One of the following tips would probably not be suggested by your attorney. Which piece of advice is **not** appropriate?

    1. Discretely chew gum to calm your nerves and dress for dinner because depositions usually take all day and you will not have time to change.

    2. Review the client's medical record and any other materials suggested by your attorney prior to your appearance for questioning.

    3. Take as much time as you need to think about your response before answering; do not let an attorney put words in your mouth.

    4. Be straightforward and truthful; remember that "I don't know" and "I don't remember" are acceptable responses.

37. Which of the following documentation tips is **not** a good idea?

    1. Carefully document your criticism of a fellow provider's clinical decision in the client's medical record. This will protect you if your treatment decisions need to be defended later.

    2. Use standard abbreviations in the medical record so that subsequent readers will have no doubt as to your meaning and intent.

    3. Document telephone conversations with the client and/or the family in the medical record. Be particularly vigilant about recording changes in the client's medications.

    4. Document noncompliant client behaviors in the medical record; be thorough yet factual.

38. In 1987, and again in 1994, Congress acted to update many of the regulations that govern the provision of long-term care services. If you are an employer or nurse manager in this environment, you need to know that:

    1. Nursing assistants working in long-term care facilities must be formally trained and certified.

    2. Clients or residents have specific rights, such as information about their physical condition, medical benefits, and associated costs.

    3. New and swifter sanctions are available to reviewers to impose upon facilities with deficiencies.

    4. All of the above.

39. You are employed as a nurse practitioner in a private medical office. You notice all the activity at the front desk, where some clients are checking in for appointments; staff are scheduling tests, and telephone advice triage is in progress. To preserve client confidentiality, you could implement which of the following changes?

    1. Orient the fax machine and computer monitor such that incoming reports or other data cannot be read by nonstaff members.

    2. Do all telephone scheduling from a more secure location, such as a conference room in the back office.

    3. Create a more private space to confer with clients who need follow-up information or explanations of tests or treatments.

    4. All of the above.

40. As a nurse-employer, you would be well-advised to have procedures in place to appropriately terminate an employee. To avoid a charge of discrimination, or a claim for wrongful termination, you should be particularly sensitive to the protections afforded to select groups. Which of the following is **not** a protected class under the antidiscrimination statutes?

    1. Pregnant women.

    2. Lesbians.

    3. Those age 40 and older.

    4. The handicapped.

41. Which activity could be considered grounds for a sexual harassment claim?

    1. A male employee tells an off-color joke to another man. The joke is overheard by a female co-worker who seems to appreciate the humor in it. The joke-telling is an isolated incident.

    2. A nurse-supervisor conducts an employee performance review. The supervisor does not mention a prior social relationship with the employee; the ratings are appropriate for the level of performance; the employee receives a salary increase.

    3. A coed locker room is decorated with multiple centerfold photos from a popular men's magazine. The female employees find this offensive and have filed several complaints.

    4. A nurse is complimented on her appearance and asked on a date by her boss. She informs the boss that she is married and not seeking another relationship. The incident is forgotten.

42. Your client is a comatose lady who needs a feeding tube inserted for long-term nutritional needs. Her husband presents you with a document that he says is his wife's living will. It is signed by him, and sets out, so he says, the wishes of his wife with respect to the feeding tube. The living will is not a legally binding document because:

    1. The wife did not sign the document.

    2. The husband is not authorized to execute a living will on behalf of his wife.

    3. This type of advance directive must be signed by the individual while he/she is legally competent to execute documents.

    4. All of the above.

43. A nurse practitioner is helping out at a clinic for homeless women. A diabetic client, in her third trimester of pregnancy, has been reasonably compliant with respect to insulin therapy. Now, however, she has announced her intent to abandon her insulin regimen because she has heard on the streets that some drugs are harmful to fetuses. Which option is not legally appropriate for the nurse practitioner, as her health care provider, to consider?

    1. Seek the support of the clinic's attorney to file a petition for court-ordered treatment for the client.

    2. Attempt to engage the client in dialogue to provide her with accurate medical information.

    3. Detain the client in the homeless shelter and administer the insulin, with or without her consent.

    4. Confer with social services to find an appropriate interim placement for the client until her medical and legal issues can be sorted out.

44. The purpose of the Americans with Disabilities Act is:

    1. To level the playing field with respect to employment and other opportunities for disabled people.

    2. To create a federal entitlement program for people with AIDS.

    3. To guarantee wheelchair access to every residential and commercial building.

    4. To authorize interpreters for deaf employees at all private businesses.

45. As a result of the U.S. Supreme Court's ruling on assisted suicide, the current state of the law on this topic is:

    1. Assisted suicide is still a criminal offense in most jurisdictions.

    2. A physician may prescribe a fatal dose of medication with the concurrence of the ethics committee.

    3. A nurse practitioner may prescribe a fatal dose of medication with the concurrence of the supervising physician.

    4. A pharmacist may instruct a client how to mix and ingest a fatal dose of prescription medication.

46. A professional negligence or medical malpractice case is a civil action. The difference between a civil lawsuit and a criminal lawsuit is:

    1. The damages sought in a civil suit are monetary; one private party sues another for money.

    2. If you are convicted in a criminal case, you are still covered by your professional liability insurer.

    3. In a criminal case, your state sues you for money; other penalties do not apply.

    4. In a civil suit, if you do not prevail you could be incarcerated.

47. Which of the following is **not** a form of alternative dispute resolution (ADR)?

    1. Mediation.

    2. Binding and nonbinding arbitration.

    3. Settlement conference.

    4. A jury trial.

48. A health care provider has a duty to disclose certain information to the client as part of the informed consent process. Exceptions to this duty would include all of the following **except**:

1. The client has waived the right to receive the data.

2. It is a bona fide emergency situation.

3. The provider believes that the information would be harmful to the client and invokes the therapeutic privilege.

4. The client is 80 years old, and the elderly are unable to comprehend complex medical facts.

49. Before contemplating providing a detailed reference on a former employee, consider the following:

    1. Check the requirements of the Human Resources Department of your employer.

    2. If the comments are perceived as negative, and the former employee becomes aware of them, you could subject yourself to suit for defamation.

    3. If the employee exhibits unsafe client care practices, it may be wiser to risk legal action from the employee than to subject future clients to this unsafe practitioner.

    4. All of the above.

50. The primary purpose of a pre-employment physical is to:

    1. Identify existing health problems that might adversely affect the company's insurance rates.

    2. Determine the mental status of the applicant.

    3. Determine if the applicant is physically capable of doing the job.

    4. Document any existing disabilities and recommend accommodations.

51. A nurse practitioner involved in work-related surveillance knows that the records related to this activity must be held for how many years after employment?

    1. 5.

    2. 25.

    3. 30.

    4. Can be destroyed only after the employee's death.

52. The nurse practitioner knows that when treating a work-related injury it is required that he/she:

    1. Document thoroughly because of the high probability of legal action.

    2. Communicate directly with the client's employer.

    3. File a report with the industrial commission documenting the injury and treatment.

    4. Notify the Occupational Safety and Health Administration.

53. Which situation would be considered reportable under the Occupational Safety and Health Act?

    1. A 3-cm abrasion of the forearm.

    2. A warehouse worker with back strain reassigned to office work for a week.

    3. A twisted ankle that responded to ice and Ace wrap.

    4. A minor closed-head injury with no loss of consciousness.

54. The purpose of an Occupational Safety and Health Administration 200 log is to record:

    1. Occupational injuries and illnesses.

    2. Only work-related deaths.

    3. Dangerous workplace situations.

    4. Lost work days.

55. The Americans with Disabilities Act (ADA) regulates how employers treat the disabled. Under the ADA, disability is defined as a physical or mental impairment that substantially limits one or more major life activities of an individual or a record of a situation in which an individual is regarded as having such an impairment. This would include:

    1. A history of addiction.

    2. Paralysis.

    3. Bipolar disorder.

    4. All of the above.

56. Bioethical practice dilemmas are best described as situations in which proposed treatment alternatives are:

    1. Ranked from most to least acceptable.

    2. Not appealing to involved parties.

    3. Lacking acceptance by anyone.

    4. Less than perfect approaches to the situation.

22 ▸ Answers & Rationales

1. **(2)** The most important advantage of an occurrence policy is that, assuming the policy is in effect at the time of the occurrence, the coverage is available regardless of how long it takes to become aware of a claim (the long "tail" of a medical malpractice claim). The limits do not automatically increase. The carrier need not be notified during the policy period as is required with claims-made coverage. The coverage under each policy may be as broad as the carrier allows.

2. **(2)** Fact witnesses and necessary paperwork are always easier to discover the closer in time you seek them after a medical misadventure. Memories are fresh and documents are less likely to be misplaced or destroyed. There is no rigid reporting window required by insurance carriers; they do want to be notified in a timely manner. Insurance premiums may be reduced if an insured's track record is clean (i.e., no claims), but not by mere compliance with policy requirements. Risk management employees prefer early notification so that damage control efforts may be implemented promptly, not for regulatory reasons.

3. **(2)** Assessment skills are presumed to be within the purview of the professional nurse, not those with fewer years of nursing education. Also, in this scenario, the LPN is an unknown entity to the delegator. Delegating to the LPN should be done cautiously after determining that person's skill level. Your license is not in jeopardy if you delegated appropriately, as in Option #1, but an error was made and is attributed to the delegatee. Activities in Options #3 and #4 are appropriate for the role.

4. **(3)** The client's capacity to consent is questionable; therefore, alternatives must be sought. If the client has a court-appointed guardian, as set out in Option #3, then that person is the decision maker. The court has already made a determination of the client's legal incapacity and appointed the person to whom you will look for consent. If there were no guardian, you would analyze whether the client herself may be able to consent or whether you would look to her mother as the most appropriate surrogate decision maker. The group home employee has no automatic legal authority to consent to treatment for any resident.

5. **(4)** Assisted suicide is still a criminal activity in most states (and in legal limbo in the others). Circumventing the client may seem to be an appealing option, but it substitutes paternalism for the autonomy we all claim as our due. A diagnosis of depression can hardly be made with inadequate data; the necessary information can only be determined by conferring with the client herself.

6. **(2)** MCOs are one group of health care organizations impacted by this law. All subscribers must be provided with the stated information at the time of enrollment. Advance directive documents, though extremely helpful in the health care setting, are never mandatory.

7. **(4)** These are the basic requirements for conducting research at health care facilities.

8. **(3)** Your insurance carrier is thoroughly familiar with the process of handling a claim. They will assist you with every step of this fearsome activity; the first significant obligation they will meet is to put you in touch with your lawyer. Conferring with the client or the client's lawyer is never a wise move. Your colleagues can only offer moral support at this stage; your lawyer is the professional of choice at this time. Never, never even think about altering a record; it can turn a defensible case into a nondefensible one.

9. **(3)** Lobbying for underserved clients is an example of justice, which is the duty to treat all clients fairly, without regard to age, socioeconomic status, or other variables. Autonomy is the client's right to self-determination without outside control. Nonmaleficence is the duty to prevent or avoid doing harm whether intentional or unintentional. Veracity is the duty to tell the truth.

10. **(4)** These are all valid reasons to protect your assets in the event of litigation. There is an opposing view regarding the need for professional liability insurance. Some professionals feel that if there are few assets to protect, insurance is an unnecessary expense. Nurses with professional liability coverage ("deep pockets") could be retained as defendants in a case for a longer period of time.

11. **(1)** Look to state law to define the circumstances under which confidential medical information may be disclosed. There may be additional requirements imposed by federal regulations (e.g., the handling of certain psychiatric records), but the bulk of the rule making on this issue is accomplished at the state level. There are exceptions to the requirement of client consent, such as communicable disease reporting to public health authorities, and court-ordered record production. Third-party payors, although powerful with their fiscal controls, must produce some proof of client consent to acquire records. An AIDS diagnosis does not shield a record from disclosure, although many states have enacted extra levels of protection for this information. Again, knowledge of state laws is helpful.

12. **(3)** The ADA does not protect this group of people. In fact, employers may test for illegal drug use; this is not considered a medical examination, which ordinarily is subject to specific requirements under the law.

13. **(4)** These are all ways to get satisfaction from a health plan. You could also offer to help explain clinical issues to plan personnel who may not be clinically oriented.

14. **(1)** Callahan believes that health care priorities need to be re-evaluated. He advocates spending first on chronic care (those who cannot be cured), then preventive care, and lastly on the high-cost, high-tech modalities that benefit few but consume enormous resources.

15. **(2)** The best immediate solution is to identify the item, and remove it from service to avoid further client injury. Then, the risk manager, in consultation with the facility's attorneys and/or insurers, will determine how to proceed with equipment analysis. Returning the item to the manufacturer removes it from your control and diminishes your opportunity to defend against a charge of user error. Immediate repair may fail to uncover the real cause of the client injury and impair a successful defense of a claim. If the litigation potential is high, the parties may wish to pool their efforts (and costs) to conduct a third-party review of the equipment. If litigation is likely, then it is also likely that the manufacturer and others in the distribution chain will be co-defendants with the facility and its staff.

16. **(2)** The level of education preferred is that of an advanced degree. The legal issues are the province of the attorneys and the judge; the nurse is expected to be the expert in the clinical issues. Published authorship on nursing issues can add credibility, but specific work experience coupled with the educational credentials are minimally required.

17. **(3)** The APA describes the workings of federal agencies, the PSDA deals with advance directives, and the OBRA changed the rules dealing with long-term care.

18. **(4)** These and other elements combine to produce a program of systematic risk identification, analysis, treatment, and evaluation, with the overall goal of loss prevention.

19. **(4)** Liability insurance is acquired to protect the organization from suits by clients arising from negligent acts of employees. Business interruption coverage is usually purchased in tandem with fire insurance. It reimburses an organization for losses sustained while the business is partially or completely shut down after a catastrophic event. The organization's management team (CEO and senior staff) is insured against losses based upon business judgment errors through directors and officers (D&O) coverage. Worker's compensation is the line of coverage that protects employees after on-the-job injuries. It is a no-fault system (negligence is not a factor) that covers employee medical bills and pays a percentage of wages while an employee is unable to work.

20. **(1)** You were driving your personal vehicle, so your own auto insurer is "primary," that is, it responds first to a loss. Since you were on company business, your injuries were sustained "within the course and scope of your employment," so there is coverage under the employer's worker's compensation policy for your medical bills and wage replacement. Depending on the circumstances and policy definitions, there could be some "excess" or additional coverage available under the employer's auto policy, but, in no event would that carrier be primarily responsible for your losses. This is not the type of incident that homeowners' insurance is intended to cover. The semitrailer, presumably in use as a business vehicle, would not be insured under a driver's personal auto policy.

21. **(1)** At this point, the mandatory reporting affects only dentists and doctors. Other licensed practitioners are subject to permissive reporting.

22. **(3)** The forwarding facility needs to know whether the receiving facility has space for the new arrival and, more importantly, the ability to treat the particular illness for which the client needs therapy. A familiar example of a client transfer is that of the burn victim for whom specialty care is mandatory and for which the locations of that specialty care are usually limited.

23. **(1)** Health care policy within the states is codified or enacted into law by the respective states' legislatures. The boards have significant input (hopefully) in the process, providing the research data and expert "testimony" that the legislatures need in order to make informed decisions. Nursing organizations should also be willing to provide background information and nurse experts to educate the lawmakers.

24. **(3)** The MCO's cost-containment strategy is enhanced if providers practice within the treatment guidelines suggested by the plans. Providers who inform clients that a certain treatment regimen is the preferred alternative create difficulties if that alternative is excluded from coverage. MCOs usually clearly set out the exclusions in the plan documents, and member services personnel are expected to be able to explain the coverage to subscribers. Experimental treatment, if excluded, would be listed as such in the plan documents.

25. **(2)** These are three of the agencies required to report. Events occurring in the other settings are exempt from reporting requirements under this federal law.

26. **(2)** This is the most factual note; the writer does not apportion blame or assume liability. The other notes would be "red flags" for a chart reviewer. The mention of an incident report makes it virtually impossible to protect these documents from disclosure, especially in those jurisdictions that still afford some protection to these internal early warning documents that seek to alert risk management personnel to a potential claim.

27. **(3)** Clients are often unable to evaluate the quality of the care they receive; however, they do react to the way in which the care is delivered. Perceptions by clients of rudeness or "uncaring" on the part of the provider often spur clients to pursue legal action. Clients tend to be more forgiving of less-than-optimal outcomes if they have been involved in the process and are treated with respect.

28. **(4)** Making one's own decisions is the basis for informed consent and the ethical underpinning of the Patient Self-Determination Act. "Doing good" (Option #1), and its corollary, "avoiding harm" (Option #3), are ethics principles usually cited as the bases for other health care activities such as maintaining professional competency. Respect for persons is a more global ethical principle supporting much of a nurse's personal philosophy of caring.

29. **(3)** Usually phrased as duty, breach, proximate cause, and damages, these are the four elements of proof required to prevail in a medical negligence action. Intentional acts are not synonymous with negligent acts. Duty presumes a professional relationship and obligation to provide services. The breach is the error or mistake ascribed to the provider that results in the harm to the client.

30. **(2)** A competent adult client is the person to whom you look for consent to treat. It is only when the client is unable to consent that surrogate decision makers are sought. Individual states' laws need to be checked for the selection and priority of surrogate decision makers.

31. **(1)** Lay jurors are not expected to know the clinical facts and circumstances involved in a professional negligence claim. The expert witness is necessary to educate the jurors about those medical facts and to testify to the standard of care to be applied. Witnesses with direct involvement in the case are no less credible because of their involvement; their testimony, and personal bias, if any, will be evaluated by the jurors in the context of their roles.

32. **(4)** With respect to nursing specialties, the standard of care is usually a national one. Facility policies, books, and journals are important to review, and physician input may be sought. In some cases, physicians may even be allowed to testify about the standard of care.

33. **(3)** One particular advantage of ADR is the flexibility of the system. In mediation, for example, the mediator can assist with crafting a solution package that meets all the needs of a party, including such things as an apology from the health care provider.

Money is not always the only answer. Insurers' goals, however, usually do focus on cash: avoiding huge damage awards to plaintiffs. If a mediator is successful in facilitating case settlements, the costs are usually significantly lower than the costs of a court trial. Insurers with an eye on the bottom line are not averse to these advantages.

34. **(1)** Statutes of limitations set out each state's rules for the timing of the filing of lawsuits, including malpractice actions. These statutes are procedural laws, in that they describe the "how-to" parameters within which legal rights may be exercised. Minority is considered a legal disability; other state laws usually define it and describe its effects. Rights to sue are not governed by statutes of limitations.

35. **(3)** Statutes may indeed differ from state to state with respect to the breadth of the protection, but most will protect a nurse who renders aid, without expectation of compensation, in a competent manner. Gross negligence will usually void the statutory protections.

36. **(1)** A professional appearance boosts your credibility as a witness. Inappropriate attire and gum-chewing detract from the professional demeanor that you will want to project. Preparation is critical before your words are recorded and transcribed as part of the official litigation transcript. Review documents as noted, but refrain from bringing any materials with you to the deposition without our attorney's approval. Always ask for clarification of ambiguous questions. Speculation is not appropriate. Your professional work history is always asked; so, a copy of your curricula vitae is a useful tool to bring along to a deposition.

37. **(1)** Jousting in the client's medical record is never a good idea. It provides fodder for plaintiffs' lawyers but does not contribute to quality nursing care. If you have a conflict with another provider, deal with the provider directly, preferably in person. Another arena for resolving such disputes is the quality review process.

38. **(4)** Long-term care is a specialized area with layers of regulatory requirements, most stemming from the federal government. Nurses who work in this environment need to be vigilant about learning the rules and maintaining compliance. Ongoing, effective communication with regulators is essential.

39. **(4)** We have a tendency to get very careless with our information management and the way we interact with clients and their very personal data. The often wide-open and very frantic front-desk atmosphere of an office does little to calm client fears that their information will be too-easily accessible to those without a need to know.

40. **(2)** Sexual preference is not a protected classification. The other options refer to different federal laws that provide varying degrees of protection to those groups. It is prudent to check with your business attorney to determine if the policies you have drafted for your office are in compliance with federal guidelines. The Equal Employment Opportunity Commission (EEOC), which enforces the laws, publishes guidelines about the various statutes. These publications are available, either free or at minimal cost, from the agency. Some may be available on the Internet.

41. **(3)** This seems to fit the criteria for a hostile environment, a form of sexual harassment. The harassment seems to be pervasive and longstanding; the women have complained and apparently no action has been taken. The isolated incident and single date request do not rise to the level of harassment. The participants did not find the actions objectionable, and job performance was not affected. In Option #2, although the potential was there for the nurse to use the prior relationship as a club to either downgrade the employee or deny a benefit, this result did not occur.

42. **(4)** Advance directives are documents crafted by individuals who personally decide how they wish their future health care decisions to be handled. The documents must be prepared while the signer is fully capable of understanding their content and importance. Since the wife in this scenario is already comatose, she has missed her opportunity to prepare advance directives. This does not mean that the spouse is unable to decide on her medical treatment, it just means that a different consent process needs to be employed.

43. **(3)** This option would create liability potential for the nurse practitioner under at least two legal theories (e.g., battery and false imprisonment). Obviously, Option #2 would be the first prong of a planned approach to convince this client that she needs the prescribed medical therapy. Option #4 would be the next choice. Court-ordered treatment is a consideration with a viable fetus.

44. **(1)** This is the overall goal of the ADA. It is not another entitlement program, and it cannot impose wheelchair ramp requirements on every building owner in America. Access ramps and interpreters may be required as a "reasonable accommodation" to qualified people in certain defined circumstances. There is no across-the-board mandate for these types of aid to the handicapped.

45. **(1)** The Supreme Court essentially deferred to the states to legislate on this topic. In most states, the activity is not permitted. In one of the states involved in the high court's case, a statute permitting assisted suicide is being challenged. Nurse practitioners need to look at their states' laws on this topic for guidance. The other providers referenced in Options #2, #3, and #4 would act at their peril if their states' laws followed the current majority view.

46. **(1)** The purpose of a medical malpractice action is to make the claimant whole by the awarding of monetary damages. The award compensates the claimant or plaintiff for the wrong (or tort) he has suffered at the hands of the defendant. On the criminal side, the state sues on behalf of society for violations of society's criminal laws. The punishment is fines, imprisonment, or both. Professional liability insurance usually excludes criminal and intentional acts; so, coverage for these types of activities is unlikely.

47. **(4)** The full-blown jury trial is what ADR seeks to avoid. Mediation and arbitration are the most well-known forms of ADR. Some jurisdictions use the settlement conference as a technique to attempt settlement after a lawsuit has been filed but before a trial begins. Another type of ADR is called a summary jury trial, which is a private, shortened version where the parties share some evidence and get a sense of the strengths and weaknesses of each side's position. There are also hybrids such as "med-arb," where a proceeding starts out as a mediation; but if the case does not settle, it is referred to an arbitrator for resolution.

48. **(4)** All clients are entitled to medical information in order to make an informed decision about treatment. Age, in and of itself, is not an exclusionary criterion. Providers may treat in the other circumstances.

49. **(4)** If the Human Resources Department has established guidelines for the handling of references, it would be wise to follow them. It is also an effective mechanism to deflect potentially problematic queries by passing requests to the department best equipped to handle them. Most employers will be very circumspect about the information released, often limiting the data to dates of employment only. Absent some protective state legislation, employers should be prudent about sharing comments on former employees' work histories.

50. **(3)** The purpose is to determine the appropriateness of the applicant for the job.

Identifying health problems to prevent hiring an individual is discriminatory. The mental status and disabilities may also be a part of the pre-employment physical but are not the primary purpose.

51. **(3)** The Occupational Safety and Health Administration requires that these records must be held for 30 years after termination of employment.

52. **(3)** It is required by law that a report of any work-related injury be filed with the industrial commission of the state in which the injury occurred.

53. **(2)** The Occupational Safety and Health Administration requires the report of any injury or illness that requires more than first aid treatment; involves loss of work time; or results in limited work status, loss of consciousness, or death.

54. **(1)** The purpose is to record occupational injuries and illnesses, which would also include death reports and lost work days; this would also reveal dangerous working conditions.

55. **(4)** All of the conditions listed would qualify under the ADA and may require accommodation in the workplace.

56. **(4)** The crux of a bioethical dilemma is that the proposed solution(s) is(are) not perfect and therefore create some aspect of moral conflict.